MANAGEMENT OF PRIMARY BONE AND SOFT TISSUE TUMORS

Proceedings of the Annual Clinical Conference on Cancer
sponsored by The University of Texas System Cancer Center
M. D. Anderson Hospital and Tumor Institute,
and published by Year Book Medical Publishers, Inc.

TUMORS OF THE SKIN

TUMORS OF BONE AND SOFT TISSUE

RECENT ADVANCES IN THE DIAGNOSIS OF CANCER

CANCER OF THE GASTROINTESTINAL TRACT

CANCER OF THE UTERUS AND OVARY

NEOPLASIA IN CHILDHOOD

BREAST CANCER: EARLY AND LATE

LEUKEMIA-LYMPHOMA

REHABILITATION OF THE CANCER PATIENT

ENDOCRINE AND NONENDOCRINE
HORMONE-PRODUCING TUMORS

NEOPLASIA OF HEAD AND NECK

RADIOLOGIC AND OTHER BIOPHYSICAL
METHODS IN TUMOR DIAGNOSIS

CANCER CHEMOTHERAPY—
Fundamental Concepts and Recent Advances

NEOPLASMS OF THE SKIN
AND MALIGNANT MELANOMA

MANAGEMENT OF PRIMARY BONE
AND SOFT TISSUE TUMORS

MANAGEMENT OF PRIMARY BONE AND SOFT TISSUE TUMORS

*A Collection of Papers Presented at the
Twenty-First Annual Clinical Conference on Cancer, 1976,
at The University of Texas System Cancer Center
M. D. Anderson Hospital and Tumor Institute,
Houston, Texas*

YEAR BOOK MEDICAL PUBLISHERS, INC.
Chicago · London

Library of Congress Catalog Card Number: 77-76915

International Standard Book Number: 0-8151-0214-3

ON THE COVER: Giant cell tumor of femoral head and neck eradicated by resection. Reconstruction was accomplished by insertion of an endoprosthesis.

Acknowledgments

FOR THEIR SUPPORT in making possible both the Twenty-First Annual Clinical Conference and the publication of this monograph, the staff of M. D. Anderson Hospital and Tumor Institute of The University of Texas System Cancer Center gratefully acknowledges the assistance of the Texas Division of the American Cancer Society, American Cancer Society, Inc., and the Division of Continuing Education of The University of Texas Health Science Center at Houston.

The program was arranged and organized by a committee composed of the following staff members of M. D. Anderson Hospital: Richard G. Martin and Alberto G. Ayala, co-chairmen; and members Robert S. Benjamin, Murray M. Copeland, Robert D. Lindberg, John A. Murray, Frank F. Parrish, Marvin M. Romsdahl, William O. Russell, Joseph G. Sinkovics, and Wataru W. Sutow.

This volume was prepared for publication in the M. D. Anderson Hospital Office of Publications by Larry W. Dybala, Susan B. Freitag and Diane C. Culhane.

Many of the illustrations were prepared by members of the M. D. Anderson Hospital Department of Medical Communications.

Foreword

The Proceedings of the Twenty-First Annual Clinical Conference, compiled here into monograph form, contain presentations made at the meeting.

In order to facilitate the earliest possible publication date of the monograph, citations in the reference list were not verified by the editors in all instances, but were, rather, published as furnished by the authors.

The material contained in the volume was submitted as previously unpublished material, except in the instances in which credit has been given to the source from which some of the illustrative material was derived.

THE EDITORS

Contents

Board of Regents

WALTER G. STERLING

Member, Board of Regents
The University of Texas System

As a MEMBER OF THE BOARD OF REGENTS of The University of Texas System, I am happy to welcome you to this conference on the management of bone and soft tissue tumors. Dr. Clark mentioned that I had been associated with Hermann Hospital for many years, and I wish to remind him that when M. D. Anderson Hospital was in the old Baker Home on Baldwin, my sister was one of the first patients. She underwent treatment with irradiated gold for her malignant disease and I believe it was one of the first treatments of this kind. Also, while M. D. Anderson Hospital was located in the Baker Home, most of the surgical procedures for cancer patients were done at Hermann Hospital.

Again, I want to welcome you to this conference; I know that you will learn many things from your fellow doctors during the meetings.

Introduction

R. LEE CLARK, M.D., M. Sc., D. Sc. *(Hon.)*

*President, The University of Texas System Cancer
Center, and Professor of Surgery, The University of
Texas M. D. Anderson Hospital and Tumor Institute,
Houston, Texas*

I WISH TO WELCOME YOU to the Twenty-First Annual Clinical Conference of The University of Texas System Cancer Center M. D. Anderson Hospital and Tumor Institute. These conferences began 20 years ago for the purpose of making current clinical cancer information available to practicing physicians in the Southwest. During the ensuing years, we have been pleased to see them acquire national and international significance. It is to those physicians who refer their patients to M. D. Anderson Hospital and with whom we cooperate in continuing to offer better care for patients with cancer that we dedicate these annual conferences.

We extend our gratitude to the cosponsors of this conference: the American Cancer Society, Inc., the National Cancer Institute, and The University of Texas Health Science Center at Houston Division of Continuing Education. We are grateful also to the American Cancer Society, Texas Division, Inc., for its support, the Texas Cancer Coordinating Commission for its endorsement, and the Board of Regents of The University of Texas.

We also thank the individuals on our staff who have worked during the past 2 years to recruit the outstanding participants and contributors to this conference on the clinical management of primary bone and soft tissue sarcomas: Dr. Richard G. Martin, Professor and Chief of the Section of General Surgery, Dr. Alberto G. Ayala, Assistant Professor of Anatomical Pathology, and their conference committee members.

3

In addition, we wish to welcome you to the Ninth Annual Special Pathology Program on Soft Tissue Neoplasms, to be presented by the M. D. Anderson Pathology Department and cosponsored by the Texas Society of Pathologists.

Although sarcomas of the bone and connective tissues are relatively rare as compared to the total number of cancers under treatment each year in the United States (approximately 6,400 newly diagnosed cases in 1976), most of the bone tumors develop in children and young adults. These tumors always represent a challenge because they are difficult to diagnose. Traditionally, a majority of patients have micrometastases at the time of first diagnosis, and pulmonary metastases develop rapidly; if aggressive, rapid, and adequate treatment is not administered, there is generally a poor prognosis. Until recently, the best overall 5-year survival rate hovered around 20%.

Traditionally, the most successful form of treatment was radical ablative surgery to remove all evidence of the primary lesion and the adjacent lymphatic drainage system, if possible, to prevent local recurrence and metastases. Such radical procedures as hip disarticulation, hemipelvectomy, and intrascapulothoracic amputations gradually were replaced by surgical excision of the bulk of tumorous tissue and attempts to establish local control of recurrences and micrometastases with radiation therapy and, still later, with drugs in combination with the other 2 modalities.

For many years, sarcomas of both bone and connective tissue, except for Kaposi's sarcoma, were considered to be radioresistant. In a report published in *The Journal-Lancet* in 1959, Clark, Martin, and White of M. D. Anderson Hospital stated:

Since most soft tissue sarcomas are radioresistant, roentgen therapy as a definitive treatment or in conjunction with surgical treatment *is not used except for Kaposi's sarcoma.* Irradiation may control a local Kaposi's sarcoma, *although it does not cure the patient.* It has been reported that liposarcomas also respond to roentgen therapy. At present, chemotherapeutic drugs are being extensively studied with regard to their effects upon the various forms of malignant disease. . . . Lesions most sensitive to irradiation seem to respond best to chemotherapy. . . . Thus far, none (i.e. no chemotherapeutic agent) has been particularly successful. At times, a temporary regression of the tumor and relief of the patient's discomfort is observed, *though the period of survival does not appear to have been prolonged.* Chemotherapy is still in the experimental stage; it is used only infrequently as a prophylactic measure. We must conclude, therefore, that, at present, *no drug is available which is both safe and reliable as a treatment for connective tissue sarcomas.*

The paper concludes:

At present, excision must be considered the treatment of choice. . . . Following local excision, local recurrence may be expected in approximately 70% of the cases, whereas, after radical operation, whether wide excision or amputation, the local recurrence rate is approximately 9%. If the tumor is eliminated entirely, including the structures of its origin, contiguous muscle bundles, fascia, periosteum, and skin, local control of the disease can be assured in approximately 90% of the patients. . . . On the whole, the 5-year survival rate of patients in this series was approximately 45.7% regardless of the classification or grading.

By 1973, Suit, Russell, and Martin of M. D. Anderson Hospital reported a series of 57 patients with soft tissue sarcomas of extremities who were treated during an 8-year period from 1961 to 1969. These patients were treated with surgical excision of most or all of their primary tumors followed, after total wound healing, with radical dose radiation therapy ranging from 6,300 to 14,000 rads. Of the 57 patients, 30 who had lesions of the elbow or below or of the knee-popliteal space or below had tourniquets applied proximal to the lesions to achieve tissue hypoxia, and then were irradiated with 8,100 to 14,000 rads in 8 to 14 fractions over 23 to 43 days. Of the 57 patients, local control was achieved in 50 (88%). Local control was achieved in all 46 patients whose primary lesions were on the elbow or more distal or the knee-popliteal space or more distal. Results were less satisfactory for the 11 patients whose lesions were on the upper arm or thigh; there were recurrences in 7 (64%). Twenty-three patients ultimately lost good use of the treated limb, but of those who sustained damage to normal tissue, all retained good function for the first 1 to 3 years posttreatment. A useful limb was retained from 2 to 10 years in 34 of the patients, and metastasis-free survival at 2 to 10 years was 58%.

In 1962 (3 years after our 1959 condemnation of chemotherapy for soft tissue sarcomas), a 12-year-old girl was referred to the pediatric section of M. D. Anderson Hospital with a diagnosis of osteosarcoma and with massive "cannonball-sized" lesions of the lungs. Following amputation of the primary lesion, Dr. W. W. Sutow and his colleagues opted to treat the lung metastases with phenylalanine mustard (PAM), and within a relatively short period of time, most of the pulmonary lesions had disappeared. Two small lesions persisting on X-ray films were excised; one was cancerous and the other, benign. Today, 14 years later, this young woman is married, the mother of a child, and has had no further evidence of cancer.

This was our first clue at M. D. Anderson Hospital that adjuvant chemotherapy might prevent lung metastases in children with osteosarcoma. Consequently, from 1962 to 1968, 14 children with no evidence of metastatic disease were treated with PAM following amputation of the primary lesion, and a 15% 5-year survival rate was achieved

(Sutow, Sullivan, Wilbur, and Cangir, 1975). Our best efforts prior to that time had yielded a 6% 5-year survival rate.

In 1968, a 3-drug regimen (vincristine, actinomycin-D, and cyclophosphamide = VAC) was effective for rhabdomyosarcoma; it was, therefore, administered to 12 patients with osteosarcoma. Four of the children survived, increasing the 5-year survival rate to 33%, which was better than any other results published in the literature to that date (Sutow, Sullivan, Wilbur, and Cangir, 1975).

In 1971, Adriamycin began to show positive results for the management of metastatic osteosarcoma in adults being treated at M. D. Anderson Hospital; thus, a new treatment regimen, CONPADRI-I, consisting of cyclophosphamide, vincristine, PAM, and Adriamycin, was developed and then adopted by the Southwest Oncology Group and administered to 18 children (17 of whom were M. D. Anderson patients). Ten of the 18 patients are still alive 49 to 72 months later—a survival rate of 56%. There are now 43 patients who have been treated with this regimen, including some adults with osteosarcoma, with a continued survival rate of 55% (Sutow *et al.*, 1975).

In 1972, the drug methotrexate (MTX) was giving good responses for metastatic osteosarcoma, so MTX with citrovorum factor rescue was added to the regimen, and the acronym was changed to COMPADRI-II. So far, the first 30 patients have been treated with this regimen and have had follow-up studies for one full year or more (Sutow *et al.*, 1976). To date, there is a 65% survival rate without evidence of disease.

Other recent approaches to the treatment of osteosarcoma have included Adriamycin alone, high-dose methotrexate with citrovorum rescue, and other types of multiple-drug regimens about which you will hear during this conference.

One of the latest reports by Dr. Gerald Rosen and his colleagues of Memorial Sloan-Kettering Institute for Cancer Research (Rosen *et al.*, 1976), which appeared in January 1976, describes the newest multimodality approach to treatment for osteosarcoma of an extremity. It includes preoperative chemotherapy, en bloc resection of the primary tumor, prosthetic replacement of the involved bone, and postoperative adjuvant chemotherapy. This technique holds promise for the retention of functional limbs and the simultaneous eradication of micrometastases. We will hear more about it from Dr. Rosen (1977, see pages 187–203, this volume).

Although the picture looks progressively brighter for the extension of survival and for much better control of local recurrence and metastases, the long-term potential for second primary tumors and the long-delayed appearance of recurrent disease warrants only cautious optimism.

REFERENCES

Clark, R. L., Jr., Martin, R. G., and White, E. C.: A critical review of the management of soft-tissue sarcomas. The Journal-Lancet, 79:327–331, July 1959.

Rosen, G.: Past experiences and future considerations with T-2 chemotherapy in the treatment of Ewing's sarcoma. In *Management of Primary Bone and Soft Tissue Tumors* (The University of Texas System Cancer Center M. D. Anderson Hospital and Tumor Institute, 21st Annual Clinical Conference on Cancer). Chicago, Illinois, Year Book Medical Publishers, Inc., 1977, pp. 187–203.

Rosen, G., Murphy, M. L., Huvos, A. G., Gutierrez, M., and Marcove, R. C.: Chemotherapy, en bloc resection, and prosthetic bone replacement in the treatment of osteogenic sarcoma. Cancer, 37:1–11, January 1976.

Suit, H. D., Russell, W. O., and Martin, R. G.: Management of patients with sarcoma of soft tissue in an extremity. Cancer, 31:1247–1255, May 1973.

Sutow, W. W., Gehan, E. A., Vietti, T. J., Frias, A. E., and Dyment, P. G.: Multi-drug chemotherapy in primary treatment of osteosarcoma. Journal of Bone and Joint Surgery, 58A:629–633, July 1976.

Sutow, W. W., Sullivan, M. P., Fernbach, D. J., Cangir, A., and George, S. L.: Adjuvant chemotherapy in primary treatment of osteogenic sarcoma. A Southwest Oncology Group study. Cancer, 36:1598–1602, November 1975.

Sutow, W. W., Sullivan, M. P., Wilber, J. R., and Cangir, A.: Study of adjuvant chemotherapy in osteogenic sarcoma. Journal of Clinical Pharmacology, 15:530–533, July 1975.

Introduction of Heath Memorial Award Recipients

ROBERT C. HICKEY, M.D.

*Director, The University of Texas System Cancer
Center M. D. Anderson Hospital and Tumor Institute,
Houston, Texas*

THE HEATH MEMORIAL AWARD has become a tradition at The University of Texas System Cancer Center Annual Clinical Conference. The award memorializes 3 brothers—Guy H., Dan C., and Gilford G. Heath—and was made possible by the late William W. Heath, former Chairman of The University of Texas System Board of Regents. The award committee carefully selects an individual who has made "outstanding contributions to the care of patients with cancer." This year, however, there are corecipients, each of whom in his own way has made major contributions to mankind; this year's recipients are Doctor Franz Michael Enzinger and Doctor Wataru W. Sutow. Doctor Franz Michael Enzinger was born in Rohrbach, Austria, and currently resides in Bethesda, Maryland. He and his wife, Inge, have 1 son, Peter. Dr. Enzinger graduated from the Staatsgymnasium Linz in Linz, Austria, and received his Doctor of Medicine degree from the University of Innsbruck, Innsbruck, Austria, although this training was interrupted by World War II. His postgraduate education was originally in the Department of Anatomy at the University of Innsbruck for 1 year, and his residency, done for the main part in the United States, was at the University of Iowa under Doctor Emory D. Warner. (On a personal note, Dr. Enzinger was one of my colleagues there.) He joined the Armed Forces Institute of Pathology (AFIP) in 1957 and became Chief of the Soft Tissue Branch in 1961. He is now

9

Chief of Division A, Armed Forces Institute of Pathology. He is head of the World Health Organization International Reference Center for the Diagnosis of Soft Tissue Tumors and has been responsible for the current classification of soft tissue tumors, especially the recognition of malignant fibrohistiocytomas. It is for these works that the Heath Committee recognizes Dr. Franz Michael Enzinger.

Doctor Wataru W. Sutow was born in Guadalupe, California. He attended a 2-room school there and collected, among other things, sea shells. He has maintained an interest in shells through adulthood, and is now a conchologist of considerable reputation.

He attended Stanford University and received his AB degree in 1939; he then began his medical training at Stanford. World War II interrupted this training and the Japanese Sutow family was evacuated to Salt Lake City. He graduated later, in 1945, with a Doctor of Medicine degree from the University of Utah School of Medicine. His internship and residency were in Pediatrics at the University of Utah.

The Atomic Bomb Casuality Commission appointed him Head of the Pediatric Department and Director of Pediatric Research. This challenge involved biomathematical studies of large patient groups with irradiation injuries, and these studies are considered significant. He continued his work as a Captain in the United States Army Medical Corps, assigned to the Atomic Bomb Casuality Commission in Japan. In 1954, he was appointed as a staff member of The University of Texas M. D. Anderson Hospital and Tumor Institute.

Doctor Sutow brought with him to M. D. Anderson Hospital a profound interest in childhood growth and development, a first-hand experience of the delayed effect of atomic irradiation, boundless energy, and an enthusiasm for intelligent systematic research. He has left his mark.

Doctor Sutow's contributions to medical research have been invaluable in the management of childhood cancer. He is cheerful, kind, and has a decisive leadership capability. His investigations of childhood neoplasms have been outstanding, and it is because of these contributions that his colleagues take justifiable pride and pleasure in presenting him as a Heath Memorial awardee.

Benign Lipomatous Tumors Simulating a Sarcoma

FRANZ M. ENZINGER, M.D.

Chief, Department of Soft Tissue Pathology,
Armed Forces Institute of Pathology,
*Washington, D.C.**

I WISH FIRST to express my appreciation for the great honor to be one of the recipients of this year's Heath Memorial Award. I am particularly honored to follow Dr. Helwig and others who have contributed so much to our knowledge of tumor pathology and oncology.

Soft tissue tumors have been a long neglected subject that still causes many problems in diagnosis and treatment. Over the past 20 years, however, much progress has been made in this field, and we are able now to interpret and diagnose many soft tissue lesions more accurately and more reliably than in the past. Especially, we have learned to distinguish between truly malignant lesions that require radical therapy and lesions that merely simulate a malignant tumor by their cellularity or immature appearance and that are readily cured by local excision. Indeed, in this group of lesions — the so-called pseudosarcomas — accurate diagnosis is superior to the best type of therapy.

The purpose of my presentation will be to elaborate on a group of lipomatous tumors that are benign but are frequently mistaken for li-

---

*The opinions or assertions contained herein are the private views of the author and are not to be construed as official or as reflecting the views of the Department of the Army or the Department of Defense.

posarcomas. The tumors that I will consider here are: (1) benign lipoblastoma and lipoblastomatosis, (2) intramuscular lipoma, (3) spindle
cell lipoma, and (4) pleomorphic lipoma.

Benign Lipoblastoma and Lipoblastomatosis

This neoplasm was described and named by Vellios in 1958
(Vellios, Baez and Schumacker, 1958), although earlier reference to
this tumor as embryonic lipoma was made by Van Meurs in 1947 (Van
Meurs, 1947). Benign lipoblastoma and lipoblastomatosis represent
the circumscribed and diffuse forms of the same tumor and may be
considered as the childhood counterpart of lipoma and diffuse lipomatosis. Because of their cellular immaturity both tumors, and especially
the diffuse or infiltrating form, have been mistaken for a sarcoma;
awareness of this entity, therefore, is all-important for correct therapy.

Under the microscope the lipoblastoma is composed of irregular
small lobules of immature fat cells separated by connective tissue trabeculae of varying thickness. The cells comprising the tumor closely
resemble the lipoblasts of myxoid liposarcoma. But unlike the latter,
the cells of each lobule are of uniform appearance and show little variation in their degree of differentiation. Sometimes, however, the cellular picture varies in different portions of the same tumor (Figs. 1 and
2), and lobules consisting entirely of primitive lipoblasts are next to
lobules showing a high degree of differentiation and approaching the
appearance of mature fat (Fig. 2).

The less differentiated lobules consist of lipoblasts intermingled
with spindle- and stellate-shaped mesenchymal cells (prelipoblasts).
The more differentiated areas are composed of a mixture of lipoblasts
and lipocytes in varying proportions. Lipoblasts containing fine vacuoles and eosinophilic granules in their cytoplasm, similar to the
brown fat cell of hibernoma, do occur but are rare (Cox, 1954). Always,
the lipoblasts are intimately associated with a mucoid matrix, the
amount of which is inversely proportional to the degree of cellular
differentiation, i.e. the least mature tumors contain most of the mucoid
material. Most lipoblastomas are richly vascular, frequently having a
plexiform capillary pattern resembling that of myxoid liposarcoma.

In our series of 35 cases, reported elsewhere (Chung and Enzinger,
1973), 88% of the tumors occurred during the first 3 years of life. The
youngest patient was a newborn and the oldest a 7-year-old boy
(median age, 1 year). Male patients outnumbered females by a ratio of
2 to 1. The upper and lower extremities were the most common sites
of the tumor (Table 1). About two thirds of the tumors were circum-

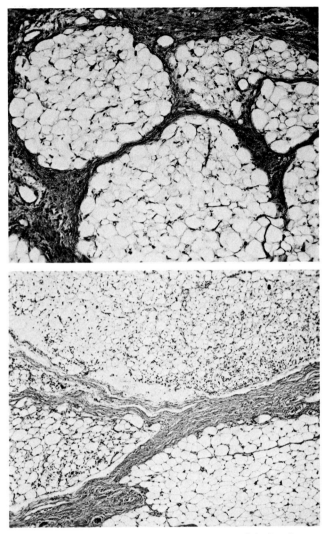

Fig. 1 (top).—Lipoblastoma showing the characteristic lobulated pattern and the immature appearance of the constituent adipose tissue cells. (×100) (AFIP Neg. No. 72-9967).

Fig. 2 (bottom).—Multiple lobules of a lipoblastoma separated by fibrous tissue septa. Note the variations in the cellular differentiation of the lipoblasts. (×80) (AFIP Neg. No. 72-9958).

TABLE 1.—CLINICAL DATA

TUMOR TYPE	NUMBER OF PATIENTS	MEDIAN AGE	MALES (PERCENT)	PREDOMINANT LOCATION
Lipoblastoma	35	1	60	Lower extremities
Intramuscular lipoma	78	44	73	Thigh, shoulder
Spindle cell lipoma	114	55	91	Posterior neck, shoulder
Pleomorphic lipoma	40	60	76	Posterior neck, shoulder

scribed and limited to the subcutis; one third were diffuse and infiltrated subcutis and muscle in the manner of lipomatosis.

Prognosis is excellent. Of the 25 patients on whom we have follow-up information, all were living and well, except 5 in whom the tumor had recurred (Table 2). Three of the 5 had diffuse forms of lipoblastomatosis. In 2, no information was available as to whether the tumors were of the circumscribed or diffuse type. In Shear's 1967 series (Shear, 1967), all 7 patients did well following local excision. Van Meurs (1947) reported progressive maturation of a lipoblastoma (embryonic lipoma) in 4 successive operations over a period of several years.

As pointed out, distinction from a myxoid liposarcoma is the main problem that faces the pathologist. Both lesions, lipoblastoma and myxoid liposarcoma, show a very similar cellular picture, with the exception that benign lipoblastoma displays a much more uniform lobular pattern and a more regular cellular population in the individual tumor lobules. Moreover, lipoblastoma occurs almost exclusively during the first 3 years of life, whereas liposarcoma in small children is exceedingly rare; in fact, among over 800 cases of liposarcoma on file at the Armed Forces Institute of Pathology, we have never encountered such a case in a child younger than 5 years.

Intramuscular Lipoma

These tumors often cause considerable concern because of their frequent large size, their deep location, and their infiltrative growth

TABLE 2.—CLINICAL BEHAVIOR

TUMOR TYPE	NUMBER OF PATIENTS	NUMBER OF FOLLOW-UP PATIENTS	RECURRENCE	
			NUMBER	PERCENT
Lipoblastoma	35	25	5	20
Intramuscular lipoma	78	46	7	15
Spindle cell lipoma	114	63	0	0
Pleomorphic lipoma	40	22	1	4.5

pattern. Most are painless and grow insidiously, replacing large portions of the affected voluntary muscle, such as the vastus lateralis or the gastrocnemius. Like other tumors that consist of mature adipose tissue cells, they are radiolucent and are readily demonstrated roentgenographically.

Microscopically, intramuscular lipoma consists of lipocytes that have infiltrated muscle tissue and have separated or replaced muscle fibers in a diffuse manner (Figs. 3 and 4). The lipocytes are fully mature and are indistinguishable from those of a lipoma or normal adipose tissue. There are no lipoblasts or giant cells. The interspersed remnants of striated muscle show varying degrees of atrophy but no evidence of reactive or reparative changes such as proliferation of sarcolemmic nuclei. Interstitial fibrosis is occasionally encountered in the vicinity of the residual muscle fibers but is never as prominent as in muscular dystrophy. There is little vascularity, a fact which has been confirmed microangiographically (Kindblom, Angervall, Stener, and Wickbom, 1974). Richly vascular intramuscular lesions diagnosed as infiltrating angiolipomas (Lin and Lin, 1974) are probably intramuscular hemangiomas in which portions of the affected muscle tissue have been replaced by fat.

The clinical parameters of our 78 patients with this tumor conformed largely with those reported in the literature (Dionne and Seemayer, 1974; Kindblom, Angervall, Stener, and Wickbom, 1974). With the exception of small children, the tumor occurred at any age. The ages of the 78 patients ranged from 4 to 74 years, with a median of 44 years. There were nearly 3 times as many males as females (57 males, 21 females). The tumor affected chiefly the muscles of the lower extremities, especially those of the thigh (35 patients), the shoulder and arm (19 patients), and the chest wall (18 patients). Three patients had tumor in the head-neck area and 1 patient each had tumor in the retroperitoneum, the hands, and the feet (Table 1). Clinically, most tumors were noted as painless, slowly growing masses which frequently became apparent only on muscle contraction. Sometimes movement caused aching or pain, but pain was rarely severe. In fact, most of the tumors had been noted to be present for several years before professional help was sought. A few were noted as an incidental finding on routine x-ray examinations. In 3 patients lipomas at other locations were associated with the tumor. At operation most involved muscle tissue, but a few were located between muscle without penetrating the muscle fascia (intermuscular lipoma). The tumors ranged in size from 1 to 27 cm , with a median of 7 cm. Obesity was mentioned in 5 patients and associated arthritis in 4 patients.

The prospect of cure is excellent if the tumor is completely removed

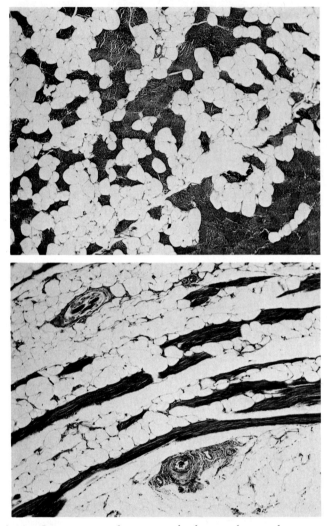

Fig. 3 (top).—Cross section of intramuscular lipoma showing lipocytes separating voluntary muscle fibers in a diffuse manner. (×50) (AFIP Neg. No. 70-8069).

Fig. 4 (bottom).—Intramuscular lipoma showing replacement of muscle fibers by infiltrating lipocytes. Note the complete absence of lipoblasts or cells with atypical nuclei. (×60) (AFIP Neg. No. 73-3200).

initially. Follow-up data were available for 46 patients. Thirty-nine (85%) of the 46 patients were well without recurrence of the tumor following local excision. In 7 (15%) the tumor had recurred; in 2 of these it had recurred twice and in 1 it had recurred 3 times (Table 2). In the series of Dionne and Seemayer (1974) (13 cases), the recurrence rate was 62.5%. In Kindblom's group (Kindblom, Angervall, Stener, and Wickbom, 1974), 33 of the 43 patients were followed; all but 1 were well after the initial excision. This tumor had recurred 17 years after its first removal. It is noteworthy that all of Kindblom's patients, except the 1 with recurrence, were initially treated by an orthopedic surgeon (B. Stener) who is particularly interested and skilled in the treatment of soft tissue tumors.

Differential diagnosis from typical examples of liposarcoma will cause few, if any, difficulties. The fat cells in intramuscular lipoma are mature and indistinguishable from those of other types of lipoma; there are neither lipoblasts nor cells with atypical hyperchromatic nuclei. Yet portions of occasional liposarcoma may be exceedingly well differentiated and may completely lack lipoblastic activity or cellular atypia. For this reason, it is mandatory to sample the tumor carefully and to prepare and study multiple sections in each case before a benign diagnosis is rendered. Diffuse rather than expansile growth, as it occurs in most well-differentiated liposarcomas, is another diagnostic point in favor of intramuscular lipoma.

Spindle Cell Lipoma

Although the less cellular examples of this tumor can be readily identified as a variant of lipoma, the more cellular variants of spindle cell lipoma may cause considerable difficulties in diagnosis. In fact, a great number of these tumors in our series (Enzinger and Harvey, 1975) were initially interpreted as liposarcoma or, when proliferated spindle cells almost completely replaced the lipomatous elements, as neurofibroma, neurilemmoma, fibrosarcoma, or neurogenic sarcoma.

The morphologic spectrum of spindle cell lipoma varies considerably (Figs. 5, 6, and 7). On one end of the spectrum there are those tumors in which only a very small portion consists of spindle cells and in which the bulk of the growth is indistinguishable from a lipoma. Usually, abundant mucoid matrix accompanies the proliferated spindle cells. At the other end of its morphological spectrum the tumor is almost completely replaced by spindle cells and there are only a few scattered lipocytes (Fig. 7). In these cases the mucoid matrix is less conspicuous and always is associated with traversing collagen fibers. In the average case spindle cells and adipose tissue cells are present in about equal proportions, but the distribution of these cells varies and the proliferation of the spindle cells may be diffuse or localized (Figs. 5 and 6). Mast cells are a prominent but nonspecific feature of this tumor. The vascular pattern tends to be inconspicuous and consists of a few thick-walled vessels of small or intermediate

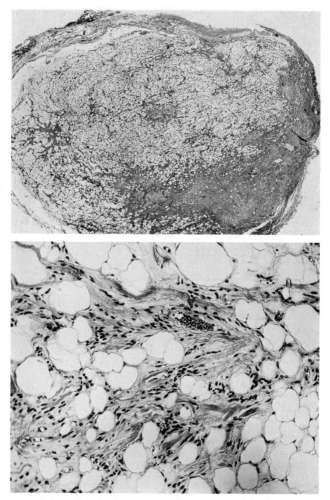

Fig. 5 (top). — Spindle cell lipoma showing the circumscription of the tumor and the uneven distribution of the spindle cells. (×5) (AFIP Neg. No. 73-3186).

Fig. 6 (bottom). — Spindle cell lipoma showing intimate mixture of lipocytes, spindle cells, and collagen fibers. (×140) (AFIP Neg. No. 74-8240).

size. Extensive vascularization, closely resembling that of a vascular tumor, is occasionally seen.

Judging from a review of 114 neoplasms of this type (Enzinger and Harvey, 1975), spindle cell lipoma has a very characteristic clinical setting: it occurs almost exclusively in male patients between 45 and 65 years of age and in nearly all cases is located in the regions of the shoulder and posterior neck (Table 1). Most of the lesions manifest as

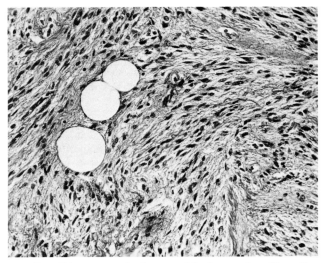

Fig. 7.—Spindle cell lipoma in which most of the fat is replaced by collagen-forming spindle cells. (×140) (AFIP Neg. No. 74-8228).

a circumscribed or encapsulated, painless, firm nodule or mass in the deep subcutis that often has been present for considerable periods of time, sometimes many years. The excised nodules are usually well circumscribed and deviate from the typical appearance of an ordinary lipoma only by the presence of grayish-white glistening areas representing the spindle cell portions and the deposited collagen. It is of interest that the diagnosis of lipoma was made more often by the surgeon, who removed the specimen, than by the pathologist, who examined the tumor.

Electron microscopic examination in 1 case (Enzinger and Harvey, 1975) suggested that the spindle cells are fibroblasts. Ultrastructurally, they showed long polar extensions and a prominent endoplasmic reticulum. Small lipid droplets in some of the cells raised the question of preadipose fibroblasts, but the absence of intermediate stages between these cells and lipocytes seems to favor cells of fibroblastic origin. Additional electron microscopic studies, however, will be required for a final determination of the exact nature of the spindle cells.

The chief problem in diagnosis, particularly in those lipomas with a marked spindle cell component, is the distinction from myxoid or spindle cell liposarcoma. A correct diagnosis should be possible if close attention is paid to the great uniformity of the spindle cells and their association with mature collagen fibers. Occasionally, spindle cells may be vacuolated, but vacuolization is much less prominent than that of the multivacuolated lipoblasts seen in liposarcoma. Focal cellular pleomorphism does not necessarily rule out a diagnosis of spindle lipoma, and we have observed transitional cases between this tumor and another tumor which we have tentatively classified as pleomorphic lipoma. Angiolipomas can be distinguished by their greater vascularity and the presence of microthrombi in the branching vascular channels. Follow-up information obtained in 63 patients with this lesion revealed an uniformly favorable clinical course without aggressive behavior or local recurrence (Table 2).

Pleomorphic Lipoma

Although we have observed examples of this tumor for many years, we were hesitant to report them as benign and specific variants of lipoma because of the great difficulty of clearly distinguishing this tumor from a fibrosing liposarcoma. Yet, from our follow-up information, there is no doubt that these tumors, despite their bizarre microscopic appearance, behave in a benign manner and are readily cured by local excision.

As the name indicates, the histologic picture is marked by a high degree of cellular pleomorphism. Scattered multinucleated giant cells are intimately associated with large amounts of mature collagen and a varying number of adipose tissue cells ranging considerably in size, probably as the result of partial cellular atrophy. Many of the giant cells have a characteristic appearance: hyperchromatic nuclei are placed at the margin of eosinophilic cytoplasm in a floret-like manner, either surrounding the entire cell or bordering it on 1 side (Figs. 8 and 9). Characteristically, these pleomorphic or giant cells are intimately associated with a matrix consisting of traversing thick bundles of mature, birefringent collagen and small amounts of mucoid material. Mast cells occur but are less common than in spindle cell lipoma. Multivaculoated cells with hyperchromatic nuclei, closely resembling lipoblasts, are encountered in some of the patients making it difficult to rule out a fibrosing liposarcoma. Yet, after studying all the cases, we have reached the conclusion that the presence of the lipoblast-like cells can be disregarded if the tumor is circumscribed and the cells are accompanied by floret-type giant cells and thick bundles of mature collagen. In a few patients, however, in whom there is a lesser amount of collagen and a greater number of lipoblast-like cells, an unequivocal diagnosis may not be possible. In such patients wide local excision is advisable as a precautionary measure rather than sim-

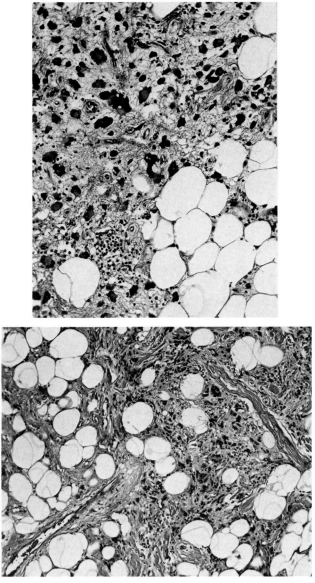

Fig. 8 (top). — Pleomorphic lipoma consisting of lipocytes and bizarre giant cells surrounded by a matrix of mucoid material and collagen. (×145) (AFIP Neg. No. 74-8232).

Fig. 9 (bottom). — Another pleomorphic lipoma showing a picture similar to Figure 8 except for a greater amount of collagen. (×90) (AFIP Neg. No. 70-8057).

ple follow-up without further surgical procedures as in the pleomorphic lipoma. Such equivocal cases were excluded from our series.

Clinically, these tumors resemble more closely a spindle cell lipoma than a liposarcoma, and in fact many of our 40 cases were initially submitted by the operating surgeon as lipomas. As in lipoma, a slowly growing mass or swelling of the affected part was usually the only complaint, except for a few cases in which recent rapid growth was noted. In 12 of the 40 patients, the tumor was known to have been present for 5 or more years without significant changes in its clinical appearance. As in spindle cell lipoma, the regions of the shoulder and posterior neck were the most common sites of occurrence. There was no tumor in children or young adults, and the greatest incidence of the tumor was in men between 50 and 70 years (Table 1). Nearly all pleomorphic lipomas were located in the deep subcutis and were partly or completely circumscribed. On cross sections they had a yellow or grayish-yellow appearance similar to that of a lipoma. The excised tumors ranged from 1 to 13 cm in diameter, with a median size of 2.8 cm.

Follow-up information was obtained from 22 patients. Nineteen of the 22 patients were well without recurrence of the tumor (Table 2). In 1 of the patients the tumor had allegedly recurred 4 times, but the previous lesions had not been examined under the microscope and there is some doubt as to the accuracy of the available data. Morphologically, this tumor shows no difference from the nonrecurrent examples of this entity. Four of the 22 patients are known to have been treated by wide local excision following the initial pathological report of liposarcoma.

Miscellaneous Benign Lesions Simulating a Liposarcoma

There are a number of secondary changes in lipoma or adipose tissue that are occasionally misinterpreted as evidence of lipoblastic activity. The exact cause of these changes is not always clear, but minor trauma or injury, with subsequent fat necrosis and inflammation, is mostly responsible for their development. In many of these cases there is myxoid degeneration of fat resulting in the accumulation of mucoid material, focal cellular atrophy, and loss of cellular cohesion. The atrophic cells often have a bizarre multivacuolated appearance and may closely resemble lipoblasts. Similar myxoid changes, probably as the result of chronic irritation, are often seen in the general area of the wrist, preceding or accompanying the formation of ganglion cysts. Lipid macrophages in a lipoma may also be mistaken for lipoblasts. These cells are usually present as small aggregates in the inter-

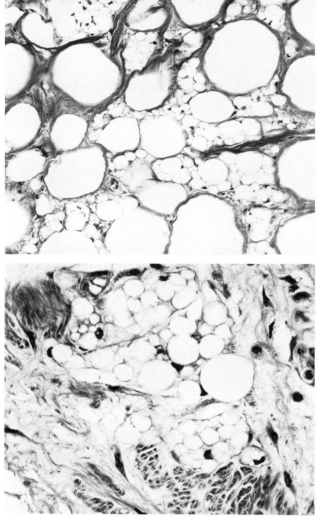

Fig. 10 (top).—Silicone granuloma in adipose tissue of breast simulating a liposarcoma. (×245) (AFIP Neg. No. 76-10623).

Fig. 11 (bottom).—Lipoblast-like macrophages secondary to injection of liquid silicone. (×530) (AFIP Neg. No. 76-19621).

stices of adipose tissue and can be readily recognized by their uniformly and finely vacuolated cytoplasm with 1 or more small and centrally placed nuclei. Lipogranulomas of the endogenous or the exogenous type have also been confused with liposarcoma. In general, they can be identified by the presence of irregularly sized, thick-walled lipid cysts and varying amounts of hyaline fibrosis in addition to scattered lipid macrophages, lymphocytes, and a varying number of foreign-body giant cells. A similar liposarcoma-like picture may be caused by the injection of liquid silicone into the breast or other tissues (Figs. 10 and 11).

Summary

Our experience with the various benign lipomatous tumors that may be confused with a liposarcoma has been reviewed. It was emphasized that such customarily malignant features as cellular immaturity, infiltrative growth, great cellularity, and cellular pleomorphism are not always evidence of malignant behavior and may be encountered in lipoblastoma, intramuscular lipoma, spindle cell lipoma, and pleomorphic lipoma, respectively. Awareness of the existence of these tumors and of their characteristic microscopic appearance is mandatory for adequate management and will prevent excessive and unnecessary surgical therapy.

REFERENCES

Chung, E. B., and Enzinger, F. M.: Benign lipoblastomatosis. An analysis of 35 cases. Cancer, 32:482–492, August 1973.

Cox, R. W.: "Hibernoma" the lipoma of immature adipose tissue. Journal of Pathology and Bacteriology, 68:511–518, October 1954.

Dionne, G. P., and Seemayer, T. A.: Infiltrating lipomas and angiolipomas revisited. Cancer, 33:732–738, March 1974.

Enzinger, F. M., and Harvey, D. A.: Spindle cell lipoma. Cancer 36: 1852–1859, November 1975.

Enzinger, F. M., and Winslow, D. J.: Liposarcoma: A study of 103 cases. Virchows Archives of Pathological Anatomy, 335:367–388, 1962.

Howard, W. R., and Helwig, E. B.: Angiolipoma. Archives of Dermatology, 82:924–931, December 1960.

Kindblom, L. G., Angervall, L., Stener, B. and Wickbom, E.: Intermuscular lipomas and intramuscular lipomas and hibernomas. A clinical, roentgenologic, histologic, and prognostic study of 46 cases. Cancer, 33:754–762, March 1974.

Lin, J. J., and Lin, F.: Two entities in angiolipoma. A study of 459 cases of lipoma with review of literature on infiltrating angiolipoma. Cancer 34: 720–727, September 1974.

Shear, M.: Lipoblastomatosis of the cheek. British Journal of Oral Surgery, 5: 173–179, November 1967.

Van Meurs, D. P.: The transformation of an embryonic lipoma to a common lipoma. British Journal of Surgery, 34:282–284, 1947.

Vellios, F., Baez, J. M., and Shumacker, H. B.: Lipoblastomatosis: A tumor of fetal fat different from hibernoma. Report of a case, with observations on the embryogenesis of human adipose tissue. American Journal of Pathology, 34:1149–1159, November–December 1958.

Perspectives in the Management of Osteosarcoma and Rhabdomyosarcoma in Children

WATARU W. SUTOW, M.D.

Department of Pediatrics,
The University of Texas System Cancer Center
M. D. Anderson Hospital and Tumor Institute,
Houston, Texas

I AM HONORED INDEED to have been designated the corecipient of the prestigious Heath Memorial Award. I take note of the obvious recognition extended to the pediatrician and to the chemotherapist in clinical areas where surgery and radiotherapy have been so preeminent. I wish to thank Dr. Clark, Dr. Hickey, and Dr. Grant Taylor, former head of the Department of Pediatrics, and through them the staff at M. D. Anderson Hospital, as well as my friends and colleagues elsewhere, for the support and cooperation given me during the past 2 decades.

The current approaches to the treatment of the major malignant neoplasms of soft tissue and bone will be discussed extensively in subsequent presentations at this conference. It is anticipated that the speakers will review the past studies as well as the results of treatments now being given. Also, the implications of the current data, no doubt, will be projected to exciting potentialities in the future.

To avoid overlap, my discussion will focus primarily on the clinical experience with which I have been personally involved, both here at

M. D. Anderson Hospital and with the Southwest Oncology Group. It will be my intent to provide perspectives for the concepts of current therapy. My comments will be restricted to 2 specific cancers, rhabdomyosarcoma and osteosarcoma. In each of these cancers there have occurred within the past few years significant and solidly established improvements in the results of therapy. A careful look at the developmental steps by which this success is being achieved seems worthwhile.

Clearly, the clinical understanding and the control of any cancer require multifaceted approaches such as those listed in Table 1. These items broadly are intended as guidelines to the study of the disease, to the study of the treatment, and to the evaluation of results of therapy.

Among the etiologic considerations are the relative incidences of the cancers and the distribution of the cases in terms of age, sex, and ethnic background. These and other factors may have implications with respect to tolerance of treatment (such as chemotherapy and radiotherapy) and to prognosis.

Of immediate and direct importance to the patient and to the physician is the identification of the clinical factors that determine the nature, direction, and intensity of the treatment program. Such factors include the histopathologic classification of the tumor, the site of the primary lesion, the extent of the disease, the response to the therapy, and the pattern of metastases.

The historical structuring of the treatment program for rhabdomyosarcoma may serve as a model to illustrate the present approach to several childhood cancers. The analysis of the M. D. Anderson Hospital experience with rhabdomyosarcoma in the Department of Pediatrics was initiated in about 1965 to determine the clinical nature of the cancer and to identify some of the factors that appeared to influence prognosis in the patient (Sutow *et al.*, 1970). Concomitantly, the status of the available therapeutic armamentarium was reviewed.

Based on experience with Wilms' tumor, the requirements for effective adjuvant therapy were formulated in 1965 as: a chemosensitive

TABLE 1.—PERSPECTIVES

Etiologic considerations
Clinical factors
Prognostic factors
Tactics of therapy
Strategy of therapy
Side effects of therapy

tumor, the availability of effective chemotherapeutic agents, and the utilization of additional effective therapeutic modalities. It seemed feasible and desirable to apply similar tactics to the management of rhabdomyosarcoma (Sutow and Sullivan, 1970). By 1967, pilot studies were under way and guidelines to the strategy of treatment had been evolved.

In the initial analysis of our patients with rhabdomyosarcoma, the extent of the disease, grossly divided into 2 categories of localized disease and extensive disease, was noted to be a major determinant of prognosis. All 24 children with extensive disease died within 30 months of diagnosis. About half of the 54 children with localized disease (including the orbital cases) survived. Recently, these cases were included in a further analysis in which the extent of the disease was estimated utilizing (retrospectively) the clinical grouping criteria of the Intergroup Rhabdomyosarcoma Study (Maurer, 1975). Inverse correlation between extent of the disease and survival was again demonstrated (Okamura, Sutow, and Moon, in press).

A number of other interactions appeared to exist—such as those between site of the primary tumor and histologic characteristics, between histologic type and prognosis, between site of primary and prognosis, and possibly between age and prognosis (Sutow *et al.,* 1970). This early study, however, preceded the consistent use of intensive multidisciplinary and multiagent therapy. It is possible that therapy will become sufficiently effective to obviate the need to consider many of these clinical factors.

Clinical investigations established the effectiveness of vincristine (Sutow *et al.,* 1966; Sutow, 1968) and of cyclophosphamide (Haddy, Nora, Sutow, and Vietti, 1967; Sutow, 1967) in the management of metastatic rhabdomyosarcoma. The dosage and schedule of administration of the drugs had been worked out and the toxicity pattern had been elucidated. By 1967, the guidelines for the strategy of treatment of rhabdomyosarcoma had been outlined (Table 2).

TABLE 2.—STRATEGY FOR THE
TREATMENT OF RHABDOMYOSARCOMA
(formulated in 1967)

Maximum utilization of effective drugs
Maximum utilization of all effective
    treatment modalities
Adequate duration of therapy
Utilization of host factors
Positive attitude
Persistent, planned all-out effort
Defined objectives

The assimilation of these principles into a practical working regimen culminated in the VAC program conceptualized 10 years ago (Sutow, 1969; Sutow and Sullivan, 1970). Obvious in the schemas were such concepts as those now termed multidrug therapy, multidisciplinary approach, adjuvant chemotherapy, and preradiotherapy (and/or preoperative) chemotherapy.

The gratifying validation of this approach to the management of rhabdomyosarcoma comes from at least 2 directions. A recent analysis (Okamura, Sutow, and Moon, unpublished data) of the survival status among children treated with these regimens confirmed and extended the previous findings of significantly improved survival rate (Wilbur, Sutow, and Sullivan, 1974; Fernandez, Sutow, Merino, and George, 1975). Secondly, the results of the Intergroup Rhabdomyosarcoma Study to be reported at this conference (see Maurer *et al.*, 1977, pages 317–332, this volume) will also indicate increased survival with systematic chemotherapy.

The story of osteosarcoma for many decades monotonously emphasized the persistent unresponsiveness of the tumor to all forms of therapy — surgery, irradiation, and drugs. The survival rate, irrespective of type of therapy, was below 20% in practically all reported series of patients (Friedman and Carter, 1972). The dramatic change that occurred recently in the attitudes towards this cancer (Jaffe, 1975) and the abrupt improvement in prognosis (Rosen, 1975; Jaffe, Frei, Traggis, and Bishop, 1974; Cortes, Holland, Wang, and Glidewell, 1975; Sutow *et al.* 1976) will be discussed in a separate paper at this conference (see Sutow, 1977, pages 163–170, this volume).

Unlike rhabdomyosarcoma, osteosarcoma had been considered to be highly resistant to chemotherapy. In 1962, however, some significant responses of metastatic tumor to the use of an alkylating agent, phenylalanine mustard (PAM) (Sullivan, Sutow, and Taylor, 1963), triggered our continuing study of this tumor. Additional investigations of dose and schedule of treatment with PAM (Sutow *et al.*, 1971a) as well as other drugs (Sutow *et al.*, 1971b; Sutow *et al.*, 1971c) have been conducted. Subsequently, several programs of adjuvant chemotherapy have been studied with the intent of eradicating micrometastases, preventing the occurrence of new metastases, and improving the cure rate (Sutow, Sullivan, Wilbur, and Cangir, 1975; Sutow *et al.*, 1975; Sutow *et al.*, 1976).

As chemotherapists began to report success in the control of osteosarcoma, questions regarding the validity of these claims have been raised (Taylor, Ivins, Dahlin, and Pritchard, in press). These questions need examination.

We have reanalyzed our own data from 1950 to 1974 on 125 patients

(Gehan *et al.*, in press). Such patients were 20 years of age or less at diagnosis. The primary lesion involved an extremity bone. All underwent amputation. None had metastases at diagnosis. Of the 125 patients, 89 did not receive any chemotherapy; 36 received multidrug adjuvant chemotherapy.

Life table analysis demonstrated no significant change in disease-free survival curves for 3 time periods: before 1963, 1963 through 1968, and 1969 through 1974 (Fig. 1). In contrast, the overall survival curve (Fig. 2) shows a distinct advantage for those who received adjuvant chemotherapy, either the CONPADRI-I or COMPADRI-II regimen (Sutow *et al.*, 1976). While the survival rate of 79% would seem impressive, the full clinical interpretation must take into account 2 facts. First, the overall survival data include those living with disease. Second, the curve also includes those living without disease but who had developed metastases (Table 3).

Thus, the overall survival curves signify both an achievement and a challenge. There have been apparent cures even though metastases had developed following primary therapy. Of the patients with metas-

Fig. 1.—Time to metastases for patients with osteosarcoma treated from 1950–1974 at M. D. Anderson Hospital. The patients were under 21 years of age, had primary tumors involving extremity bones, underwent amputation, and had no metastases at diagnosis. (Courtesy of Gehan *et al.*, in press.)

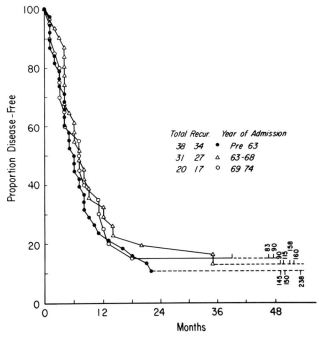

Total	Recur.		Year of Admission
38	34	•	Pre 63
31	27	△	63-68
20	17	○	69 74

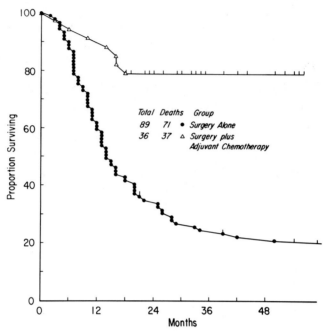

Fig. 2.—Survival of patients with osteosarcoma treated from 1950 to 1974 at M. D. Anderson Hospital. The surviving population includes those with no evidence of disease and those living with disease. The adjuvant chemotherapy consisted of CON-PADRI-I and COMPADRI-II regimens. (Courtesy of Gehan *et al.*, in press.)

tases, many had undergone thoracic surgery, some more than once. All had received radiation therapy and chemotherapy. The challenge stems from the probability that those living with disease will die and that more effective therapy for metastatic disease still must be developed.

TABLE 3.—SURVIVAL AFTER
FAILURE ON ADJUVANT
THERAPY FOR OSTEOSARCOMA

LIVING NED° (MONTHS)	LIVING WITH DISEASE (MONTHS)
12+	18+
27+	20+
41+	24+
41+	34+
52+	41+
56+	

°NED—no evidence of disease.

At the present time, the progress in the clinical management of osteosarcoma can be measured by at least 4 parameters. First, there has been a significant improvement in long-term control rates, and it is hoped that long-term control can be equated with cure. Second, the disease-free interval has been prolonged in those who develop metastases. Third, increased ability to control metastatic disease is being documented. Fourth, evidence strongly indicates that duration of survival, even with metastases, has been lengthened (Cortes, Holland, Wang, and Glidewell, 1975; Jaffe, 1972; Rosen *et al.*, 1975; Sutow *et al.*, 1975). Additionally, with effective chemotherapy, still another accomplishment is being exploited—that of tumor resection and prosthetic bone replacement, permitting the preservation of limb (Rosen *et al.*, 1976).

The treatment of patients with osteosarcoma has been discussed principally in terms of the 3 major modalities of surgery, radiation therapy, and chemotherapy. Other approaches are under investigation. Adoptive immunotherapy (Neff and Enneking, 1975), the use of autogenous tumor vaccines (Southam *et al.*, 1973), and the administration of transfer factor (Levin *et al.*, 1975) have been reported. Exogenous use of interferon has also been tried (Strander *et al.*, 1974). To date, it has not been possible to produce sound evidence for the clinical effectiveness of any of these measures comparable to that already available for surgery, chemotherapy, and, to some degree, radiotherapy.

In summary, it is clear that current treatment programs have significantly improved the clinical ability to control such cancers as rhabdomyosarcoma and osteosarcoma. The increased effectiveness of therapeutic strategies results from a number of factors. Diagnosis is becoming more precise. Staging and grouping techniques now permit accurate assessment of the extent of the disease in a patient at any particular time. The treatment regimen can be manipulated for specific treatment objectives. Among the significant tactics are the use of drugs in combination (multiagent chemotherapy) and the programming of multimodal or multidisciplinary therapy.

Finally, of growing importance as more and more patients survive is the need for recognition of the nature and significance of side effects of therapy, particularly the late, delayed consequences.

REFERENCES

Cortes, E. P., Holland, J. F., Wang, J. J., and Glidewell, O.: Adriamycin (NSC-123127) in 87 patients with osteosarcoma. Cancer Chemotherapy Reports, (Part 3) 6:305–313, October 1975.

Fernandez, C. H., Sutow, W. W., Merino, O. R., and George, S. L.: Childhood rhabdomyosarcoma. Analysis of coordinated therapy and results. American Journal of Roentgenology, Radium Therapy and Nuclear Medicine, 123: 588–597, March 1975.

Friedman, M. A., and Carter, S. K.: The therapy of osteogenic sarcoma: current status and thoughts for the future. Journal of Surgical Oncology, 4: 482–510, October 1972.

Gehan, E. A., Sutow, W. W., Uribe-Botero, G., Romsdahl, M., and Smith, T. L.: Osteosarcoma: The M. D. Anderson experience, 1950–1974. (In press.)

Haddy, T. B., Nora, A. H., Sutow, W. W., and Vietti, T. J.: Cyclophosphamide treatment for metastatic soft tissue sarcoma. Intermittent large doses in the treatment of children. American Journal of Diseases of Children, 114: 301–308, September 1967.

Jaffe, N.: Recent advances in the chemotherapy of metastatic osteogenic sarcoma. Cancer, 30:1627–1631, December 1972.

————: The potential of combined modality approaches for the treatment of malignant bone tumors in children. Cancer Treatment Reviews, 2:33–53, 1975.

Jaffe, N., Frei, E., III, Traggis, D., and Bishop, Y.: Adjuvant methotrexate and citrovorum-factor treatment of osteogenic sarcoma. New England Journal of Medicine, 291:994–997, November 7, 1974.

Levin, A. S., Byers, V. S., Fudenberg, H. H., Wybran, J., Hackett, A. J., Johnston, J. O., and Spitler, L. E.: Osteogenic sarcoma. Immunologic parameters before and during immunotherapy with tumor-specific transfer factor. Journal of Clinical Investigation 55:487–499, March 1975.

Maurer, H. M.: The Intergroup Rhabdomyosarcoma Study (NIH): Objectives and clinical staging classification. Journal of Pediatric Surgery, 10:977–978, December 1975.

Maurer, H. M., Moon, T., Donaldson, M., Fernandez, C., Gehan, E. A., Hammond, D., Hays, D. M., Lawrence, W., Jr., Ragab, A., Raney, B., Soule, E. H., Sutow, W. W., and Tefft, M.: Preliminary results of the Intergroup Rhabdomyosarcoma Study (IRS). In *Management of Bone and Soft Tissue Tumors* (The University of Texas System Cancer Center M. D. Anderson Hospital and Tumor Institute, 21st Annual Clinical Conference on Cancer). Chicago, Illinois, Year Book Medical Publishers, Inc., 1977, pp. 317–332.

Neff, J. R., and Enneking, W. F.: Adoptive immunotherapy in primary osteosarcoma. An interim report. Journal of Bone and Joint Surgery, 57A: 145–148, March 1975.

Okamura, J., Sutow, W. W., and Moon, T. E.: Prognosis in children with metastatic rhabdomyosarcoma. Medical and Pediatric Oncology. (In press.)

Rosen, G.: The development of an adjuvant chemotherapy program for the treatment of osteogenic sarcoma. Frontiers of Radiation Therapy and Oncology, 10:115–133, 1975.

Rosen, G., Murphy, M. L., Huvos, A. G., Gutierrez, M., and Marcove. R. C.: Chemotherapy, en bloc resection, and prosthetic bone replacement in the treatment of osteogenic sarcoma. Cancer, 37:1–11, January 1976.

Rosen, G., Tefft, M., Martinez, A., Cham, W., and Murphy, M. L.: Combination chemotherapy and radiation therapy in the treatment of metastatic osteogenic sarcoma. Cancer 35:622–630, March 1975.

Southam, C. M., Marcove, R. C., Levin, A. G., Buchsbaum, H. J., and Miké, V.: Clinical trial of autogenous tumor vaccine for treatment of osteogenic sarcoma. In *Seventh National Cancer Conference Proceedings.* Philadelphia, Pennsylvania and Toronto, Canada, J. B. Lippincott Company, 1973, pp. 91–100.

Strander, H., Cantell, K., Jakobsson, P. A. Nilssone, U., and Söderberg, G.: Exogenous interferon therapy of osteogenic sarcoma. Acta Orthopaedica Scandinavica, 45:958–959, 1974.

Sullivan, M. P., Sutow, W. W., and Taylor, G.: L-phenylalanine mustard as a treatment for metastatic osteogenic sarcoma in children. Journal of Pediatrics 63:227–237, August 1963.

Sutow, W. W.: Chemotherapeutic management of childhood rhabdomyosarcoma. In *Neoplasia in Childhood* (The University of Texas M. D. Anderson Hospital and Tumor Institute at Houston, 12th Annual Clinical Conference on Cancer). Chicago, Illinois, Year Book Medical Publishers, Inc., 1969, pp. 201–208.

————: Chemotherapy in the management of osteosarcoma. In *Management of Primary Bone and Soft Tissue Tumors* (The University of Texas System Cancer Center M. D. Anderson Hospital and Tumor Institute, 21st Annual Clinical Conference on Cancer). Chicago, Illinois, Year Book Medical Publishers, Inc., 1977, pp. 163–170.

————: Cyclophosphamide (NSC-26271) in Wilms' tumor and rhabdomyosarcoma. Cancer Chemotherapy Reports, 51:407–409, October 1967.

————: Vincristine (NSC-67574) therapy for malignant solid tumors in children (except Wilms' tumor). Cancer Chemotherapy Reports, 52:485–487, June 1968.

Sutow, W. W., Berry, D. H., Haddy, T. B., Sullivan, M. P., Watkins, W. L., and Windmiller, J.: Vincristine sulfate therapy in children with metastatic soft tissue sarcoma. Pediatrics, 38:465–472, September 1966.

Sutow, W. W., Fernandez, C. H., Mountain, C. F., King, O. Y., Rivera, R. L., and Mumford, D. M.: Multimodal treatment of pulmonary metastases in osteogenic sarcoma (Abstract). Proceedings of American Association for Cancer Research, 16:39, 1975.

Sutow, W. W., Gehan, E. A., Vietti, T. J., Frias, A. E., and Dyment, P. G.: Multidrug chemotherapy in primary treatment of osteosarcoma. Journal of Bone and Joint Surgery, 58A:629–633, July 1976.

Sutow, W. W., and Sullivan, M. P.: Successful chemotherapy for childhood rhabdomyosarcoma. Texas Medicine, 66:78–81, April 1970.

Sutow, W. W., Sullivan, M. P., Fernbach, D. J., Cangir, A., and George, S. L.: Adjuvant chemotherapy in primary treatment of osteogenic sarcoma. A Southwest Oncology Group Study. Cancer, 36:1598–1602, November 1975.

Sutow, W. W., Sullivan, M. P., Ried, H. L., Taylor, H. G., and Griffith, K. M.: Prognosis in childhood rhabdomyosarcoma. Cancer, 25:1384–1390, June 1970.

Sutow, W. W., Sullivan, M. P., Wilbur, J. R., and Cangir, A.: Study of adjuvant chemotherapy in osteogenic sarcoma. Journal of Clinical Pharmacology, 15:530–533, July 1975.

Sutow, W. W., Sullivan, M. P., Wilbur, J. R., Vietti, T. J., Kaizer, H., and Nagamoto, A.: L-phenylalanine mustard (NSC-8806) administration in osteogenic sarcoma: An evaluation of dosage schedules. Cancer Chemotherapy Reports, 55:151–157, April 1971a.

Sutow, W. W., Wilbur, J. R., Vietti, T. J., Vuthibhagdee, P., Fujimoto, T., and Watanabe, A.: Evaluation of dosage schedules of mitomycin C (NSC-26980) in children. Cancer Chemotherapy Reports, (Part 1) 55:285–289, June 1971b.

Sutow, W. W., Vietti, T. J., Fernbach, D. J., Lane, D. M., Donaldson, M. H., and Lonsdale, D.: Evaluation of chemotherapy in children with metastatic Ewing's sarcoma and osteogenic sarcoma. Cancer Chemotherapy Reports, (Part I) 55:67–78, February 1971c.

Taylor, W. F., Ivins, J. C., Dahlin, D. C., and Pritchard, D. J.: *Osteogenic Sarcoma Experience at Mayo Clinic, 1963–1974.* (In press.)

Wilbur, J. R., Sutow, W. W., and Sullivan, M. P.: The changing treatment of rhabdomyosarcoma in children, particularly in treatment for inoperable rhabdomyosarcoma of the nasopharynx and oropharynx. In *Neoplasia of Head and Neck* (The University of Texas System Cancer Center M. D. Anderson Hospital and Tumor Institute, 17th Annual Clinical Conference on Cancer). Chicago, Illinois, Year Book Medical Publishers, Inc., 1974, pp. 281–288.

Development of a Clinical Staging System for Primary Malignant Tumors of Bone: A Progress Report

MURRAY M. COPELAND, M.D., GUY F. ROBBINS, M.D., and MAX H. MYERS, Ph.D.

Cochairman, The Task Force on Malignant Bone Tumors, American Joint Committee for Cancer Staging and End Results Reporting, The University of Texas System Cancer Center M. D. Anderson Hospital and Tumor Institute, Houston, Texas; Cochairman, The Task Force on Malignant Bone Tumors, American Joint Committee for Cancer Staging and End Results Reporting, Memorial Hospital for Cancer and Allied Diseases, New York, New York; and Statistician Consultant, Head, End Results Section, Biometry Branch, National Cancer Institute, Bethesda, Maryland

PRIMARY MALIGNANT LESIONS of the bone present important diagnostic and treatment problems. Vital to making a diagnosis are both the interpretation of radiograms and the analysis of histopathologic features of the disease. In clinically appraising a patient for therapy, it is necessary to know the natural history of the disease, the clinical characteristics, the extent of disease, the essential histopathology, and what influence a specific therapy may have upon the disease.

Increasingly sophisticated diagnostic techniques and more intensive study of each patient have enhanced our ability to determine the extent of each bone neoplasm with knowledge of the essential pathology. This assessment aids in the selection of the most effective treatment and indicates the attendant prognosis.

It was believed by the American Joint Committee Task Force on Malignant Bone Tumors that an abstract form (or protocol) with instructions for use (see Appendix and Table 1) would be essential in developing a comprehensive analysis of a large series of cases, and

TABLE 1.—CLASSIFICATION OF MALIGNANT BONE TUMOR

PATIENT IDENTIFICATION AND HISTORY

Name _____   Institution _____
Age _____ /__/ Male /__/ Female /__/ Unknown   Hospital No. _____
/__/ White /__/ Black /__/ Other /__/ Unknown   Source of Case _____
   (Prior cancer? /__/ Yes /__/ No Date _____)   Date of Admission _____
   (Site & Type _____)   Date of Diagnosis _____
   (Treatment _____)

SYMPTOMS (Check all applicable)

	Duration
/__/ Pain	_____
/__/ Swelling	_____
/__/ Weight loss	_____
/__/ Functional impairment	_____
/__/ Fever	_____
/__/ Malaise	_____
/__/ Other, specify	_____

CLINICAL FINDINGS (Check all applicable)
Location of Primary __R__ __L__
Clinical Size ____ cm /__/ Not palpable

	Yes	No
Skin temperature elevation	/__/	/__/
Systemic fever (1st examination)	/__/	/__/
Tenderness	/__/	/__/
Venous distention	/__/	/__/
Lymphedema	/__/	/__/
Fracture	/__/	/__/
Ecchymosis	/__/	/__/
Muscle atrophy	/__/	/__/
Lymph node evaluation	/__/	/__/
Specify node(s) _____		

LABORATORY FINDINGS (1st admission)

	Normal	Elevated	Decreased
Alkaline phosphatase	/__/	/__/	/__/
Hemoglobin	/__/	/__/	/__/
Calcium	/__/	/__/	/__/
Phosphorous	/__/	/__/	/__/
Total proteins	/__/	/__/	/__/
WBC	/__/	/__/	/__/
Differential count _____			

RADIOGRAPHIC FINDINGS

/__/ Radiogram /__/ Angiogram /__/ Tomogram
/__/ Bone scan (type _____)
Quality _____ Date _____
....
Specific Location of Tumor within Bone
Long bone, specify __R__ __L__
/__/ Epiphysis /__/ Metaphysis /__/ Proximal
/__/ Distal /__/ Diaphysis (central) /__/ Periosteal
....
/__/ Pelvic bone __R__ __L__ _____
/__/ Cranium _____
                    (Bone and Site)
/__/ Mandible __R__ __L__
/__/ Spine __C__ __T__ __L__ __S__ __Co.__
/__/ Scapula __R__ __L__
/__/ Rib __R__ __L__
/__/ Soft tissue mass, specify _____

....
Extent of Involvement
/__/ Single primary tumor
/__/ Multifocal primary within one bone
/__/ Multiple primaries in more than one bone
Size: Longitudinal ____ cm Transverse ____ cm
Lesion Edge:
   /__/ sharp edge with sclerosis
   /__/ sharp edge without sclerosis
   /__/ ill-defined

Abbreviations:

   R — Right; L — Left
   C — Cervical
   T — Thoracic
   L — Lumbar
   S — Sacral
   Co. — Coccyx

Character of Bone Involvement
/__/ sclerotic
/__/ lytic
/__/ medullary involvement
Cortical involvement:
   /__/ thickening   /__/ thinning   /__/ perforation
Periosteal reaction:
   /__/ lamellation   /__/ spiculation
   /__/ solid sclerosis   /__/ amorphous
/__/ soft parts
   specify type _____

....

X-ray Evidence of Metastases (1st examination)
                        Positive Negative Not Done
Chest film: /__/   /__/   /__/
Chest tomogram: /__/   /__/   /__/
Bone survey:
   /__/ complete   /__/   /__/   /__/
   /__/ partial   /__/   /__/   /__/
   /__/ isotope bone scan /__/   /__/   /__/
   Type isotope _____

==

PATHOLOGIC FINDINGS OBTAINED BY:

Biopsy of Primary
   This institution /__/ Yes
   Tourniquet used /__/ Yes
   Type of biopsy: /__/ Excisional /__/ Incisional
                    /__/ Trochar   /__/ Needle
....
Histologic type
Source: /__/ Pathology report /__/ Review slides
Type _____
   _____
   _____

==

DEFINITIVE SURGERY

Gross Size _____ × _____ × _____
                  Dimensions in cm
Location within bone (Long bones only)
   /__/ Proximal /__/ Distal /__/ Central
Final Diagnosis _____
                  (Histopathology)

/__/ No treatment prescribed   Date _____
   Reason, specify _____
   _____

Surgery   /__/ no surgery
Amputation: /__/ through involved bone
   /__/ through bone above /__/ disarticulation
   /__/ local resection   /__/ curretage
   /__/ other, specify _____
....
Radiation
   Date started _____ Completed _____
....
Chemotherapy   /__/ no chemotherapy
   Date started _____ Completed _____
   Type: /__/ Systemic   /__/ Regional
....
Immunotherapy   /__/ no immunotherapy
   Date started _____ Completed _____
   _____

==

FOLLOW-UP

Recurrence   /__/ none
   /__/ never free
   /__/ local recurrence _____
                                   Date
   /__/ metastasis, specify _____
                                   Date
   _____
....
Last Known Vital Status _____
                                   Date
   /__/ Alive   /__/ Dead
Cancer status:
   /__/ not present   /__/ probably present
   /__/ cancer confirmed   /__/ unknown
....
Cause of death, specify _____
   _____

==

Autopsy   /__/ Yes /__/ No

   /__/ free of bone cancer

   /__/ bone cancer present

   /__/ other cancer present

   /__/ no information

_____

that a preliminary field trial on retrospective cases could establish the useful components of the protocol and identify the lack of available information in such a retrospective study. If the records available for study proved inadequate, it would become necessary to obtain appropriate information from a prospective study in order to develop a significant end results study and/or clinical classification.

Accordingly, the Task Force on Malignant Bone Tumors organized such a pilot study to determine the adequacy of an abstract form (protocol) for assessing the availability of essential data retrospectively. Six Task Force members, representing institutions with large bone tumor registries, were asked to complete abstracts for approximately 10 or more consecutive bone cancer cases each, working back in time from patients diagnosed in December 1965.

Of a total of 64 abstracts presented, 6 did not meet the necessary selection criteria specified in the protocol instructions, thus leaving 58 case abstracts suitable for inclusion in the analysis.

Certain basic information such as age, sex, race, date of diagnosis, and date of admission to the reporting hospital was routinely available, together with information pertaining to histologic diagnosis and patient follow-up. However, much of the requested clinical and radiographic data considered by the Task Force members as absolutely essential was unreported (Tables 2, 3, and 4).

TABLE 2.—MALIGNANT BONE TUMORS:
HISTOLOGIC TYPE DISTRIBUTION

HISTOLOGIC TYPE	NUMBER OF CASES	PERCENT
Osteosarcoma	23	40
Chondrosarcoma	12	21
Ewing's sarcoma	8	14
Fibrosarcoma	4	7
Primary reticulum cell sarcoma	3	5
Malignant giant cell tumor	2	3
Other specified types	5	9
Type not specified	1	2
Total	58	101°

°Percentages sum to 101 due to rounding.
American Joint Committee feasibility study.

TABLE 3.—MALIGNANT BONE TUMORS:
CLINICAL FINDINGS

CLINICAL FINDINGS	DATA GIVEN	NO ANSWER
Tumor size	35	23
Skin temperature elevation	26	32
Tenderness	52	6
Venous distention	20	38
Lymphedema	24	34
Fracture	40	18
Ecchymosis	21	37
Muscle atrophy	29	29

American Joint Committee feasibility study.

TABLE 4. – MALIGNANT BONE TUMORS:
RADIOGRAPHIC FINDINGS

RADIOGRAPHIC FINDINGS	DATA GIVEN	NO ANSWER
Localization	48	10 (17%)
Tumor size	30	28 (48%)
Lesion edge	38	20 (34%)
Cortical involvement	42	16 (28%)
Medullary involvement	18	40 (69%)
Fracture	20	38 (66%)
Periosteal involvement	18	40 (69%)
Soft part involvement	34	24 (41%)
Multiple primary areas	4	54 (93%)
Character of bone involvement	50	8 (14%)
Evidence of metastases	53	5 (9%)

American Joint Committee feasibility study.

Protocol Analysis

Of the 58 evaluable malignant bone tumor patients, 35 (60%) were male. Thirteen patients (22%) were under 15 years of age, 23 (40%) were between 15 and 24 years, and 11 (19%) were 55 years and over. Histologic diagnoses (Table 2) were available in 57 cases and revealed a 40% incidence of osteosarcoma, 21% chondrosarcoma, and 14% Ewing's sarcoma. The other diagnoses consisted of fibrosarcoma (4 cases), primary reticulum cell sarcoma (3 cases), malignant giant cell tumor (2 cases), and 1 case for each of the following histologic types: chordoma, adamantinoma, malignant hemangioendothelioma, plasmacytoma, and a mixed tumor with areas of osteosarcoma, fibrosarcoma and malignant giant cells.

Data concerning symptoms prior to bone tumor diagnosis were generally unavailable in the medical charts reviewed. The protocol requested information on the duration prior to admission of tenderness, pain, swelling, weight loss, functional impairment, fever, and malaise. The presence or absence and duration of pain were recorded for 56 of the 58 patients; however, information on the remaining symptoms was not recorded for 30% or more of the patients. We were generally unwilling to assume that failure to mention any single symptom or finding meant that it was not present.

Tables 3 and 4 show the frequencies with which clinical and radiographic findings, respectively, were recorded in hospital charts. Of the clinical parameters, tenderness was the only one with a level of available information (90% of the patients) acceptable for statistical analysis. Clinical tumor size, for example, was recorded for only 60% of patients. Radiographic findings, considered by our consultants to be indispensable, were generally not recorded in a high enough percentage of patients to conduct a meaningful study of prognostic factors from the radiological point of view. Similarly, data were not mentioned or were unknown for cortical involvement in 28% of the abstracts, for medullary involvement in 69%, for periosteal involvement in 69%, and for soft part involvement in 41%. Radiographic findings were based on a review of radiographs in 24 of the 58 cases and, for these, the data were generally available. The Task Force consultants, however, reported that the important information from radiographs was not routinely available for review.

The information obtained at the time of primary therapy was recorded for all but 1 patient, and the follow-up on living patients was good. Only 3 of 23 patients alive at last contact had been followed for less than 4 years, thus permitting, via actuarial survival analysis, valid estimation of the 5-year survival rate for patients in different histopathological categories. For example, in a review of 700 cases of primary bone sarcoma seen by the senior author in the past 35 years, the end results reported on cases classified histopathologically reveal a 5-year survival rate as noted in Table 5.

In addition, the protocol requested data on acid phosphatase, alkaline phosphatase, hemoglobin, calcium, phosphorus, total proteins, white blood cell count, differential count, and platelet count. Data were submitted on hemoglobin for 57 patients and on white blood cell count for 54 patients; differential counts were submitted for 53 patients. For the remaining items in this category, the percentage of cases with missing data ranged from 33% to 79%. While the laboratory factors were not considered absolutely necessary for a staging field trial on malignant bone tumors, they were considered potentially important and should not be excluded simply because they did not prove useful for staging other forms of cancer.

TABLE 5. – MALIGNANT BONE TUMORS: 5-YEAR SURVIVAL

Primary chondrosarcoma	15%
Secondary chondrosarcoma	38%
Malignant chondroblastoma	0%
Osteogenic sarcoma sclerosing	20%
Parosteal osteoma	50%
(Parosteal osteogenic sarcoma)	
Ewing's sarcoma	4%
Reticulum cell sarcoma of bone	35% – 42%

Comment

The data examined for this feasibility study illustrate some of the problems encountered in attempting to answer scientific questions by utilizing information recorded in patients' records as a part of routine medical care. If, for example, the clinicians and diagnostic radiologists who were involved in the management of these patients had realized the need for carefully recording detailed information and had had a guide showing what specifically to record, the data needed for a field trial on malignant bone tumors would have been available. It is very probable that information on bone tumor patients currently being entered into medical records is no more specific than that observed in this study. This is not meant as a critical reflection on the medical community, but rather as a recognition of the fact that data are usually recorded for a specific purpose. Therefore, if it is desirable to use field trial data to assist in the development of a staging classification for malignant bone tumors, there is no alternative to designing a study to intentionally collect the required data for a prospective study.

The Task Force on Malignant Bone Tumors has concluded that the future of the classification of primary bone tumors lies in prospective studies and has recommended that the existing protocol (abstract form and instructions) be utilized by interested institutions and individuals that have access to a large number of bone cancer patients.

The American Joint Committee believes that establishing an accurate diagnosis, with extent of disease, is absolutely essential for the evaluation of a bone tumor classification and staging for end results reporting. The Committee, therefore, does not recommend a clinical classification for staging and end results reporting of primary malignant tumors of bone based on current information available, but believes that in 5 to 10 years, through prospective field trials, the appropriate data on a sufficient number of patients with follow-up could be available for an adequate field trial analysis.

At a recent meeting of the Executive Committee of the American Joint Committee it was decided that the Task Force on Malignant Bone Tumors should not become involved in such a study, but rather that an appropriate institution or group of institutions would be better suited to carry out a prospective study where rigid controls of patient records, diagnostic procedures (especially radiographic studies), laboratory studies, treatment, and follow-up could be carried out over a long time interval (5 to 10 years). The protocol and instructions herein presented will be made available through the American Joint Committee for Cancer Staging and End Results Reporting, 55 East Erie Street, Chicago, Illinois 60610 (Copeland *et al.* 1976).

It seems appropriate, however, to identify certain histopathologic classifications as examples, and to discuss their use in classifying the bone neoplasms according to specific types which follow a definite clinical course. An evaluation of the treatment of these specific types of tumors reflects the effectiveness of the therapy used.

The histopathologic classifications recommended are to be found in the following:

1. Histological Typing of Primary Bone Tumors and Tumor-like Lesions (Schajowicz *et al.* 1972). This classification was adopted by the Task Force as a reasonable compromise among its members (Table 6).

2. Classification of Bone Tumors (Geschickter and Copeland, 1949) (Table 7).

3. Classification of 3,987 Primary Tumors of Bone (Dahlin, 1967).

4. Histogenesis of Bone Tumors (Jaffe, 1965).

Such classifications reflect the histologic tissue pattern which remains the decisive factor in the diagnostic interpretation of the neoplasm. In certain cases, however, judgement is based on the dominant histologic appearance of tissue taken from various parts of the lesion.

TABLE 6.—HISTOLOGICAL TYPING OF PRIMARY BONE TUMORS AND TUMOR-LIKE LESIONS* (WHO)

I. BONE-FORMING TUMORS

A. *Benign*
1. Osteoma
2. Osteoid osteoma and osteoblastoma (benign osteoblastoma)

B. *Malignant*
1. Osteosarcoma (osteogenic sarcoma)
2. Juxtacortical osteosarcoma (parosteal osteosarcoma)

II. CARTILAGE-FORMING TUMORS

A. *Benign*
1. Chondroma
2. Osteochondroma (osteocartilaginous exostosis)
3. Chondroblastoma (benign chondroblastoma, epiphyseal chondroblastoma)
4. Chondromyxoid fibroma

B. *Malignant*
1. Chondrosarcoma
2. Juxtacortical chondrosarcoma
3. Mesenchymal chondrosarcoma

III. GIANT-CELL TUMOR (OSTEOCLASTOMA)

IV. MARROW TUMORS
1. Ewing's sarcoma
2. Reticulosarcoma of bone
3. Myeloma

*Schajowicz, *et al.*: *Histological Typing of Bone Tumours.* Geneva, Switzerland, World Health Organization, 1972, 59 pp.

TABLE 7.—CLASSIFICATION OF BONE TUMORS*

TUMORS OF OSSEOUS ORIGIN

Cartilaginous	*Osseous*	*Resorptive*
Osteochondroma, solitary and multiple	Osteomas and ossifying fibromas of skull and jaws	Bone cyst
Chondroma	Osteoid-osteoma	Diffuse osteitis fibrosa (parathyroidism)
Chondromyxoid fibroma	Osteogenic sarcoma, sclerosing and osteolytic	Fibrous dysplasia, polyostotic or monostotic
Chondroblastoma, benign and malignant	Parosteal osteoma and myositis ossificans	Giant cell tumor
Chondrosarcoma, primary or secondary		

TUMORS OF NONOSSEOUS ORIGIN

Marrow and Haversian Systems	*Metastatic Deposits*	*By Inclusion or Direct Invasion*
Ewing's sarcoma	Carcinoma of prostate, breast, kidneys, etc.	Chordoma
Primary reticulum sarcoma	Metastatic lymphomas, neuroblastoma, and sarcomas	Angioma, angiosarcoma
Multiple myeloma		Fibroma and fibrosarcoma, fascial or nerve sheath
Chloroma and leukemia of bone		Myosarcoma
Reticuloendotheliosis		Liposarcoma
Xanthomas and granulomas of bone		

*C. F. Geschickter and M. M. Copeland: Embryogenesis of bone and its relationship to skeletal tissue. In *Tumors of Bone*. Philadelphia, J. B. Lippincott and Co., 1949, p. 27.

In addition, the clinical findings may be of help, but the radiographic studies, often regarded as a part of the gross pathologic picture, frequently afford important evidence as to the malignant or benign nature of the lesion. Laboratory studies are of little aid in diagnosing the average primary malignant bone tumor (an exception is in diagnosing multiple myeloma). The pathologist, the surgeon, or the radiologist dealing with bone tumors should view the diagnostic problem not only from his own standpoint but also from that of the other disciplines concerned.

No doubt, prospective clinical trials will be enhanced by more adequate case records and will permit a satisfactory clinical classification for staging and end results reporting of primary malignant bone tumors. In the interim, however, we have pointed out effective tools and mechanisms for evaluating patients for treatment and for determining survival rates based on the clinicopathologic analysis of the patient's type of disease.

Acknowledgments

This study was done in connection with activities of the Task Force on Malignant Bone Tumors of the American Joint Committee for Cancer Staging and End Results Reporting.

The participants in this pilot study included: David C. Dahlin, M.D., Mayo Clinic; Jack Edeiken, M.D., Jefferson Medical School; Richard G. Martin, M.D., M. D. Anderson Hospital; Crawford J. Campbell, M.D., Albany Medical College; Theodore B. Miller, M.D., Memorial Sloan-Kettering Cancer Center; and Michael Bonfiglio, M.D., The University of Iowa Medical School.

Appendix

INSTRUCTIONS FOR USE OF PROTOCOL
FOR
CLASSIFICATION OF MALIGNANT BONE TUMORS

The purpose of this study is to develop and test a method for a meaningful staging classification for primary malignant bone tumors. The malignant tumors qualifying for this study include all primary malignant tumors of skeletal tissues of the body. Extraskeletal malignant bone tumors are to be excluded.

For the correct interpretation of the collected data, it is necessary to have a description of the material supplied by each institution. In order to have this description, each responsible individual who fills out the checklist should provide the following complete information.

PATIENT IDENTIFICATION AND HISTORY

All patients with histologically confirmed primary malignant disease of bone and who received their first treatment in the reporting institution are to be included. Patients who had a previous biopsy (including excisional biopsy) elsewhere within an interval of 3 months and were then treated at the reporting institution also are to be included.

Adequate follow-up information on the group of cases is essential, and every effort should be made to obtain such information, if possible. Any institution which is not able to provide current follow-up information on at least 90% of its cases should not participate in this study.

DATE OF ONSET OF DURATION PRIOR TO ADMISSION.—Symptoms or other findings after the initiation of treatment should not be included (exception: histopathology).

DEFINITION OF STARTING TIME.— In considering the definition of starting time for reporting of cancer survival and end results, the date of initiation of treatment is to be used as the starting time for evaluation of therapy. Thus, the starting point from which survival rates are calculated is defined as the date, in treated patients, when first definitive tumor-directed treatment was commenced and, in untreated patients, as the date on which it was decided that no tumor-directed treatment would be given. This definition is used since it will usually coincide with the date of clinical staging of the cancer. All dates in the treatment section of the protocol are to be filled in if possible.

INITIAL TREATMENT. — Any treatment initiated within 4 months of initial diagnosis is to be included.

CLINICAL FINDINGS

Clinical findings are defined as the clinical evaluation of the lesion at the time of initial work-up in the hospital.

LOCATION OF PRIMARY TUMOR. — The specific bone involved should be indicated in those locations where the bones are listed under the general anatomical classification, such as metatarsal bone, etc. Also identify left as L and right as R, when appropriate.

TUMOR SIZE. — Specific dimensions, determined by palpation, should be listed.

RADIOGRAPHIC FINDINGS

EXTENT OF INVOLVEMENT. — Extension beyond tissue of origin into surrounding periosteal zone or soft parts should be indicated.

SPECIFIC LOCATION WITHIN BONE. — Tumors should be specifically located as to the diaphysis, metaphysis, epiphysis, or combinations. Localization of the tumor should be specified as involving the proximal or distal end for long bones. If more than 1 area is involved (i.e., diaphysis and metaphysis) check each appropriate block. In certain instances in flat bones it will be necessary to define the location with reference to the proximity to the joint.

LAMELLATED PERIOSTEAL REACTION (ONIONSKIN). — One or more strips of new bone laid down adjacent to the cortex a millimeter or less in width, with each strip separated by a radiolucent line.

SPICULATED PERIOSTEAL REACTION. — Thin strips of new bone formation laid down at approximately 90 degrees to the cortex and separated by radiolucent bands.

SOLID SCLEROSIS (PERIOSTEAL REACTION). — New bone laid down adjacent to the cortex and greater than 1 mm.

AMORPHOUS PERIOSTEAL REACTION. — Irregular deposits of new bone formation adjacent to the cortex but still within the bone. This is usually identified by the presence of Codman's triangles indicating elevation of the periosteum.

Pathologic Findings

Gross findings obtained at definitive surgery should be recorded according to size (3 dimensions) and location (in long bone). Those lesions 5 cm or less from the joint line should be designated as proximal or distal.

Histologic Type

There is an understandable variation in the terms used by different pathologists in describing the histology of this group of lesions. The histologic types to be included are the following: osteosarcoma, parosteal osteosarcoma, chondrosarcoma, fibrosarcoma, malignant giant cell tumor, primary reticulum cell sarcoma (lymphosarcoma), Ewing's sarcoma, and other (specify by diagnosis). Terms such as periosteal sarcoma, periosteal osteosarcoma, undifferentiated round cell sarcoma, hemangiosarcoma (or its synonyms), "adamantinoma," etc., should be entered as given in the pathologic reports where they differ from the classification given above. Include undifferentiated bone sarcoma under "other." DO NOT include chordoma of bone or myeloma.

At times there is some variation in the diagnostic label which a particular neoplasm is given during its course. The Task Force recommends that the *Histologic Typing of Primary Bone Tumours and Tumour-Like Lesions* published by the World Health Organization, Geneva, 1972, be used for specific definition of histologic typing. A Task Force review committee will have responsibility for reviewing the clinical, radiographic, and histologic data accumulated during the first year of the study in order to standardize reporting.

The recorder must sign the abstract form and indicate the date.

References

Copeland, M. M., Bonfiglio, M., Campbell, C. J., Dahlin, D. C., Edeiken, J., Latourette, H. B., Martin, R. B., Miller, T. R., Mountain, C. F., Raventos, A., Robbins, G. F., and Myers, M.: Staging of primary malignant bone tumors. In *Classification and Staging of Cancer by Site, A Preliminary Handbook.* Chicago, Illinois, The American Joint Committee for Cancer Staging and End Results Reporting, 1976, pp. 249–260.

Dahlin, D. C.: Introduction and scope of study: Classification of 3,987 primary tumors of bone. In *Bone Tumors.* Springfield, Illinois, Charles C Thomas, Publisher, 1967, pp. 3–15

Geschickter, C. F., and Copeland, M. M.: Embryogenesis of bone and its relationship to skeletal tissue. In *Tumors of Bone.* Philadelphia, Pennsylvania, J. B. Lippincott and Company, 1949, p. 27.

Jaffe, H. L.: Histogenesis of bone tumors. In *Tumors of Bone and Soft Tissue* (The University of Texas M. D. Anderson Hospital and Tumor Institute, 8th Annual Clinical Conference on Cancer). Chicago, Illinois, Year Book Medical Publishers, Inc., 1965, pp. 41–44.

Schajowicz, F., Ackerman, L. F., Sissons, H. A.: *Histological Typing of Bone Tumours.* Geneva, Switzerland, World Health Organization, 1972, pp. 19–20.

The Radiologic Approach to Bone Tumors

JACK EDEIKEN, M.D.

Professor of Radiology, Jefferson Medical College, Philadelphia, Pennsylvania, and Consultant in Radiology, The University of Texas System Cancer Center M. D. Anderson Hospital and Tumor Institute, Houston, Texas

IN THE CARE of a patient with a bone tumor, there must be close cooperation among the pathologist, the orthopedic surgeon, and the radiologist. The radiologist's role in the evaluation of the patient is to arrive at a diagnosis which will be compatible with the later histologic diagnosis. No experienced bone pathologist will review the histopathology of a patient without studying the roentgenograms. The radiologist provides a statistical evaluation, and by studying various aspects of the roentgenograms and the patient's history, an accurate histologic diagnosis may often be made.

Clinical History

Pain is a frequent symptom of bone tumor, and its character often aids in distinguishing benign from malignant processes. The pain of tumor begins as mild, aching pain, usually a deep bone pain which can be relieved initially by mild analgesics; but later the pain becomes unrelenting. Pain occurring at rest almost invariably distinguishes the pain of tumor from pain secondary to degenerative disease or trauma. Inflammatory disease may also be relieved by rest, but not commonly, and it is more often easily controlled with analgesics. Pain from bone tumors is usually worse at night because there are fewer external stimuli.

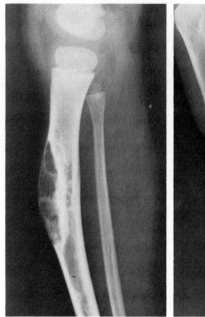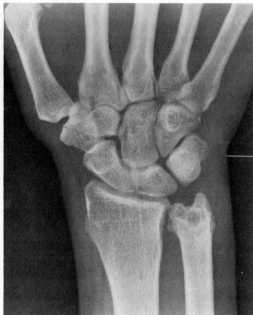

Fig. 1 (left).—Fibrous dysplasia of the tibia. Note the sharp transition between the lesion and the normal bone. There is a thick sclerotic rim on the inner aspect. Notice that the rim is smooth both on the inside and outside of the lesion, indicating lack of aggression.

Fig. 2 (right).—Interosseous ganglion of the ulna. Notice that the sclerotic rim around the lesion is not as thick as in Figure 1, but the inside and outside of the sclerosis are well-defined and indicate a lack of aggression.

The patient's appearance may often distinguish tumors such as Ewing's sarcoma from reticulum cell sarcoma. Patients with Ewing's sarcoma look sick, feel sick, and act sick. Those with reticulum cell sarcoma often look very well in spite of the presence of a large tumor. Certainly, elevation of temperature and an increase in white blood cell count are characteristic of most bone infections, but these symptoms may also appear with some bone tumors, particularly Ewing's sarcoma, although the fever is not as elevated or spiked as in infection.

The roentgenographic features that help distinguish bone tumors from other lesions are the aggressiveness of the lesion, indicated by the edge of the lesion or transition zone between the lesion and normal bone, and the type of periosteal reaction. The transition zones are most helpful in distinguishing aggressive from nonaggressive lesions, and may be grouped into 3 general categories: those with a sclerotic rim and a short transition zone, those with the lesion well-defined from the normal bone, and those with an ill-defined or long transition zone.

The sclerotic rim must be evaluated for sharpness on both the inside and the outside of the lesion, i.e. the margin adjacent to the lesion and the margin adjacent to the normal bone. If both are clearly defined, this indicates a long-standing, inactive lesion, usually benign (Figs. 1 and 2). The single exception is a cartilaginous lesion which may have been present and nonaggressive within the bone for many years. When it exhibits its malignant characteristics, the first sign is pain, and the roentgen features lag considerably. Therefore, lesions in bone with a sharply defined sclerotic margin on both the tumor and normal-bone side are usually benign and inactive, with the exception of some chondrosarcomas.

The bone lesion with no sclerotic rim but with a well-defined or short transition zone is usually benign (Fig. 3). Occasionally there will be an increased density surrounding the lesion, suggesting a sclerotic

Fig. 3 (left). – Unicameral bone cyst of calcaneus. There is no definite sclerotic rim, but there is a very sharp transition between the abnormal and the normal bone, indicating a lesion with slightly more aggressiveness than the lesion with a sclerotic margin.

Fig. 4 (right). – Chondroblastoma of tibia. Note that the lesion is well-defined with a sclerotic margin. However, the margin fades off into the normal bone, indicating aggressiveness.

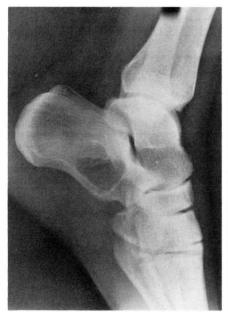 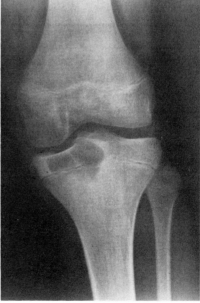

rim, but the density on the normal-bone side fades off, which is an indication of aggression (Fig. 4). Most lesions with a short transition zone are benign, but there are occasional exceptions such as malignant giant cell tumor, chondrosarcoma, and fibrosarcoma. However, usually these malignant lesions have a very long transition zone and are easily differentiated.

The ill-defined or very long transition zone is an indication of marked aggressiveness and usually indicates malignant disease. However, some benign aggressive conditions can produce this characteristic; these include infection, eosinophilic granuloma, aneurysmal bone cyst, and benign giant cell tumor (Figs. 5 and 6).

Periosteal reactions also help differentiate aggressive from nonaggressive lesions. The 2 types of periosteal reactions are the solid, which almost always indicates benignancy, and the interrupted, which indicates aggressiveness. Some benign aggressive conditions are infection, eosinophilic granuloma, giant cell tumor, and aneurysmal bone cyst.

Fig. 5 (left).—Osteosarcoma of the tibia. Notice that the osteolytic lesion fades into the normal bone and that the transition zone is long. This indicates aggression and usually malignant disease. However, infections and other granulomatous lesions also may exhibit this aggressiveness.

Fig. 6 (right).—Reticulum cell sarcoma of the humerus. There is a long transition zone between the osteolytic area and the normal bone. This indicates marked aggressiveness and usually is present in malignant disease.

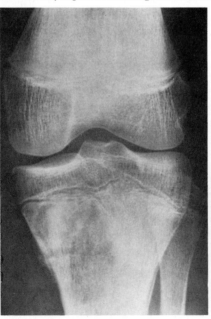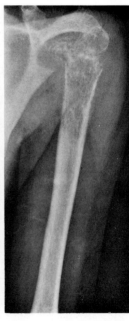

The solid periosteal reaction is more than 1 mm in width and is usually attached to the cortex, although occasionally a thin line separates them (Fig. 7). It almost invariably indicates benignancy, and there are only 2 infrequent exceptions. The first is in the case of certain long-standing malignant tumors which are asymptomatic until the patient sustains a pathologic fracture or complains of mass. This may occur in osteosarcoma or Ewing's sarcoma, but only rarely. The second type is not a diagnostic problem (since the diagnosis has been made previously) and appears in a malignant tumor that has been treated with irradiation or chemotherapy. If the tumor growth has stopped, periosteal reaction may consolidate and present a nonaggressive or benign appearance.

The interrupted periosteal reaction may be the sunburst type (Fig. 8) or the lamellated (onionskin) type (Fig. 9). These reactions are an indication of aggression and usually malignancy, but infection and

Fig. 7 (left).—Infantile cortical hyperostosis of the tibia and fibula. There is a solid periosteal reaction on the medial aspect of the tibia, indicating a benign lesion.

Fig. 8 (center).—Ewing's sarcoma of the femur. There is a sunburst or right angle periosteal reaction on the anterior surface of the femur. This indicates an aggressive lesion, but it may also be seen in benign disease such as infection.

Fig. 9 (right).—Ewing's sarcoma of the femur. There is a lamellated periosteal reaction at the distal end of the lesion on the medial aspect. This indicates aggression, but not necessarily malignant disease. There is also some right angle periosteal reaction in the center of the lesion medially.

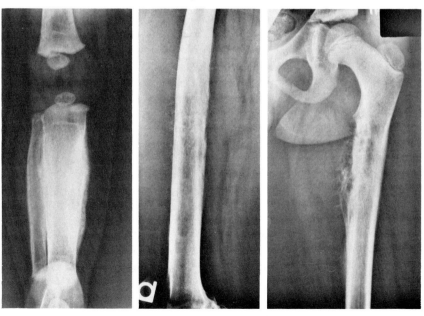

certain benign tumors such as hemangioma, eosinophilic granuloma, pulmonary osteoarthropathy, or others may show this interruption early in their course.

The age of the patient is the most useful indication of the type of malignant disease. If the patient has a known malignant lesion of bone, then age alone can aid in the diagnosis in approximately 85% of cases. In children less than 6 months of age, malignant lesions of bone are almost invariably the result of neuroblastoma. Among older children, Ewing's sarcoma is more common in the first decade than it is in higher age groups, but osteosarcoma is still the most common tumor. In teenagers or patients in their second decade, osteosarcoma is by far the most common tumor. In the third and fourth decades, lymphomas and other round cell tumors are the most common lesions. From the fourth decade onward, metastatic malignant disease and multiple myeloma are the most frequent diseases. Therefore, one begins with the age of the patient and tries to fit the tumor into the roentgenographic features.

There are 2 major pitfalls in the histologic diagnosis of bone tumors:

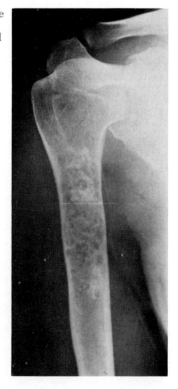

Fig. 10.—Chondrosarcoma of the humerus. The lesion is well-defined in the humerus and shows circles of calcification, especially at the distal end of the lesion, indicating the cartilaginous nature. There is no other change to suggest malignant disease. There is no destruction of bone, periosteal reaction, or soft tissue mass. However, this patient had pain and the histologic diagnosis was chondrosarcoma.

(1) the impossibility of distinguishing many cartilaginous malignancies from benign cartilaginous lesions; and (2) the formation of a periosteal reaction or reactive new bone in benign conditions, which may be easily mistaken for osteosarcoma. In these 2 conditions, the roentgenographic appearance is most helpful to the histopathologist.

In certain chondroid tumors, there is no way to distinguish the benign from the malignant either roentgenographically or histopathologically. In this instance, a cartilaginous tumor in an older patient, in an extremity other than the small bones of the hands and feet, and with a history of pain, is almost certainly a chondrosarcoma, even if the appearance is benign both roentgenographically and histiologically (Fig. 10).

Certain lesions such as fatigue fractures, stress fractures, desmoids, and the brown tumors of hyperparathyroidism may be mistaken for malignant disease. The first 3 are usually mistaken for osteosarcoma, while brown tumors may be mistaken for malignant giant cell tumors. The history and chemical studies will allow one to correct the latter, while the roentgen appearance will usually lead to the proper diagnosis in the case of fractures and desmoids.

Summary

Evaluation of a patient with malignant tumor requires the cooperation of the pathologist, the orthopedic surgeon, and the roentgenologist in evaluating the history, histologic appearance, and roentgenographic features. With this group corroboration, the diagnosis can usually be clearly established.

Histologic Classification of Primary Tumors of Bone

HARLAN J. SPJUT, M.D.

Department of Pathology, Baylor College of Medicine, and St. Luke's Episcopal Hospital, Houston, Texas

THE CLASSIFICATION OF TUMORS of the bone, both in the past and in the present, is based upon histological patterns. The patterns, in turn, correlate in general with the gross appearance, the radiographic features, and the biological behavior of the tumor. A classification based upon etiological factors might be more meaningful, but these factors are known in only a few instances; thus, at the moment, this form of classification is not practical. A classification based upon the skeletal location of a tumor has been suggested. This has some merit, in the sense that many tumors of bone have a predilection for certain locations. For example, a large number of chondrosarcomas occur in the pelvic bones, and giant cell tumors often are epiphyseal-metaphyseal in the long bones. Due to a considerable overlapping of the location of the various tumors, however, this form of classification would break down, and it is somewhat cumbersome. If the factor of age is inserted, there is a further refinement as to possible histologic type of tumor in certain locations. Again, the sites are not always specific, making this form of classification nonworkable.

The weakness of classification based on histological features has been pointed out by Johnson (1953). Basically, if one considers that tumors of bone are of single cell (mesenchymal cell) origin, then one can understand that there is potential for considerable intermixture of cell patterns in a tumor. Johnson (1953) believes that the various types of patterns that develop do so on the basis of influence of the environment in which they developed; for example, the growth rates of the bones in which they occur, the growth rates and metabolic gradients within a bone, and of course the numerous biochemical factors that would influence the growth of bone. With this potential in direction of differentiation available it is easy to understand why an occasional Ewing's sarcoma, for example, may contain both cartilage and bone. The mixtures of components are seen throughout many of the tumors of bone, both benign and malignant.

Recognizing the weakness of the classification based almost entirely upon morphological features, it is of interest to note how this type of classification has changed over the years. In 1940, James Ewing published a classification that consisted of 7 major groups of tumors (Table 1). One notes that chondroblastoma, for example, is absent from the classification and is included under the benign category as an epiphyseal giant cell tumor. Ewing's sarcoma does not appear, but is synonymous with diffuse endothelioma. In 1954, Ackerman and del Regato published a classification of tumors of bone (Table 2) that, in contrast to that presented by Ewing, shows a remarkable increase in the number of recognized lesions. For example, benign chondroblastoma, chondromyxoidfibroma, osteoid osteoma, nonossifying fibroma, osteogenic fibromas, and the adamantoma of the tibia all appeared in the classification. The World Health Organization (WHO) published a classification (Table 3) in 1972 (Schajowicz, Ackerman, and Sissons, 1972) that is similar to that in Table 2. Again, new tumors have been

TABLE 1.—REVISED CLASSIFICATION OF BONE TUMORS, 1939

	MALIGNANT	BENIGN
1. Osteogenic series	Medullary and subperiosteal Telangiectatic Sclerosing Periosteal Fibrosarcoma, medullary, subperiosteal	Exostosis Osteoma
2. Chondroma series	Chondrosarcoma Myxosarcoma	Chondroma
3. Giant-cell tumors	Benign, malignant	Epiphyseal giant-cell tumor
4. Angioma series	Angio-endothelioma Diffuse endothelioma	Cavernous angioma Plexiform angioma
5. Myeloma series	Plasma-cell Myelocytoma Erythroblastoma Lymphocytoma	
6. Reticulum-cell sarcoma 7. Liposarcoma		

(From Ewing, 1940.)

TABLE 2.—CLASSIFICATION OF TUMORS OF BONE, 1954

	BENIGN TUMORS OF BONE	MALIGNANT COUNTERPART	MALIGNANT TUMORS OF BONE
Of cartilage-cell or cartilage-forming connective tissue derivation	Peripheral-osteocartilaginous exostosis (Multiple exostosis)	Peripheral chondrosarcoma	Chondrosarcoma
	Central — Enchondroma (skeletal enchondromatosis)	Central chondrosarcoma	
	Benign chondroblastoma	Not known	
	Chondromyxoid fibroma	Not known	
Of osteoblastic derivation	Osteoma	Not known	
	Osteoid-osteoma	Not known	
	Osteogenic fibroma	Not known	
	Other osteoid-tissue-forming tumors	Osteogenic sarcoma	Osteogenic sarcoma
Of nonosteoblastic connective tissue derivation	Nonosteogenic fibroma	Not known	Fibrosarcoma
	Least aggressive giant-cell tumor	Malignant variety	Malignant giant-cell tumor
Of mesenchymal connective tissue origin	———————	———————	Ewing's sarcoma
Of hematopoietic origin	———————	———————	Multiple myeloma / Leukemia / Reticulum-cell sarcoma / "Lymphosarcoma" / Hodgkin's disease
Of nerve origin	Neurofibroma / Neurilemoma	Malignant Schwannoma	
Of vascular origin	Hemangioma	Angiosarcoma (hemangioendothelial sarcoma)	Hemangioendothelial sarcoma
Of fat-cell origin	Lipoma	———————	Liposarcoma (?)
Of notochordal derivation	———————	———————	Chordoma
Of adamantine or possibly basal-cell derivation	———————	———————	So-called adamantinoma

(From Ackerman and del Regato, 1954.)

defined and appear in the WHO classification: mesenchymal chondrosarcoma, juxtacortical osteosarcoma, juxtacortical chondrosarcoma, and malignant mesenchyma. Two tumors that do not appear in the preceding classifications are periosteal osteosarcoma and malignant fibrous histiocytoma. The former is similar to, if not the same as, the WHO juxtacortical chondrosarcoma.

Tumor-like lesions form part of the classification and include fibrous dysplasia, aneurysmal bone cysts, various reactive lesions, solitary bone cysts, and the histiocytoses. These lesions are not necessarily neoplasms, but they are inextricably part of the differential diagnosis of neoplastic disease of bone from the clinical, radiographic, and

TABLE 3.—WHO CLASSIFICATION OF TUMORS OF BONE

I. Bone-forming tumors
   A. Benign
      1. Osteoma
      2. Osteoid osteoma and osteoblastoma (benign osteoblastoma)
   B. Malignant
      1. Osteosarcoma (osteogenic sarcoma)
      2. Juxtacortical osteosarcoma (parosteal osteosarcoma)
II. Cartilage-forming tumors
   A. Benign
      1. Chondroma
      2. Osteochondroma (osteocartilaginous exostosis)
      3. Chondroblastoma (benign chondroblastoma, epiphyseal chondroblastoma)
      4. Chondromyxoid fibroma
   B. Malignant
      1. Chondrosarcoma
      2. Juxtacortical chondrosarcoma
      3. Mesenchymal chondrosarcoma
III. Giant cell tumor (osteoclastoma)
IV. Marrow tumors
      1. Ewing's sarcoma
      2. Reticulosarcoma of bone
      3. Lymphosarcoma of bone
      4. Myeloma
V. Vascular tumors
   A. Benign
      1. Hemangioma
      2. Lymphangioma
      3. Glomus tumor (glomangioma)
   B. Intermediate or indeterminate
      1. Hemangioendothelioma
      2. Hemangiopericytoma
   C. Malignant
      1. Angiosarcoma
VI. Other connective tissue tumors
   A. Benign
      1. Desmoplastic fibroma
      2. Lipoma
   B. Malignant
      1. Fibrosarcoma
      2. Liposarcoma
      3. Malignant mesenchymoma
      4. Undifferentiated sarcoma
VII. Other tumors
      1. Chordoma
      2. "Adamantinoma" of long bones
      3. Neurilemoma (schwannoma, neurinoma)
      4. Neurofibroma
VIII. Unclassified tumors
IX. Tumor-like lesions
      1. Solitary bone cyst (simple or unicameral bone cyst)
      2. Aneurysmal bone cyst
      3. Juxta-articular bone cyst (intra-osseous ganglion)
      4. Metaphyseal fibrous defect (non-ossifying fibroma)
      5. Eosinophilic granuloma
      6. Fibrous dysplasia
      7. "Myositis ossificans"
      8. "Brown tumor" of hyperparathyroidism

TABLE 4.—MODIFIED WHO CLASSIFICATION
OF TUMORS OF BONE

I. Bone-forming tumors
   A. Benign
      1. Osteoma
      2. Osteoid osteoma and osteoblastoma (benign osteoblastoma)
   B. Indeterminate
      1. Aggressive osteoblastoma
   C. Malignant
      1. Osteosarcoma (osteogenic sarcoma)
      2. Juxtacortical osteosarcoma (parosteal osteosarcoma)
      3. Periosteal osteosarcoma
II. Cartilage-forming tumors
   A. Benign
      1. Chondroma (enchondroma)
      2. Osteochondroma (osteocartilaginous exostosis)
      3. Periosteal chondroma
      4. Chondroblastoma (benign chondroblastoma, epiphyseal chondroblastoma)
      5. Chondromyxoid fibroma
   B. Malignant
      1. Chondrosarcoma
      2. Mesenchymal chondrosarcoma
      3. Dedifferentiated chondrosarcoma
III. Giant cell tumor (osteoclastoma)
IV. Marrow tumors
      1. Ewing's sarcoma
      2. Malignant lymphoma
      3. Myeloma
V. Vascular tumors
   A. Benign
      1. Hemangioma
      2. Lymphangioma
      3. Glomus tumor (glomangioma)
   B. Intermediate or indeterminate
      1. Hemangioendothelioma
      2. Hemangiopericytoma
   C. Malignant
      1. Angiosarcoma
VI. Other connective tissue tumors
   A. Benign
      1. Desmoplastic fibroma
      2. Lipoma
   B. Malignant
      1. Fibrosarcoma
      2. Malignant fibrous histiocytoma
      3. Liposarcoma
      4. Malignant mesenchymoma
      5. Undifferentiated sarcoma
VII. Other tumors
      1. Chordoma
      2. "Adamantinoma" of long bones
      3. Neurilemoma (schwannoma, neurinoma)
      4. Neurofibroma

(continued)

TABLE 4.—MODIFIED WHO CLASSIFICATION
OF TUMORS OF BONE *(cont.)*

VIII. Unclassified tumors
  IX. Tumor-like lesions
     1. Solitary bone cyst (simple or unicameral bone cyst)
     2. Aneurysmal bone cyst
     3. Juxta-articular bone cyst (intra-osseous ganglion)
     4. Metaphyseal fibrous defect (non-ossifying fibroma)
     5. Eosinophilic granuloma
     6. Fibrous dysplasia and ossifying fibroma
     7. "Myositis ossificans"
     8. "Brown tumor" of hyperparathyroidism

pathological standpoints. The aneurysmal bone cyst is a somewhat controversial lesion, in that whether it is neoplastic or not is not certain. Many observers believe that aneurysmal bone cyst is a lesion that is engrafted upon a pre-existing neoplasm of bone, for example, chondroblastoma. Whether this is true for all aneurysmal bone cysts is difficult to prove. There are other lesions of bone such as osteomyelitis, hyperparathyoidism, and metastases that may add confusion to the differential diagnosis. Radiographically, these diseases may impart a suggestion of a primary malignant disease or a benign tumor of bone.

We have modified the WHO classification for our use (Table 4). We have added aggressive osteoblastoma, periosteal osteosarcoma, periosteal chondroma, dedifferentiated chondrosarcoma, malignant fibrous histiocytoma, and ossifying fibroma. Reticulosarcoma and lymphosarcoma have been combined into malignant lymphoma of bone.

Tumors of Osteoblastic Derivation

With one exception, there does not appear to be a benign counterpart of an osteosarcoma (Fig. 1). The exception may be the benign osteoblastoma that, in recent years, has been observed to undergo malignant transformation in rare examples (Seki *et al.*, 1975). Occasionally, osteoblastoma manifests a locally aggressive course (Marsh *et al.*, 1975).

Of the benign osteoblastic lesions, the osteoid osteoma and the benign osteoblastoma are the common ones. Both are histologically similar, that is, composed of irregularly shaped and oriented osteoid and calcified bony trabeculae. Osteoblasts are prominent and are seen along with occasional osteoclasts. The stroma between the trabeculae is fine areolar and very vascular; inflammatory components are not seen. The osteoid osteoma is reasonably well-defined radiographi-

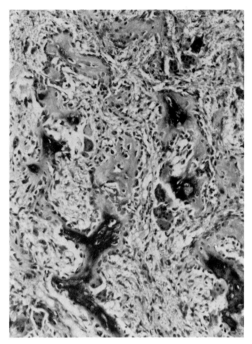

Fig. 1.—Benign osteoblastoma. Osteoid and mineralized osteoid with numerous osteoblasts. The stroma is loose, fibrous and appears benign. (×125).

cally, but the osteoblastoma is less so, being a larger lesion and provoking less of a bony reaction about it. Whether the 2 lesions are the same, except for size, is open to question. Generally the osteoid osteoma measures a centimeter or less in greatest dimension, whereas the benign osteoblastoma measures more than 1 cm and usually more than 2 cm in its greatest dimension. Osteomas are composed of dense cortical bone with little osteoblastic activity. Osteomas of long bones are uncommon with this lesion, being most frequently located in the skull, particularly the frontal sinuses.

Osteosarcomas, by definition, consist of malignant osteoid or bone associated with a malignant stroma (Fig. 2). From this there are many variants, including those that are dominantly composed of malignant cartilage or a malignant fibrous stroma. On this basis Dahlin and Coventry (1967) have subclassified osteosarcomas into osteoblastic, chondroblastic, and fibroblastic. Recently Scranton and associates (Scranton, De Cicco, Totten, and Yunis, 1975) have subclassified osteosarcoma into 6 histologic forms: (1) chondromyxoid, (2) sarcoma-

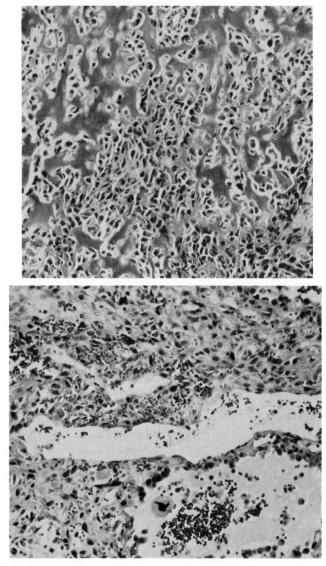

Fig. 2 (top).—Osteosarcoma. Malignant osteoid with an irregular poorly oriented pattern. The osteoblasts are cytologically malignant. (×175).

Fig. 3 (bottom).—Osteosarcoma that is richly vascular; sometimes designated as telangiectatic. The stroma is malignant with osteoid formation. (×200).

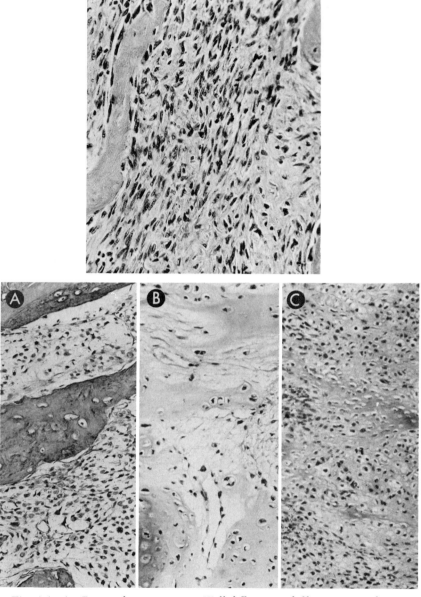

Fig. 4 (top).—Parosteal osteosarcoma. Well-differentiated fibrous stroma between bony trabeculae. (×100).

Fig. 5 (bottom).—Periosteal osteosarcoma. The varied malignant components are seen: **A**, stromal, **B**, cartilaginous, and **C**, osteoid. (×75).

tous, (3) endocrine, (4) classical, (5) microtrabecular sclerosing, and (6) massive osteoid. The subclassifications are related somewhat to expected prognosis. A small number of osteosarcomas are richly vascular with large and small vascular spaces (Fig. 3). This histological type may have a worse prognosis than other types (Dahlin, 1976 b).

Two variants of osteosarcoma are the parosteal (juxtacortical) osteosarcoma and the periosteal osteosarcoma. The former is diagnosable radiographically as a lobular, radiodense lesion arising on the posterior surface of the distal femoral metaphysis. Ordinarily it does not involve the medullary cavity. Histologically, parosteal osteosarcoma consists of well-differentiated bony, fibrous, and cartilaginous components (Fig. 4). The differentiation may be such that on examination of a biopsy specimen the pathologist may be lulled into a sense of security in diagnosing a benign lesion such as osteochondroma or fibrous dysplasia. It is important to differentiate this tumor from intramedullary osteosarcoma, since the expected survival is considerably better. In contrast to the parosteal osteosarcoma, periosteal osteosarcoma frequently involves the tibia, and radiographically appears to be a superficial lesion arising from the periosteum. With proper radiographic studies, the medullary cavity can be shown to be uninvolved (Unni, Dahlin, and Beabout, 1976). These lesions are not as dense radiographically as parosteal osteosarcomas and, radiographically, tend to produce coarse spiculation. Evidence of cartilaginous calcification may be noted. Grossly, periosteal osteosarcoma appears confined by the periosteum, which is attenuated, and to the cortex, which may appear thickened in the region of the tumor. On cut surface, bone and cartilage are usually identifiable, and in some lesions the suggestion of spiculation may be appreciated. The medullary bone appears spared. Histologically, such tumors present a varied pattern, often being composed of malignant bone, osteoid, cartilage, and a malignant stroma (Fig. 5A, B, and C). The degree of pleomorphism and the differentiation of these components vary considerably. It should be pointed out that periosteal osteosarcoma is designated as periosteal chondrosarcoma in the WHO classification. Osteosarcomas complicating Paget's disease of bone, irradiation, and infarction are histologically similar to those arising de novo. It is true, however, that many of the tumors are undifferentiated sarcomas.

Tumors of Cartilage Cell Origin

Chondrosarcoma can be subclassified into 2 types that reflect a gross pattern, i.e. peripheral and central. The peripheral type grows out-

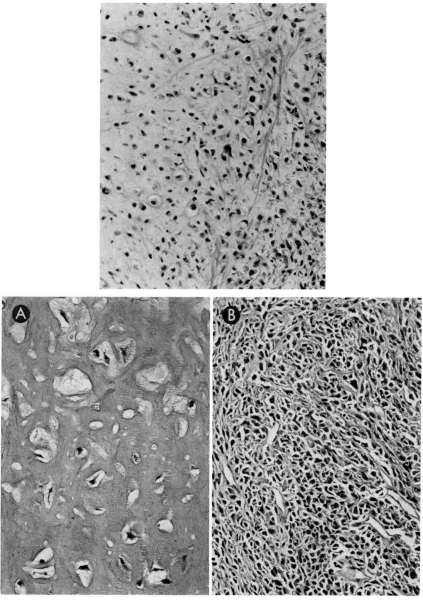

Fig. 6 (top).—Chondrosarcoma. Pleomorphic chondrocytes are readily apparent in a hyaline matrix. (×100).

Fig. 7 (bottom).—A dedifferentiated chondrosarcoma. **A,** Well-differentiated chondrosarcoma forms part of the tumor and **B,** poorly differentiated fibrosarcoma forms another portion of the tumor. (×150).

ward from the surface of a bone. The implications often are that this lesion was preceded by an osteochondroma. The central type of chondrosarcoma occupies the medullary cavity and, in some instances, may have arisen from a preexisting enchondroma. Histologically, both lesions may be identical. The well-differentiated forms resemble normal hyaline cartilage, and the pathologist is relegated to searching for a rather subtle nuclear alteration such as binucleate cells and slightly enlarged chondrocytic nuclei (Fig. 6). Multiple sections are necessary in order to confirm that the lesion is malignant. The chondrosarcomas that are less well-differentiated are easily diagnosed as being composed of malignant cartilage and ordinarily present little histologic problem. The majority of chondrosarcomas are well-differentiated.

Two variants of chondrosarcomas have been identified: (1) mesenchymal chondrosarcoma and (2) dedifferentiated chondrosarcoma (Dahlin, 1976a). Mesenchymal chondrosarcoma may have a radiographic pattern that is similar to that of chondrosarcoma. Histologically it is differentiated from chondrosarcoma by a malignant cartilage that blends with an undifferentiated mesenchymal component which, in some areas, resembles Ewing's sarcoma. The survival for patients

Fig. 8.—Benign chondroblastoma. The uniform cellularity of the chondroblasts is noted. Multinucleated giant cells are present. (×190).

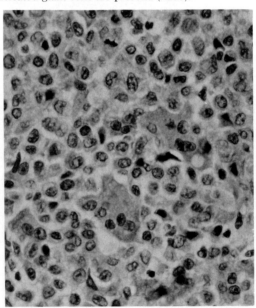

with mesenchymal chondrosarcoma may be long, but metastases and death may occur years after primary treatment.

The dedifferentiated chondrosarcoma is a lesion that ordinarily follows a well-differentiated chondrosarcoma (Fig. 7A and B). In this lesion, well-differentiated areas of chondrosarcoma may be identified; in other lesions, there will be a malignant mesenchymal component that may resemble a fibrosarcoma, for example. Dedifferentiated chondrosarcoma should be suspected in a patient who has a well-differentiated chondrosarcoma which, in a short period of time, suddenly recurs and grows rather rapidly. The survival of these patients has been poor.

Osteochondromas, enchondromas, periosteal chondromas, benign chondroblastoma (Fig. 8), and chondromyxoid fibroma are benign cartilaginous tumors that may enter into the differential diagnosis of tumors of bone. Enchondromas and periosteal chondromas, in particular, present diagnostic problems because of cellularity and nuclear atypia.

Tumors of Connective Tissue Origin

Of the benign lesions in this category, the nonossifying fibroma and the ossifying fibroma are the commonest, with nonossifying fibroma by far the more frequent of the 2. Nonossifying fibroma occurs in the metaphysis of long bones, is eccentrically located, and is readily identified radiographically. Histologically, it is composed of a fibrous stroma with multinucleated giant cells, collections of histiocytes, and hemosiderin. The stromal pattern is that of a palisading of the spindle cells, imparting a feature that is common to the lesions and helps to identify them. Ossifying fibroma is possibly related to fibrous dysplasia and is an uncommon lesion in the long bones, being most frequently seen in the facial bones. This lesion consists of a mature fibrous stroma with a bony component that is lamellar bone, in contrast to the woven bone of fibrous dysplasia. Osteoblasts are prominent, whereas fibrous dysplasia, is not prominent.

Fibrosarcoma primary in bone has the same histologic pattern as do the lesions that occur in the body soft tissues (Fig. 9). They are often metaphyseal and, radiographically, are destructive and radiolucent. By strict definitions these lesions do not contain malignant osteoid or bone, thus differentiating them from the fibroblastic form of osteosarcoma.

A recently delineated lesion of bone is primary malignant fibrous histiocytoma that has the same histological pattern as those lesions

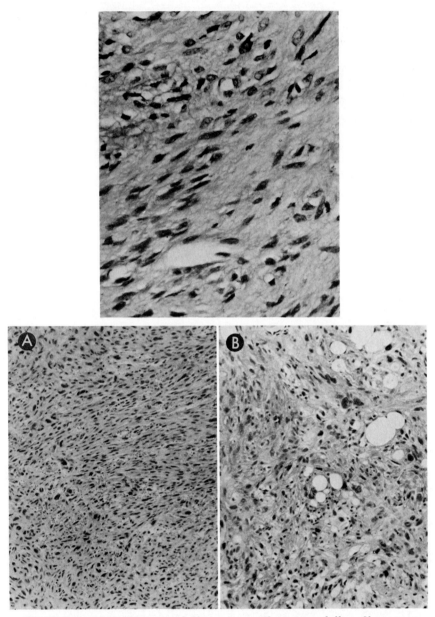

Fig. 9 (top).—Well-differentiated fibrosarcoma. The intramedullary fibrosarcomas are histologically similar to those of the somatic soft tissues. (×150).

Fig. 10 (bottom).—Malignant fibrous histiocytoma. **A,** Spindle cell stroma producing interlacing bundles. (×75). **B,** pleomorphic cells, foamy cells, and inflammatory cells. (×150).

occurring in the somatic soft tissues. It is possible that it has been included formerly among the fibrosarcomas. The stromal pattern consists of spindled to round cells that have been demonstrated by electron microscopy apparently to be of histiocytic origin. The more mature portions of the stroma will have a pattern that resembles that seen in the nonossifying fibroma (Fig. 10A and B). A so-called storiform pattern of the nuclei is seen. Other components of the lesion are the Touton giant cells, bizarre giant cells, bizarre mitotic figures, and an inflammatory component. Differentiation of benign from malignant fibrous histiocytoma at times is difficult, as bizarre nuclei also may be seen in the benign forms. This lesion may be difficult to differentiate from the more poorly differentiated fibrosarcomas and from fibroblastic osteosarcomas. Malignant fibrous histiocytomas are known to metastasize to the lungs and occasionally to lymph nodes (Spanier, Enneking, and Enriquez, 1975).

The giant cell tumor of bone is a fairly well-defined lesion from the radiographic standpoint. It occurs dominantly in the distal ends of long bones. An epiphyseal-metaphyseal component is expected in the giant cell tumor. Radiographically, it is generally a destructive lesion of the medullary cavity, often resulting in attenuation of the cortex; it abuts upon the articular cartilage of the long bone involved. Histologically, the diagnostic feature is an abundance of multinucleated giant cells associated with a stroma that varies from rounded to spindle cells. In contrast to the malignant fibrous histiocytoma, the stroma does not, except for focal areas, present the storiform pattern. Giant cell tumors have been subclassified according to differentiation by a grading system which includes Grades I, II, and III lesions. The better differentiated lesions have a stroma that is histologically malignant. Generally, the nuclei of the giant cells participate in the variations in grade.

Tumors of the Primitive Mesenchyme

The major lesion in this category is Ewing's sarcoma. It was considered originally by Ewing to be of endothelial origin; hence, the name diffuse endothelioma (Table 1). However, electron microscope studies have indicated that the cells are not endothelial, and that they seem to arise from primitive mesenchymal cells. Ewing's sarcoma is generally a tumor of young persons, with at least 80% of the tumors occurring before the age of 30. They tend to be diaphyseal or metaphyseal in the long bones and are often sclerotic roentgenographically. Histologically, the cells are uniform, imparting a somewhat monotonous pattern. The cells have indistinct cytoplasm, an ovoid nucleus, and nucleoli that are not prominent. This latter feature is helpful in distinguishing Ewing's tumor from malignant lymphomas of bone, since nucleoli are prominent in lymphomas. Ewing's sarcoma is bone-destructive and provokes considerable periosteal reaction. In most instances there is an extraosseous component of the lesion.

Since the lesion occurs commonly in the pediatric age group, it must be differentiated from metastatic neuroblastoma. At times this is difficult, but, generally, metastatic neuroblastoma forms rosettes and a glial-type stroma may be identified.

A stain, periodic acid-Schiff (PAS), is helpful in differentiating Ewing's sarcoma from other small round cell lesions. It has been demonstrated that the cytoplasm of Ewing's sarcomas often contains PAS-positive granules. This is in contrast to the rare PAS-positive granules in neuroblastoma and their absence in malignant lymphomas. It is true that the staining characteristics are not uniform, and all lesions designated as Ewing's sarcoma do not contain PAS-positive granules; however, when positive, this is a helpful means of differentiating it from the other tumors.

Tumors of Hematopoietic Origin

The major lesions in this group that are usually considered among primary tumors of bone are malignant lymphoma and plasma cell myeloma. Histologically, the malignant lymphomas have much the same pattern as is seen in the extraskeletal lymphomas. The majority have a pattern consistent with histiocytic lymphoma or a mixed histiocytic and lymphocytic lymphoma (Fig. 11). Primary Hodgkin's disease of bone is rare. Histologically, the lesion may be difficult to differentiate from a Ewing's sarcoma. The differentiation is aided by the presence of reticulin in malignant lymphomas and the absence of PAS-positive granules in the cytoplasm of the malignant lymphomas. In contrast, the Ewing's sarcomas have little, if any, reticulin between the individual cells. (PAS-positive granules have been described above.) Another feature of malignant lymphoma that is helpful in distinguishing it from Ewing's sarcoma is the presence of enlarged and rather obvious nucleoli in many of the neoplastic cells. A sprinkling of mature lymphocytes is a common feature. With the diagnosis of this lesion, it is imperative that the patient be examined for extranodal origin of the lesion in order to rule out, as well as one can, secondary involvement of bone.

Plasma cell myeloma is usually readily identifiable as such. The le-

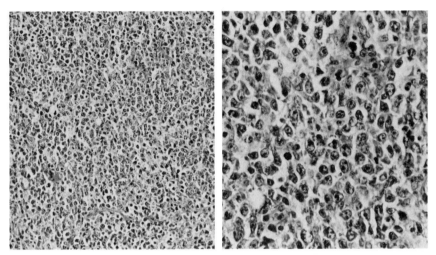

Fig. 11.—Malignant lymphoma. At the 2 magnifications the uniform pattern of lymphoma is evident and at the higher magnification (**right**) nucleoli are evident. (×75 and ×180).

sions that are poorly differentiated may mimic other neoplasms such as undifferentiated carcinomas or malignant lymphomas. The methyl green-pyronine stain may be helpful in diagnosing lesions that do present a differential diagnostic problem, with the cystoplasm of plasmacytic cell taking on a red color. The presence of amyloid may be helpful in the differentiation of myeloma from other neoplastic diseases.

Tumors of Vascular Origin

The major benign lesions in this category are the hemangiomas and lymphangiomas. They are histologically identical to those seen in the extraskeletal soft tissues and viscera, with the majority being of the cavernous type. Occasional glomus tumors appear to originate in the skeleton.

Angiosarcomas, often referred to as hemangioendotheliomas, are tumors with identifiably malignant endothelial cells. A feature that should lead one to suspect an angiosarcoma is complex anastomosing channels. Even though these may be present, one should still endeavor to identify neoplastic endothelial cells. Rare hemangiopericytomas primary in bone have been described. Histologically, they are identical to those arising in the somatic soft tissues.

Neurogenic Tumors

Neurilemomas and neurofibromas involve the skeleton. They are histologically similar to those seen elsewhere. Neurilemomas are uncommon and usually, if not always, solitary. Neurofibromas are often seen as an accompaniment to neurofibromatosis.

Tumors of Fat Cell Origin

Both the lipoma and the liposarcoma are rare as primary neoplasms of bone. Histologically, they again are similar to those seen in the somatic soft tissues. There is no evidence to indicate that lipoma transforms into liposarcoma.

Tumors of Unknown Origin

The major lesion in this category is adamantinoma of the tibia. Only occasionally does this lesion occur in bones other than the tibia (Moon, 1965). This, of course, is exclusive of the mandibular and maxillary lesions. Histologically, these tumors are similar to odontogenic adamantinoma. However, there are variations. Some of these lesions have a pattern that suggests a vascular tumor, with little evidence of elements that are comparable to the adamantinoma, leading to the suggestion that this lesion is of vascular origin. A few electron microscope studies support, but perhaps do not prove, an epithelial origin for this tumor (Albores-Saavedra, Diaz-Gutierrez, and Altimirano-Dimas, 1968).

Discussion and Conclusions

The classification of tumors of bone remains based upon morphological features, primarily histologic. Even though this means of classification is not always satisfactory, it does in general correlate with an expected biological behavior of the neoplasms. There is no doubt that it is at times difficult, and perhaps impossible, to classify all lesions precisely, because there is considerable overlapping and potential for varied patterns. It might be that with ultrastructural studies, histochemical determinations, tissue cultures, attempts at isolation of potential etiological agents such as viruses, and immunopathological studies, a more precise classification of tumors of bone will evolve.

Numerous studies have appeared describing the ultrastructural features of the various tumors of bone. These have served to verify con-

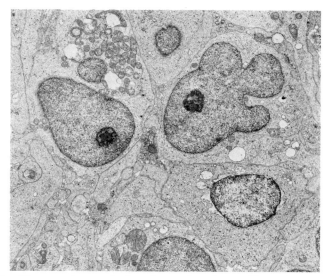

Fig. 12. — Electron micrograph of a malignant lymphoma of bone. Prominent nucleoli and nuclear irregularity are seen. Cytoplasmic organelles are sparse and glycogen is absent. (×6,800). (Courtesy of Dr. A. G. Ayala, Department of Pathology, M. D. Anderson Hospital.)

Fig. 13. — Electron micrograph of a Ewing's sarcoma. Nucleoli and organelles are inconspicuous. The nuclear chromatin tends to be finely granular and uniformly dispersed. Glycogen, indicated as unstained cytoplasmic areas, is present. (×6,200). (Courtesy of Dr. A. G. Ayala, Department of Pathology, M. D. Anderson Hospital.)

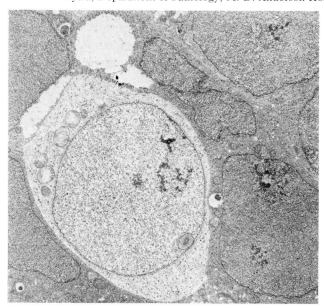

cepts as to cell origin and, in some instances, have clarified controversial lesions. For example, electron microscope studies have shown that Ewing's sarcoma and primary lymphoma of bone are distinct entities (Figs. 12 and 13). These 2 tumors are at times difficult to distinguish by light microscopy (Steiner, Ghosh, and Dorfman, 1972; Erlandson and Huvos, 1974; Hou-Jensen, Priori, and Dmochowski, 1972).

Although the emphasis in this presentation has been on the histological features of the various tumors of bone, I have not meant to minimize the importance of the clinical data or the radiographic and gross features in the diagnosis of tumors of bone. The importance of the radiographic features and the location in the diagnosis of neoplasms of bone cannot be overemphasized. In effect, the radiographic features represent the only means by which a pathologist can study the gross configuration of many neoplasms.

Addendum

Another variant of chondrosarcoma has been reported recently. This is clear cell chondrosarcoma that resembles chondroblastoma radiographically. It has a tendency to recur locally and may metastasize to the lungs (Unni, Dahlin, Beabout, and Sim, 1976).

Acknowledgment

The author gratefully acknowledges Mrs. Alice Haydon for printing the photomicrographs.

REFERENCES

Ackerman, L. V., and del Regato, J. A.: *Cancer. Diagnosis, Treatment, and Prognosis.* 2nd edition. St. Louis, Missouri, C. V. Mosby Co., 1954, 1201 pp.

Albores-Saavedra, J., Diaz-Gutierrez, D., and Altimirano-Dimas, M.: Adamantinoma de la tibia. Observaciones ultraestructurales. Revista Medica del Hospital General, Mexico City, 31:241–252, 1968.

Dahlin, D. C.: Chondrosarcoma and its "variants." International Academy of Pathology Monograph. Bone and Joints. Baltimore, Maryland, The Williams and Wilkins Co., 1976a.

Dahlin, D. C.: Comments, Third Annual International Skeletal Society Meeting. Montreal, 1976 b.

Dahlin, D. C., and Coventry, M. B.: Osteogenic sarcoma. A study of six hundred cases. Journal of Bone and Joint Surgery, 49A:101–110, January 1967.

Erlandson, R. A., and Huvos, A. G.: Chondrosarcoma: a light and electron microscopic study. Cancer, 34:1642–1652, November 1974.

Ewing, J.: *Neoplastic Diseases*. 4th edition. Philadelphia, Pennsylvania and London, England, W. B. Saunders Co., 1940, 1160 pp.

Hou-Jensen, K., Priori, E., and Dmochowski, L.: Studies on ultrastructure of Ewing's sarcoma of bone. Cancer, 29:280–286, February 1972.

Johnson, L. C.: A general theory of bone tumors. Bulletin of the New York Academy of Medicine, 29:164–171, 1953.

Marsh, B. W., Bonfiglio, M., Brady, L. P., and Enneking, W. F.: Benign osteoblastoma: range of manifestations. Journal of Bone and Joint Surgery, 57A:1–9, January 1975.

Moon, N. F.: Adamantinoma of the appendicular skeleton. Clinical Orthopaedics, 43:189–213, 1965.

Schajowicz, F., Ackerman, L. V., and Sissons, H. A.: *Histological Typing of Bone Tumours*. Geneva, Switzerland, W.H.O., 1972, 59 pp.

Scranton, P. E., Jr., De Cicco, F. A., Totten, R. S., and Yunis, E. J.: Prognostic factors in osteosarcoma. Cancer, 36:2179–2191, 1975.

Seki, T., Fukuda, H., Ishii, Y., Hanaoka, H., Yatabe, S., Takano, M., and Koide, O.: Malignant transformation of benign osteoblastoma. A case report. Journal of Bone and Joint Surgery, 57A:424–426, April 1975.

Spanier, S. S., Enneking, W. F., and Enriquez, P.: Primary malignant fibrous histiocytoma of bone. Cancer, 36:2084–2098, December 1975.

Steiner, G. C., Ghosh, L., and Dorfman, H. D.: Ultrastructure of giant cell tumors of bone. Human Pathology 3:569–586, December 1972.

Unni, K. K., Dahlin, D. C., and Beabout, J. W.: Periosteal osteogenic sarcoma. Cancer, 37:2476–2485, May 1976.

Unni, K. K., Dahlin, D. C., Beabout, J. M., and Sim, F. H.: Chondrosarcoma: clear cell variant. Journal of Bone and Joint Surgery, 58A:676–683, 1976.

Periosteal Osteosarcoma

HARLAN J. SPJUT, M.D.,* ALBERTO G. AYALA,
M.D., LUIS A. DE SANTOS, M.D., and JOHN A.
MURRAY, M.D.

*Department of Pathology, Baylor College of Medicine
and St. Luke's Episcopal Hospital*; Departments of
Pathology, Radiology, and Surgery (Orthopedic Service),
The University of Texas System Cancer Center
Texas System Cancer Center M. D. Anderson
Hospital and Tumor Institute, Houston, Texas*

PERIOSTEAL OSTEOSARCOMA is a lesion that has been defined recently by Unni, Dahlin, and Beabout (1976). The importance of the
delineation of this lesion lies in a biological behavior that differs
from intramedullary and parosteal osteosarcoma. Periosteal osteosarcoma has a predilection for a tibial or femoral location. As the name
suggests, this tumor is confined to the periosteum and cortex without a
medullary component. For this study, we have reviewed the case histories of 13 patients whose lesions fulfill the radiographic and pathologic criteria for the diagnosis of periosteal osteosarcoma. Care has
been taken to eliminate patients with parosteal osteosarcoma and
intramedullary osteosarcomas from the study. The cases are from The
University of Texas System Cancer Center M. D. Anderson Hospital
and Tumor Institute and a consultation file (H.J.S.).

Clinical Data

The average age of the 13 patients was 29.3 years, with an age range
of 14 to 62 years. Seven patients were younger than 21 years of age.
The group included 9 males and 4 females (Table 1). The signs and
symptoms of the lesion were nonspecific except for pain and swelling

TABLE 1.—CLINICAL AND PATHOLOGICAL DATA

CASE #	AGE AT DIAGNOSIS SEX	SITE	HISTOLOGY	SURGERY	METASTASES	CHEMO-THERAPY	SURVIVAL
1	14 M	Humerus, lower metaphysis	Large chondrosarcomatous component plus anaplastic sarcoma, focal permeation of cortex	Left middle humerus amputation 4-17-63	None	None	N.E.D. 13 years
2	15 M	Femur, upper diaphysis	Large ossified component Large anaplastic component Little cartilage permeation of cortex	Left hip disarticulation 1-13-72 thoracotomies right 10-9-73 left 12-11-73	Lungs, right and left	Actinomycin, melphalan, vincristine, Cytoxan, Adriamycin-DIC, C-parvum	N.E.D. 4 years, 7 months
3	16 M	Femur, diaphysis. Large tumor enveloping diaphysis	Abundant ossified and abundant anaplastic stroma. Little cartilage. Permeation of cortex	Right hip disarticulation 12-2-68	Lungs at 2 years supraclavicular lymph nodes	Vincristine, actinomycin, Cytoxan	Died 3 years, 6 months
4	19 M	Femur, diaphysis. Similar to previous	Abundant ossified material Abundant cartilage Little anaplastic sarcoma No permeation of cortex	Left hip disarticulation 1-22-70	None	None	N.E.D. 6 years, 6 months
5	19 M	Tibia, tibial tubercle	Central ossified and cartilaginous area surrounded by anaplastic sarcoma.	Local resection 9-13-73	None	None	N.E.D. 2 years, 4 months
6	19 F	Tibia, similar to previous	No permeation of cortex Similar to case 5	Above-the-knee amputation 8-15-69	None	None	N.E.D. 4 years. Lost to follow-up in 1973

No.	Age/Sex	Site	Histology	Surgery	Metastases	Chemotherapy	Status
7	62 M	Femur, diaphysis	Large anaplastic sarcomatous component. Cartilaginous and ossified background	Right hip disarticulation 3-8-76	None	Prophylactic Adriamycin, vincristine	N.E.D. 3 months
8	40 F	Mid-shaft femur	Dominantly cartilaginous	Hip disarticulation 11-18-75	None	Methotrexate Citrovorum factor	N.E.D. 6 months
9	39 M	Mid-shaft fibula	Dominantly osteoblastic	Local resection 1965. Recurrence 1968 and above-the-knee amputation 1968	Lungs	Irradiation and chemotherapy 1971	Died 1972 7 years
10	24 M	Mid-shaft tibia	Dominantly cartilaginous with osteoblastic component	Above-the-knee amputation 1969	None	None	N.E.D. 1975
11	49 F	Femur	Dominantly fibroblastic and hyalinized. Focally malignant. Abnormal bone	Local resect and bone graft October 1975	None	None	N.E.D. Sept. 1976
12	50 M	Femur	Poorly differentiated osteoblastic	Disarticulation	Lungs	None	Died 4 months
13	15 F	Femur	Osteoblastic and fibroblastic				N.E.D. 3 months

M – male.
F – female.

in the area of the tumor. Four of the patients had a history of trauma that preceded the diagnosis of the lesion. Pain in the thigh had been present in 1 of the patients for 8 months. In 1 other patient, the pain was referred to the knee, which lead to her being treated for arthritis prior to diagnosis of tumor. The laboratory data were noncontributory. Three of the tumors were located in the tibia; 8 in the femur; 1 in the humerus; and 1 in the fibula. All of the lesions were located in the metaphysis or the diaphysis of the long bone. Three femoral lesions were located in the lower one third of the bone, 1 posteriorly and 2 anteriorly.

Roentgenographic Findings

As a group, periosteal osteosarcomas were radiographically exophytic cortical lesions involving a long bone, and presenting as a visible mass of osseous matrix associated with an area of periosteal cortical

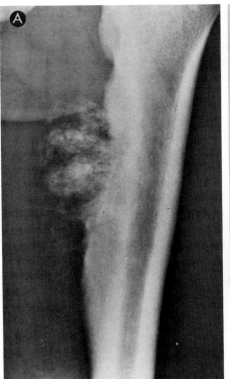
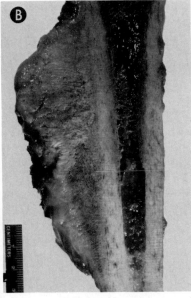

Fig. 1.—Periosteal osteosarcoma of the femur from a 15-year-old male. **A**, cortical sclerosis is present. The heavily calcified osteoid matrix is seen easily, as is coarse spiculation. **B**, a sagittal section of the tumor seen in **A**. Its cortical-periosteal localization is evident. The outline is somewhat lobular with radiation of tissue components from the cortex.

thickening. The cortical nature of the lesions was apparent in plain x-ray films in most cases. Tomography, when available, was of considerable assistance in defining the cortical origin and demonstrating lack of medullary extension by the tumor. Dense periosteal and cortical thickening was seen radiographically in 50% of the lesions at the site of origin (Fig. 1A). Codman's triangles were seen in 2 lesions.

The matrix of the tumor varied from a few spicules to coarse calcification and/or ossification, but in no case was this as dense or as uniform as the usual parosteal sarcoma. On the contrary, the matrix was nonhomogeneous with mixed areas of density and lucency. The density of the matrix calcification tended to decrease from the center to the periphery of the tumor (Table 2). A soft tissue component representing noncalcified matrix was seen at the periphery of the lesions in approximately 70% of the tumors.

Femoral Lesions

The femur was the most common location of the periosteal osteosarcomas in this series. The lesions ranged from 27.0 × 12.5 cm to 7.0 × 1.0 cm. Two were metaphyseal, 1 proximal, 1 distal; 6 involved the medial diaphyseal third of the femur, with 2 being slightly proximal, 1 slightly distal, and the rest strictly diaphyseal. Three of the lesions wrapped around the femoral shaft and, at 90°-angle projections, calcified matrix was seen at both sides of the femoral shaft (Fig. 2A). Tomography, when available, demonstrated the lack of medullary extension.

All but 3 of the lesions had heavy, coarse calcification; the remainder had scanty to moderate calcification. One of the lesions differed from the others in that it presented posteriorly a thick pedicle in the mid-third of the shaft. This tumor was more homogeneous than the rest, and resembled mature myositis ossificans or parosteal sarcoma.

Tibial Lesions

The tibial tumors ranged from 8.0 × 5.5 cm to 3.0 × 1.0 cm. These were all anterior lesions, 2 in the proximal metaphysis and 1 in the mid-shaft. The metaphyseal tumors showed fine osteoid spiculation (Fig. 3A); the diaphyseal tumor presented as an area of saucerization of the outer cortex with Codman's triangles. All the lesions showed a moderate degree of cortical thickening, but to a lesser degree than the femoral tumors.

TABLE 2.—PERIOSTEAL OSTEOSARCOMAS—RADIOGRAPHIC FINDINGS

CASE	LOCATION	SIZE	CORTEX	SIDE	MATRIX	SOFT TISSUE
1	Distal left humerus underside	4.0 cm × 1.0 cm	Superior and inferior Codman's triangles	Strictly medial cortex	Very scanty, only 2 or 3 osteoid spicules	Mild component
2	Proximal left femur	Vertical 13.0 cm, Horizontal 5.0 cm	Thickened locally under the lesion and extending 2–3 cm beyond	Medial cortex only, lateral cortex intact	Coarse osteoid matrix with coarse spiculation, denser center than periphery	Moderate component
3	Proximal femur	19 cm		Medial cortex only marked	Coarse osteoid spiculation	
4	Proximal + mid-left femoral shaft	27.0 cm × 12.5 cm	Normally thickened under the lesion	Wraps around bone, point of origin cannot be determined radiographically	Coarse matrix with areas of actual ossification, coarse spiculation, denser center than periphery	Moderate component
5	Proximal right tibia	8.0 cm × 5.5 cm	Thickened locally under lesion	Lesion wraps around anterior medial and lateral cortex	Medium to fine spiculations	Mild component
6	Left proximal tibia	7.0 cm × 2.0 cm	Minimally thickened	Anterior cortex	Fine osteoid spiculation	Mild component
7	Mid-left femoral	10.0 cm × 3.0 cm	Only minimal thickening	Posterior medial cortex	Scanty osteoid matrix with more calcified matrix between, few spiculations	Significant component

8	Left mid-shaft femur posterior	15.0 cm × 2.5 cm	Thickened only at point of origin	Posterior cortex only	Exophytic lesion with areas of dense homogeneous ossification. Inferior area non-homogeneous with osteoid spiculation localized	Moderate component
9	Mid-shaft left fibula	2.0 cm × 0.5 cm	Intact	Lateral cortex only	Fine spiculations, denser at center than periphery	None
10	Mid-shaft left tibia	3.0 cm × 1.0 cm Approx.	Superior and inferior Codman's triangles	Medial side only marked	Very scanty, no matrix seen	Minimal
11	Distal 1/3 right femur, anterior	12.0 cm × 3.0 cm	Minimally thickened	Mainly anterior, but same degree of wrapping laterally and medially	Coarse spiculation. ? cartilage matrix	Mild component
12	Upper femoral metaphysis	19 cm	Slightly thickened intact	Lesion wraps around femur	Fine streaming and spiculation appear to radiate from the cortex	Minimal
13	Distal mid-shaft left femur	12.0 cm × 6.0 cm	Not thickened	Lesion wraps around shaft, point of origin not determined	Fine osteoid spiculation	Significant soft tissue component

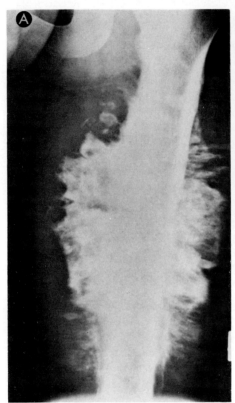

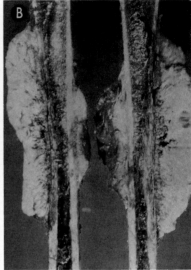

Fig. 2.—A large periosteal sarcoma that varies from the expected pattern. This tumor occurred in a 16-year-old man. **A,** spiculation is prominent and the lines did not infringe upon the medullary portion of the underlying femur. **B,** hemisection of the lesion seen in **A.** The well-outlined tumor that is seen distorts the cortex but does not involve medullary bone.

Other Lesions

One was located in the mid-shaft of the fibula. It measured 2.0×0.5 cm and was the smallest of the group; otherwise, it was quite typical in its cortical location, slight cortical thickening, and exophytic osteoid spiculation. The second was a humeral tumor located at the medial aspect of the distal metaphysis; this was similar in configuration to the mid-tibial lesion, presenting with Codman's triangles and an area of subperiosteal cortical erosion with a few spicules of osteoid in the center.

As a generalization, a diagnosis of periosteal osteosarcoma should be suggested radiographically when a lesion involves the cortex of a long bone with an exophytic form and spiculation and is confined to the cortex. It is important that the medullary bone be demonstrably free of tumor.

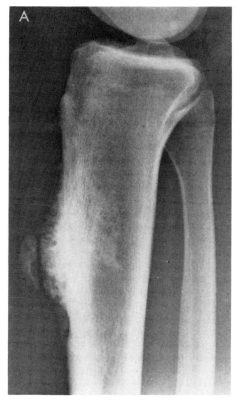

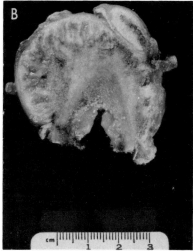

Fig. 3.—Periosteal osteosarcoma of the tibia in a 19-year-old man. **A,** the cortical thickening and sclerosis, the spiculation, and the variegated sclerotic and radiolucent mass are seen. **B,** a cross-section of the tumor seen in **A.** The intimate relationship to the cortex and the suggestive radiating pattern are notable.

Gross Pathological Features

In correlation with the radiographic findings, the medullary cavity in all cases studied was free of tumor. The cortex was involved, but the bulk of the tumor was subperiosteal. The site of origin, i.e. cortex or periosteum, could not be ascertained, as the tumor blended with both structures (Figs. 1B, 2B, and 3B). The expanding tumor impinged upon the surrounding skeletal muscle. The cut surfaces of the lesions were granular, with obvious evidence of ossification, particularly centrally. These areas were firm to hard. Interspersed gray, shiny lobular areas consistent with cartilage were common. In most of the lesions, the bony arrangement imparted a spiculated pattern to give the impression of tissue radiating from the superficial portions of the cortex. Peripherally, the sarcomas were somewhat lobulated with smooth margins; the surrounding soft tissues separated easily from the tumor.

Histological Findings

Histologically, the tumors showed a varied pattern, usually a combination of cartilage, bone, osteoid, and a fibrous component (Figs. 4–12). Five of the cases were predominantly cartilaginous and the others were predominantly osteoblastic. In those cases in which osteoid and bone were major components, there appeared to be a radiation of the spicules from the cortex. Where cartilage was the predominant pattern, a lobular contour was prominent. In 1 of the lesions, there was extensive necrosis and hyalinization with only a few small areas that were identifiable as residual sarcoma. At the junction of tumor and periosteum, there was often intense proliferation of immature cells between the periosteum and the underlying neoplasm, suggesting a transition from periosteum to tumor. In 1 of the cases, extensive cartilage imparted to the tumor an appearance resembling mesenchymal chondrosarcoma. In 2 of the cases, tumor penetrated the periosteum and invaded the adjacent skeletal muscle. Vascular invasion was noted in 1 of the specimens. No attempt was made to grade the lesions; however, there was considerable variation in the differentiation of the components.

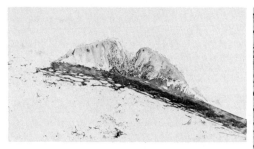

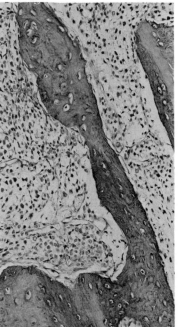

Fig. 4 (above).—A scanning view of a periosteal osteosarcoma. The radiating features, its central osseous component, and its relationship to cortex and medullary bone are seen. (H & E ×5).

Fig. 5 (right).—Undifferentiated malignant stroma beneath spicules of periosteal bone. (H & E ×75).

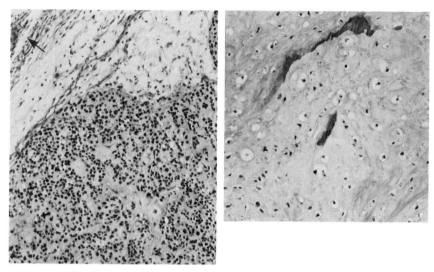

Fig. 6 (left).—Periosteum is seen at the *arrow*. The tumor has a lobular outline and illustrates the poorly differentiated element of the cartilaginous component. (H & E ×75).

Fig. 7 (right).—Spicules of bone surrounded by well-differentiated malignant cartilage that made up 1 component of the tumor. (H & E ×80).

Fig. 8.—Poorly differentiated malignant cartilage. (H & E ×200).

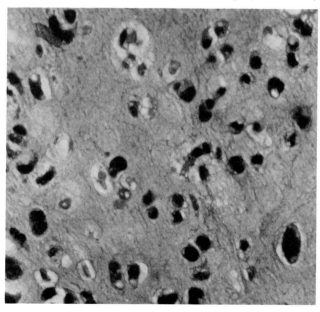

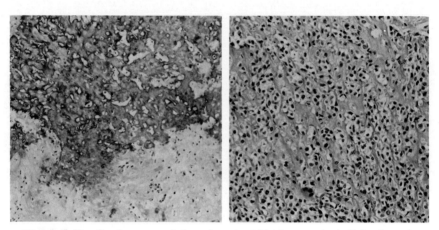

Fig. 9 (left).—Poorly oriented, heavily mineralized, sparsely cellular bone in a periosteal osteosarcoma. (H & E ×50).
Fig. 10 (right).—Malignant osteoid similar to that which might be seen in an intramedullary osteosarcoma. (H & E ×100).

Pulmonary metastases were resected from the 1 patient; histologically, they were identical to the primary lesion. This sarcoma was predominantly osteoblastic and had a lobular appearance which persisted in the metastases (Fig. 13).

Permeation of the cortex was occasionally observed, and in 1 lesion there was involvement of the immediately subjacent medullary cavity. This tumor, grossly and radiographically, appeared to be confined to the periosteum and cortex.

Treatment and Follow-up

Nine of the patients underwent amputation or hip disarticulations and 4 were known to have had local resections. One patient had local recurrence following partial resection of the fibula; an above-the-knee amputation was then done. This patient survived 7 years, dying of pulmonary metastases. Five of the patients received chemotherapy, 3 as treatment for metastases and 2 as adjunctive therapy. The agents included actinomycin, vincristine, Cytoxan, Adriamycin, and methotrexate with citrovorum factor.

Of the 13 patients, 3 are known to have died: 1 at 3½ years, 1 at 7 years, and 1 at 4 months after primary surgical therapy (Table 1). One patient underwent bilateral thoracotomies, with resection of the metastases, followed by chemotherapy and is living with no evidence of

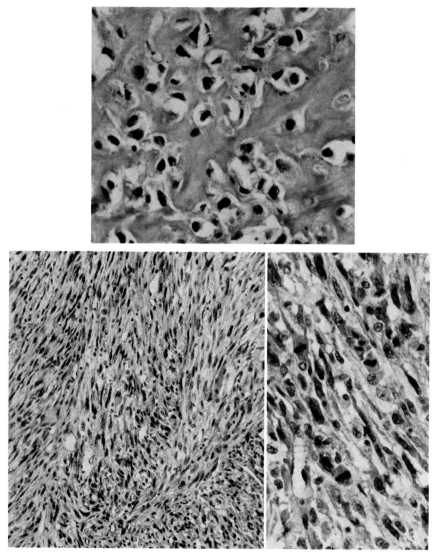

Fig. 11 (top).—Higher magnification of malignant ·osteoid from a periosteal osteo-sarcoma. (H & E ×190).

Fig. 12 (bottom).—A fibroblastic component of a periosteal osteosarcoma. Nuclear pleomorphism and mitotic figures are evident. (H & E *(left)* ×100 and *(right)* ×190.)

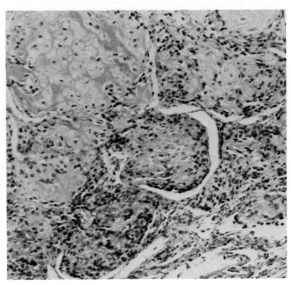

Fig. 13. — Pulmonary metastases from the case in Figures 2A and 2B. The metastases are histologically similar to the primary tumor. (H & E ×175).

disease after 4 years and 7 months. The remaining patients are living without evidence of disease for periods ranging from 3 months to 13 years. The patient with the largest femoral tumor has had no further complaints after amputation, and is living with no evidence of disease at 78 months.

Discussion

Although periosteal osteosarcoma is considered to be a newly de-fined entity, there is evidence that it was recognized earlier. Mention of a periosteal variant of osteogenic sarcoma was included in a classifi-cation of tumors of bone by Ewing in 1940. However, a description was not included in the text. In Jaffe's book, published in 1958, Ew-ing's classification was included, but the lesion was not described in the text. But, in 1960, Jaffe published a paper entitled "Intracortical Osteogenic Sarcoma" that describes a lesion radiographically, grossly, and histologically similar to periosteal osteosarcoma. In the 1972 World Health Organization classification, periosteal osteosarcoma is designated as a juxtacortical chondrosarcoma under the heading of Malignant Cartilage-Forming Tumors. Because of the histological components described by us and by Unni, Dahlin, and Beabout

(1976), we cannot consider periosteal osteosarcoma as a form of chondrosarcoma.

Lichtenstein recognized periosteal fibrosarcoma, chondrosarcoma, and osteogenic sarcomas in 1955. He illustrated an example of periosteal osteosarcoma in an 18-year-old boy. The tumor involved the distal one third of the femur. In 1972, Lichtenstein recorded 2 other patients as having periosteal osteosarcoma, 1 tibial in a 5-year-old child and 1 femoral in a 15-year-old girl.

In 1975, Aegerter and Kirkpatrick mentioned the possibility of periosteal osteosarcoma, but expressed doubt as to the existence of such a lesion with the phrase "if there be such an entity." The first diagnosis of periosteal sarcoma made in our group was in 1963 when a lesion of the lower end of the humerus of a 14-year-old girl was interpreted as "osteogenic sarcoma, periosteal type." Three other of the lesions in our series were diagnosed as osteogenic sarcomas and 1 as parosteal osteosarcoma. The fibular tumor was originally considered to be an atypical form of myositis ossificans, but the submitting pathologist had considered it to be a form of osteogenic sarcoma. The remaining lesions were primarily diagnosed as periosteal osteosarcomas. From the preceding facts, it becomes evident that periosteal sarcomas have been previously recognized, although, until the paper by Unni, Dahlin, and Beabout (1976), the lesion had not been clearly defined.

Although not specific, the radiographic features of periosteal sarcoma should enable one to make a preoperative diagnosis of or a least give strong consideration to the diagnosis of periosteal osteosarcoma. Pathologically, the lesion is fairly distinctive and distinguishable from intramedullary osteosarcoma and parosteal osteosarcoma. It is usually not difficult to distinguish intramedullary osteosarcoma from periosteal osteosarcoma. The former results in sclerosis of medullary bone, cortical erosion, obliteration, and periosteal reaction characteristic of a malignant tumor. In contrast, periosteal osteosarcoma does not have a radiographically demonstrable medullary component. Histologically, the 2 may be indistinguishable. Parosteal osteosarcoma is more likely to be a differential diagnostic problem. In this lesion, the radiographic features are distinctive and an integral part of the diagnosis. The most common location is the lower end of the femur, posteriorly; radiographically, it forms a dense, lobular, well-outlined mass, often with a radiolucent line between a portion of the major part of the tumor and the underlying cortex. Histologically, parosteal osteosarcomas show well-differentiated bone, fibrous stroma, and cartilage. On the basis of a biospy, a diagnosis of benign lesion is made often, e.g. osteochondroma, fibrous dysplasia, or healing fracture. Localized myositis ossificans during its early development may mimic periosteal osteosarcoma radiographically, but its outlines are usually smooth and the spiculation characteristic of a malignancy is not observed. Histologically, with an adequate biopsy, myositis ossificans shows the zoning phenomenon, i.e. central immaturity and peripheral maturity of bone and stroma. This would not be seen in periosteal osteosarcoma.

Although we recognize the need for a clear-cut definition of periosteal osteosarcoma, Case 10 (Table 2), in which minimal medullary involvement was found histologically, could not be excluded. It is acceptable for periosteal osteosarcoma to invade adjacent soft tissues and the underlying cortex. Thus, it seems reasonable that a malignant tumor could be expected to infringe upon the medullary bone at times. This should be seen histologically as a minimal component so as to exclude intramedullary osteosarcomas. It is of interest that Unni, Dahlin, Beabout, and Ivins (1976) accept medullary involvement in parosteal osteosarcoma but not in periosteal osteosarcoma (Unni, Dahlin, and Beabout, 1976).

If we combine information from the present study with that reported by Unni and co-workers, we find that among the 36 patients, 21 were male and 15 were female, with an age range of 9 to 62 years. Twenty-three of the patients were younger than 21 years. The age grouping differs from that of intramedullary osteosarcoma in which the peak incidence is in the teenager. The anatomical distribution of the 36 tumors is: tibia 17, femur 15, humerus 2, ilium 1, and fibula 1.

Conclusions

Periosteal osteosarcoma is a fairly distinct radiographic, pathologic, and biological entity. It is a lesion that should be distinguished from intramedullary and parosteal osteosarcomas, since the biological behavior differs from these 2 lesions. The average age at which the lesion occurs is older than that for intramedullary osteosarcoma and younger than for parosteal osteosarcoma. In addition, periosteal osteosarcoma seems to have a predilection for the tibia and femur. It is possible that in a well-selected case this lesion can be properly treated with wide local resection and restitution with bone graft or a prosthesis. However, in others, the location and size of the tumor is such as to require amputation or disarticulation. Each case must be individualized in regard to treatment. Whether chemotherapy or radiation therapy will play a role in the treatment of patients with this tumor remains to be determined. In those tumors that are anaplastic, prophylactic chemotherapy may be given and is more certainly indicated in the event of metastases.

Of the 23 patients reported by Unni, Dahlin, and Beabout (1976), 8 died of their disease. However, 2 of these patients died as late as 16 and 29 years after diagnosis, apparently of unrelated causes. Of our 13 patients, 3 are known to be dead; the others are alive, apparently without evidence of disease. These results, although based on relatively few cases, suggest that periosteal osteosarcoma deserves to be distinguished from intramedullary osteosarcoma.

Acknowledgments

We gratefully acknowledge the following physicians who furnished data and permitted us to use their cases in this study: R. E. Fechner, Houston, Texas; O. A. Severance, San Antonio, Texas; L. J. Williams, Jr., Houston, Texas; M. M. Salisnjak, Rochester, New York; and R. N. Gidwani, Ontario, Canada.

REFERENCES

Aegerter, E., and Kirkpatrick, J. A., Jr. *Orthopedic Diseases.* 4th edition. Philadelphia, Pennsylvania, W. B. Saunders Company, 1975.

Ewing, J.: *Neoplastic Diseases.* 4th edition. Philadelphia, Pennsylvania, and London, England, W. B. Saunders Company, 1940, 1160 pp.

Jaffe, H. L.: *Tumors and Tumorous Conditions of the Bones and Joints.* Philadelphia, Pennsylvania, Lea and Febiger, 1958, 629 pp.

Jaffe, H. L.: Intracortical osteogenic sarcoma. Bulletin of the Hospital for Joint Diseases, 21:189–197, 1960.

Lichtenstein, L.: Tumors of periosteal origin. Cancer, 8:1060–1069, September–October 1955.

Lichtenstein, L.: *Bone Tumors.* 4th edition. St. Louis, Missouri, C. V. Mosby Company, 1972, 441 pp.

Schajowicz, F., Ackerman, L. V., and Sissons, H. A.: *Histological Typing of Bone Tumours.* Geneva, Switzerland, World Health Organization, 1972, 59 pp.

Unni, K. K., Dahlin, D. C., and Beabout, J. W.: Periosteal osteogenic sarcoma. Cancer, 37:2476–2485, May 1976.

Unni, K. K., Dahlin, D. C., Beabout, J. W., and Ivins, J. C.: Parosteal osteogenic sarcoma. Cancer, 37:2466–2475, May 1976.

Radionuclide Bone Imaging in Primary Bone Tumors

THOMAS P. HAYNIE, III, M.D.

Section of Nuclear Medicine, Department of Medicine,
The University of Texas System Cancer Center
M. D. Anderson Hospital and Tumor Institute,
Houston, Texas

ONCOLOGY HAS RECENTLY SEEN a rapid increase in the popularity of bone scanning (Lentle *et al.*, 1976). This increase follows the introduction of ^{99m}Tc-phosphorus complexes which permit rapid total-body surveys to be performed, with a low radiation dose to the patient. In addition, improvements in instrumentation have greatly increased the ease with which the surveys may be accomplished. Two factors seem paramount in prompting this more widespread use of bone scanning. The first is the relative ease with which radionuclide bone scans may be performed and interpreted compared to a radiographic bone survey. The second is the discovery that the bone scan is a more sensitive indicator of abnormality than the X-ray bone survey in the detection of metastatic bone disease (Pistenma, McDougall, and Kriss, 1975). In the process of using bone scans, it has been found that this greater sensitivity applies also to infectious, metabolic, traumatic, and benign neoplastic disease in the same way as it does to malignant disease, and this nonspecificity has created problems in diagnosis which demand careful clinical and X-ray correlation of bone scan results in clinical use (O'Mara, 1974).

This paper reviews the current state of knowledge of the use of bone scanning in primary bone tumors and briefly covers the technique and the preliminary results obtained in patients with primary bone tumors who undergo work-up at M. D. Anderson Hospital.

Materials and Methods

RADIOPHARMACEUTICALS

The wide variety of ^{99m}Tc-phosphorus complexes available has created confusion regarding the relative merits and mechanism of action of these many agents (Jones, Francis, and Davis, 1976). The technetium-tin-phosphorous agents are divided into 2 main classes: those complexed with phosphates and those complexed with phosphonates. The most widely accepted view of the mode of action of this group of scanning agents is that they react to the phosphorous groups by absorption into the calcium of hydroxyapatite in bone. Recent work, however, suggests they may also interact in vivo with certain large molecules such as fibrous or globular proteins (Davis and Jones, 1976). The radiopharmaceutical used at M. D. Anderson Hospital is technetium-tin-pyrophosphate, an agent chosen because of its stability in vitro and its good localizing properties in vivo. A dose of 15 mCi is administered intravenously, and scanning is begun 3 hours after administration. The only preparation is to have the patient void immediately prior to beginning the scan.

INSTRUMENTATION

There are a variety of instruments available for performing bone scans. Originally, the instrumentation used at M. D. Anderson Hospital consisted of dual 5-inch detector rectilinear scanners for total-body imaging, supplemented with gamma camera views of suspicious areas and areas of high incidence of metastases. More recently, newer instrumentation (a hybrid between the traditional rectilinear scanner and the gamma camera) has been employed which permits more rapid scanning, with resolution equal to that of the rectilinear scanner. Gamma cameras may still be useful, however, for close inspection of suspicious areas, and when fitted with pin-hole collimation, may elucidate abnormalities not apparent on a survey scan. In most instances, however, the survey film suffices. Anterior and posterior total-body views are obtained; generally, these require about 20 minutes at a speed of 5 to 10 cm/min.

INDICATIONS AND LIMITATIONS OF BONE SCANS IN PRIMARY BONE TUMORS

Review of the literature indicates that experience with bone scanning in primary bone tumor is still limited, although a number of small series have been published (Gilday and Ash, 1976; Goldman and Braunstein, 1975; Harmer, Burns, Sams, and Spittle, 1969; Holsti and Patomaki, 1967; McNeil *et al.*, 1973; Moon, Dworkin, and LaFleur, 1968; Wanken, Eyring, and Samuels, 1973; Shirazi, Rayudu, and Fordham, 1973; Spencer, Herbert, Rish, and Little, 1967), many of which were done with older radiopharmaceuticals such as ^{18}F and ^{87m}Sr. Although these studies have pointed out potential areas of use, a number of limitations have become evident, many of which relate to the nonspecificity of the technique. These indications and limitations are:

DIFFERENTIAL DIAGNOSIS.—Primary malignant bone tumors have usually been found to be abnormal on bone scanning. This includes the primary lesion, which in most cases will also be abnormal on radiograph, and, particularly in the case of Ewing's sarcoma, metastatic sites which may be detected on bone scanning prior to the development of abnormalities visible on X-ray film. In contrast, various types of benign bone tumors, including simple and aneurysmal bone cysts, fibrous cortical defects, and nonossifying fibromas, generally have minimal or no increased uptake of radiopharmaceutical unless traumatized. Osteochondromas and enchondromas show varied accumulation of activity, and osteoid osteomas and fibrous dysplasia generally demonstrate marked activity. At times, osteoid osteomas have been detected in symptomatic patients prior to the development of X-ray film changes. This may require high resolution gamma camera images (Gilday and Ash, 1976). The limitation of bone scanning in differential diagnosis relates to the fact that the scan may be abnormal any time there is active tumor growth, whether benign or malignant. The predictive value of the test for malignancy, therefore, is dependent on the prevalence of the various types and stages of tumors in the population.

TREATMENT PLANNING.—Even when the primary lesion is quite evident on X-ray examination, a bone scan may show the extent of involvement more accurately and thus be a better guide to surgical and radiotherapeutic treatment planning (Spencer, Herbert, Rish, and Little, 1967). In the case of lung metastases being considered for resection, it is important to be sure that further unsuspected metastases have not occurred, and the bone scan is a rapid method for performing this type of bone and soft tissue survey. The limitation that exists for this indication is that there are secondary changes, usually thought to be hyperemic, in uninvolved adjacent bone which may cause abnormal radionuclide uptake and thereby cause one to overestimate the extent of tumor (Thrall, Geslien, Corcoron, and Johnson, 1975). Sometimes the distinction between secondary benign changes and multicentric disease can be based on the location and pattern of abnormal uptake.

FOLLOW-UP OF THE PRIMARY LESION.—Where radiation therapy or chemotherapy is selected as the primary treatment of a malignant primary bone tumor, the uptake of radiopharmaceutical at the site of the primary lesion can be used to monitor local progression of disease (McNeil *et al.*, 1973). A caution in this instance is that uptake in a radiated area several months after radiation therapy may not mean tumor recurrence or persistence, but rather infection or pathologic fracture. Correlation with clinical signs and symptoms and X-ray film changes may help to resolve this question.

DETECTION OF BONE METASTASIS.—Bone scans appear to have greater sensitivity than skeletal X-ray surveys in the detection of bone metastasis. The problem is, however, that degenerative, inflammatory, traumatic, and dystrophic bone diseases may cause abnormal bone scan, and it is often unwise to diagnose metastases without roentgenographic confirmation (Bessler, 1968). Provided a normal base-line scan has been obtained, these other etiologies can often be excluded on follow-up examinations. The bone scan then becomes a very valuable procedure for following patients posttherapy. In osteosarcoma, it is said that bony metastases are rarely preceded by lung metastases, but since no large series of patients has been followed with the more recent bone scanning techniques, this concept needs further investigation.

DETECTION OF SOFT TISSUE METASTASIS OF OSTEOGENIC SARCOMA.—The phenomenon of calcification of metastatic osteogenic sarcoma in lung and other soft tissue sites leading to abnormal localization of bone-seeking radiotracers in these sites has been recognized since 1967 (Woodbury and Beierwaltes, 1967). It now appears that occasionally bone scanning may detect some of these metastases prior to their presentation on X-ray film (Samuels, 1968). Metastatic soft tissue sites outside the lungs may also be detected first by bone scanning (Shirazi, Rayudu, and Fordham, 1974). Since other primary and metastatic tumors may show uptake in soft tissue sites, caution will have to be used in ascribing these to metastatic osteosarcoma (Richman *et al.*, 1975). In such cases, the presence of a normal base-line study will be useful.

Results

At M. D. Anderson Hospital, the great majority of bone scans have been performed in searches for metastatic lesions from those primary tumors known to metastasize commonly to bone, such as breast, lung, kidney, and prostate. Only about 5% or less of bone scans have been in primary bone tumors. In the first 6 months of this year, we performed 14 bone scans in patients with osteosarcoma, 11 in patients with Ewing's sarcoma, and 8 in patients with miscellaneous other primary malignant bone tumors, such as chondrosarcomas, malignant giant cell tumors, and synovial sarcomas. Only 1 patient had a bone scan for a benign bone tumor, which turned out to be an aneurysmal bone cyst, and the scan was normal. Of the patients with osteosarcomas, only 1 patient was studied prior to amputation, and showed no metastatic disease. Twelve patients were examined in follow-up, and metastatic lesions were detected in 8. In patients with Ewing's sarcoma, 9 were scanned prior to treatment, and metastatic disease was seen in 1; 2 patients were scanned in follow-up after initial therapy, and metastatic disease was detected in both. Among the patients in the miscellaneous group, 2 were examined prior to therapy, and no metastatic disease was found. Six scans were performed posttherapy, and metastatic disease was revealed in 3 scans. Overall, metastatic disease detected prior to initial therapy was found in 1 of 12 (8%) patients, and after therapy, in 13 of 20 (65%). The latter figure is biased by the fact that the majority of patients scanned posttherapy were already known or strongly suspected to have metastatic disease.

Two illustrative cases will be presented to demonstrate some of the results obtained thus far in bone scanning of primary bone tumors at M. D. Anderson Hospital.

CASE 1, EWING'S SARCOMA. — This 17-year-old man developed pain in the right hip, and an X-ray film revealed a probable Ewing's sarcoma of the proximal right femur. There were questionable X-ray film changes in the proximal left femur which were nondiagnostic. A bone scan was performed (Fig. 1) which showed marked abnormal uptake in the proximal right femur and other areas of abnormality in the proximal right humerus, in the skull, and in the thoracic spine. There were also nonspecific hyperemic changes in the right acetabulum, in the bones surrounding the right knee, and in the right ankle. Biopsy of the right femur revealed Ewing's sarcoma. The patient received X-ray therapy to the right hip and was subsequently placed on chemotherapy. No follow-up bone scans have been obtained.

CASE 2, OSTEOGENIC SARCOMA. — This 47-year-old woman developed a lesion of the left fibula in 1970 which, on X-ray film, was shown to be osteogenic sarcoma. The left lower extremity was amputated at midthigh. No further therapy was given. In 1974 she developed a lesion of the right buttock which was resected; she was referred to M. D. Anderson Hospital, where X-ray films revealed a metastasis in the left ilium. A bone scan (Fig. 2A) revealed abnormal up-

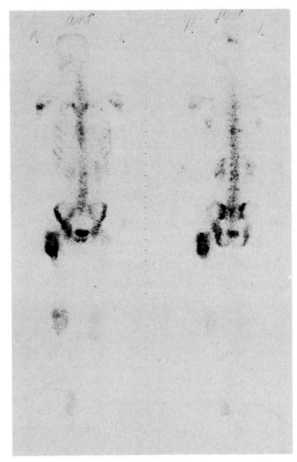

Fig. 1.—Case 1, ⁹⁹ᵐTc-Sn-pyrophosphate bone scan in a 17-year-old man with Ewing's sarcoma, primary in proximal right femur. Clinically and by X-ray examination occult metastases are noted in skull, proximal right humerus and spine. Secondary benign hyperemic uptake is seen in right pelvis (acetabulum) and in the right knee and ankle. *Left*, anterior view; *right*, posterior view. Right side of patient is to reader's left in both views.

take in the left ilium; 2 areas of abnormality were seen in the right upper abdomen, one which appeared to correspond to the lower pole of the right kidney, the other which appeared to lie anterior to the upper pole of the right kidney. X-ray films at this time were nondiagnostic for disease outside the bones. She was placed on multidrug chemotherapy; however, she continued to experience progression of her disease and X-ray films the following year demonstrated calcified

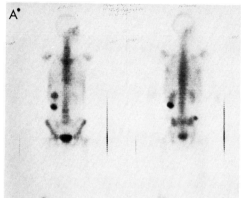
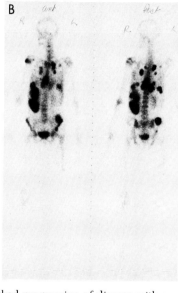

Fig. 2.—A, Case 2, ^{99m}Tc-Sn-pyrophosphate bone scan performed in September 1975, in a 47-year-old woman with osteogenic sarcoma primary in the left fibula (postamputation). Metastasis is seen in the left ilium and in soft tissues of the right abdomen. Orientation of views is the same as in Figure 1. **B,** Case 2, follow-up scan performed in July 1976 reveals marked progression of disease with enlargement of left ilial and right abdominal lesions. New lesions have appeared in both lungs and the right proximal humerus. Orientation of views is same as in Figure 2A.

masses in the kidney, lungs, and liver. The bone scan (Fig. 2B) also demonstrated additional areas of abnormal uptake in these organs. When last seen, she continued to have progressive disease in spite of treatment.

Discussion

It is too soon to attempt to outline a definitive role for bone scanning in the management of primary bone tumors. Preliminary results suggest that the technique may find an important role in the management of these tumors, just as it has in monitoring metastatic disease from nonosseous primaries. This role will become better defined in the future, as the procedure is used more commonly in the work-up and follow-up of these patients. At present, it appears that bone scanning's most important contribution to the management of the patient with primary bone malignancy is surveying for metastatic disease in treatment planning and in follow-up posttherapy. Usually its use should be as an adjunct to chest X-ray films for radiographic imaging of lung lesions. X-ray examination should also be used to further evaluate those areas found to be abnormal on bone scanning, and wherever symptoms exist without bone scan abnormality.

Summary and Conclusion

Bone scanning with newer radiopharmaceuticals and instrumentation has been reviewed, with attention given to the current clinical indications and limitations of their use in primary bone tumors. A number of areas of potential value for bone scanning have been discussed, with the conclusion that, although it is early to make definitive statements, it appears that total body radionuclide bone imaging offers a useful supplement to the work-up of the primary bone tumor patient, and may be of most value in posttherapy follow-up.

Acknowledgments

The author gratefully acknowledges the valuable assistance of Howard J. Glenn, Ph.D., Monroe F. Jahns, Ph.D., and James E. Seabold, M.D., the resident physicians in the Section of Nuclear Medicine, and the technologists in the radiopharmaceutical and radioisotope laboratories of M. D. Anderson Hospital for the performance and analysis of the patient bone scintigrams.

REFERENCES

Bessler, W. T.: Skeletal scintigraphy as an aid in practical roentgenographic diagnosis. The American Journal of Roentgenology, Radium Therapy and Nuclear Medicine, 124:899–907, April 1968.

Davis, M. A., and Jones, A. G.: Comparison of ^{99m}Tc-labeled phosphate and phosphonate agents for skeletal imaging. Seminars in Nuclear Medicine, 6: 19–31, January 1976.

Frankel, R. S., Jones, A. E., Cohen, J. A., Johnson, K. W., Johnston, G. S., and Pomeroy, T. C.: Clinical correlations of ^{67}Ga and skeletal whole-body radionuclide studies with radiography in Ewing's sarcoma. Radiology, 110: 597–603, March 1974.

Gilday, D. L., and Ash, J. M.: Benign bone tumors. Seminars in Nuclear Medicine, 6:33–46, January 1976.

Goldman, A. B., and Braunstein, P.: Augmented radioactivity on bone scans of limbs bearing osteosarcomas. Journal of Nuclear Medicine, 16:423–424, May 1975.

Harmer, C. L., Burns, J. E., Sams, A., and Spittle, M.: The value of flourine-18 for scanning bone tumors. Clinical Radiology, 20:204–212, April 1969.

Holsti, L. R., and Patomaki, L. K.: [18]F scanning of primary and metastatic bone tumors. Annals of Internal Medicine (Finland), 56:131–135, January 1967.

Jones, A. G., Francis, M. D., and Davis, M. A.: Bone scanning: Radionuclidic reaction mechanisms. Seminars in Nuclear Medicine, 6:3–18, January 1976.

Lentle, B. C., Russell, A. S., Percy, J. S., Scott, J. R., and Jackson, F. I.: Bone scintiscanning updated. Annals of Internal Medicine, 84:297–303, March 1976.

McNeil, B. J., Cassady, J. R., Geiser, C. F., Jaffe, N., Traggis, D., and Treves, S.: Flourine-18 bone scintigraphy in children with osteosarcoma or Ewing's sarcoma. Radiology, 109:627–631, December 1973.

Moon, N. F., Dworkin, H. J., and LaFleur, P. D.: The clinical use of sodium flouride F 18 in bone photoscanning. Journal of the American Medical Association, 204:116–122, June 10, 1968.

O'Mara, R. E.: Bone scanning in osseous metastatic disease. Journal of the American Medical Association, 229:1915–1917, September 30, 1974.

Pistenma, D. A., McDougall, I. R., and Kriss, J. P.: Screening for bone metastases. Are only scans necessary? Journal of the American Medical Association, 231:46–50, January 6, 1975.

Richman, L. S., Gumerman, L. W., Levine, G., Sartiano, G. P., and Boggs, S. S.: Localization of ^{99m}Tc-polyphosphate in soft tissue malignancies. The American Journal of Roentgenology, Radium Therapy and Nuclear Medicine, 124:577–582, August 1975.

Samuels, L. D.: Lung scanning with ^{87m}Sr in metastatic osteosarcoma. The American Journal of Roentgenology, Radium Therapy and Nuclear Medicine, 104:766–769, December 1968.

Shirazi, P. H., Rayudu, G. V., and Fordham, E. W.: Extraosseous osteogenic sarcoma of the small bowel demonstrated by ^{18}F scanning. Journal of Nuclear Medicine, 14:295–296, May 1973.

Shirazi, P. H., Rayudu, G. V. S, and Fordham, E. W.: ^{18}F bone scanning: Review of indications and results of 1,500 scans. Radiology, 112:361–368, August 1974.

Spencer, R., Herbert, R., Rish, M. W., and Little, W. A.: Bone scanning with ^{85}Sr, ^{87m}Sr and ^{18}F. Physical and radiopharmaceutical considerations and clinical experience in 50 cases. The British Journal of Radiology, 40: 641–654, January 1967.

Thrall, J. H., Geslien, G. E., Corcoron, R. J., and Johnson, M. C.: Abnormal radionuclide deposition patterns adjacent to focal skeletal lesions. Radiology, 115:659–663, June 1975.

Wanken, J. J., Eyring, E. J., and Samuels, L. D.: Diagnosis of pediatric bone lesions: Correlation of clinical, roentgenographic, ^{87m}Sr scan, and pathologic diagnoses. Journal of Nuclear Medicine, 14:803–806, November 1973.

Woodbury, D. H., and Beierwaltes, W. H.: Flourine-18 uptake and localization in soft tissue deposits of osteogenic sarcoma in rat and man. Journal of Nuclear Medicine, 8:646–651, September 1967.

The Surgical Management of Primary Neoplasia of Bone

JOHN A. MURRAY, M.D.

Clinical Associate Surgeon (Orthopedics),
Department of Surgery,
The University of Texas System Cancer Center
M. D. Anderson Hospital and Tumor Institute,
Houston, Texas

ALTHOUGH THE MOST COMMON NEOPLASM of bone encountered in the practice of orthopedic surgery is metastatic carcinoma, the management of this entity will not be included in this presentation on primary bone tumors.

The basic approach to the treatment of primary neoplasia of bone can be summarized by 3 basic goals: 1) eradicate the tumor; 2) avoid amputation when possible; and 3) preserve maximum function. There can be no compromise with the first of these basic goals. Unless the neoplasm is completely eradicated at its site of origin, the extremity and/or the individual remains at risk. Any procedure that is not designed to satisfy this goal should be abandoned from its onset.

To avoid associated pitfalls, a diagnosis should be established, thus enabling the surgeon to plan any necessary eradication procedure, aided by the classification of the neoplasia involved (Table 1). This classification is clinically very functional and differs little from most other classifications (Dahlin, 1967; Spjut, Dorfman, Fechner, and Ackerman, 1971).

It is, of course, desirable to avoid the mutilative result of amputation of an extremity whenever possible. Regardless of the quality and advanced technical improvement in prostheses of today, they are not a satisfactory substitute for the original extremity, in which sensation

TABLE 1.—PRIMARY NEOPLASIA OF BONE

BENIGN	AGGRESSIVE	MALIGNANT

Cartilage
  Osteochondroma
  Enchondroma
  Chondromyxoid fibroma
  Chondroblastoma
	Cartilage
	  Chondroma
		Cartilage
		  Chondrosarcoma

Bone
  Osteoid osteoma
  Osteoblastoma
	Bone
	  Giant cell tumor
	  Adamantinoma
	  Parosteal osteosarcoma
		Bone
		  Osteosarcoma
		  Periosteal osteosarcoma

Fibrous
  Nonossifying fibroma
  Fibrous dysplasia
  Ossifying fibroma
  Desmoplastic fibroma
		Fibrous
		  Fibrosarcoma
		  Fibrohistiocytoma

Neural
  Neurofibroma
		Neural
		  Neurosarcoma

Vascular
  Hemangioma
		Vascular
		  Hemangiosarcoma

Aneurysmal Bone Cyst		

		Small Round Cell
		  Ewing's sarcoma
		  Lymphoma
		  Leukemia
		  Myelomatosis

and motor power can be preserved. By the same token, the useless extremity, i.e. that which has a marked decrease in sensation and/or motor power, can be a hazard to the patient.

Ideal management of primary neoplasia of bone by the orthopedic surgeon is obviously controlled by the histopathology of the lesion involved and the exact anatomical site and physical size of the lesion. Available clinical or radiographic data should be incorporated into the planning of this management of the lesion, since the histopathology alone does not always convey the biological behavior of a given lesion. There is no substitute for using good, sound clinical judgement in treating these lesions and individualizing the treatment of each. (Note: Just what constitutes preservation of maximum function is the single area in which surgeons experienced in the management of neoplasms differ most in their opinions regarding treatment technique. The surgical technique of reconstruction after eradication of a neoplasm of bone in the extremity is beyond the scope of this presentation. You are referred to the abundant orthopedic literature covering reconstruction of major bone and joint defects.)

The following is a brief generalization regarding the surgeon's role in the management of each of the following: small cell sarcoma, frankly malignant lesions, locally aggressive lesions, and benign lesions of bone (Table 2).

Small round cell lesions, as listed in the classification of neoplasia of bone, do not afford the surgeon much opportunity to apply his expertise in their overall care. The surgeon's initial responsibility is to recognize the lesion as a possible small round cell tumor and to supply the pathologist with adequate material for both light and electron microscopic studies.

Basic principles in the management of neoplasia of bone can be satisfied without further surgical intervention (Fernandez, Lindberg, Sutow, and Samuels, 1974) except in specific individual cases, e.g. Ewing's sarcoma of the foot. The surgeon does become involved in the management of the complications involving the bone, secondary to the disease or its treatment (radiation necrosis with fracture and fracture through biopsy site).

In considering surgical management of other primary malignant tumors of bone (osteosarcoma, chondrosarcoma, and fibrosarcoma), it is obvious that the aggressive forms of these diseases can be eradicated only by ablative surgery. Experience collected to date demon-

TABLE 2.—GENERAL SCHEMA OF SURGICAL PROCEDURES
BY CLASSIFICATION

I. Small round cell lesion
  A. Biopsy
  B. Amputation for lesions not amenable to x-ray therapy
  C. Surgical management of the complications of the lesion or treatment
II. Frankly malignant lesion
  A. Amputation
III. Locally aggressive lesion (late metastases)
  A. Wide local excision
  B. Amputation
IV. Benign lesion
  A. Curettage and pack
  B. Excision—no reconstruction
    1. No disability
    2. With disability
  C. Excision—with reconstruction
    1. Autograft alone
    2. Autograft with allograft supplement
    3. Endoprosthesis
    4. Endoprosthesis with allograft
    5. Allograft replacing joint surface
      a. Partial
      b. Whole

strates that no procedure short of ablation will eradicate or control these lesions (Dahlin and Coventry, 1967). Again, the exact histopathology, the anatomical site, and the size of the lesion significantly affect the necessary level of amputation for tumor control. Axial skeletal lesions present unique and difficult problems, with treatment frequently directed at palliation only.

The group we have labeled "Locally Aggressive Lesion (late metastasizing)" (Table 2) is managed surgically by radical bone resection, while at the same time, attempts are made to salvage the essential soft tissues in order to preserve necessary function in the extremity and, thus, avoid amputation (Enneking, Personal Communication). In this particular group, the exact histopathology, site, and size of each lesion require careful individualization and sound clinical judgement (Spjut, Dorfman, Fechner, and Ackerman, 1971). In addition to those lesions listed in the classification of neoplasia as locally aggressive, well-differentiated chondrosarcoma and fibrosarcoma confined to bone also are amenable to treatment by wide local resection.

The time-honored surgical procedure for nonmalignant neoplasia of bone is to curettage and pack the resultant defects with bone chips, either autografts or allografts. Our experience has led us to believe that a change in this form of management is needed. We believe that many of these lesions are better managed by total excision with an adequate margin of normal tissue. Again, we stress obtaining exact histopathology, anatomical site, and size of the lesion, which dictate what resection and reconstruction problems will be encountered. Some lesions remain that can be managed, based on past experience and their natural history, by curettage and packing (Fig. 1).

The best results for the patient in the management of benign lesions of bone are obtained in clinical situations in which the lesion can be resected with no reconstructive procedure required and which leave the patient with no significant disability. Osteochondroma and benign proximal and mid-shaft fibular lesions fall most frequently into this category (Fig. 2).

Following this, the best results for the patient are obtained in clinical situations in which the lesion lends itself to eradication by resection and does not require reconstruction, but which leave the patient with some disability. Lesions that fall into this category are those in the anterior pelvis which can be resected *in toto*, although this is a procedure that often sacrifices the obturator nerve function to the adductor muscle mass (Fig. 3).

Next are lesions whose histopathology, site, and size do lend themselves to resection but also require reconstruction. Those that can be

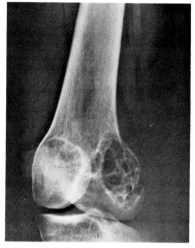

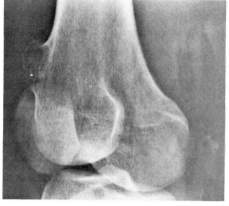

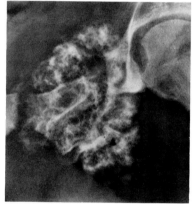

Fig. 1 (above left).—Chondroblastoma of the medial distal femoral epiphysis and metaphysis eradicated by curettage and autograft chips.

Fig. 2 (above).—Osteochondroma of the distal lateral femoral condyle eradicated by excision without reconstruction and with no resultant disability.

Fig. 3 (left).—Sarcomatous transformation in an osteochondroma of the pubic ramus eradicated by excision without reconstruction. The obturator nerve was sacrificed, thus denervating the adductor muscle mass.

resected and managed by autograft, either by bone chips from the pelvis or by cortical-cancellous graft from the fibula or rib, fall into this category. Distal radial lesions and small lesions in the shaft of long bone also fall into this category (Fig. 4).

Lesions that require reconstruction by the use of autografts and that are supplemented by allografts after eradication by adequate resection are treated in clinical situations in which the next best results for the patient are obtained. Extensive diaphyseal lesions and some upper extremity lesions are representative of this category.

The third type of lesion requiring reconstruction, but the least desirable for the patient, is that lesion best managed by resection and the use of a prosthesis secured by methylmethacrylate, but requiring no

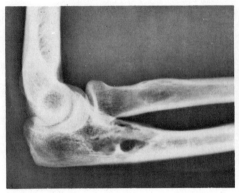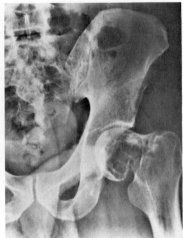

Fig. 4 (left).—Chondromyxoid fibroma of the ulna resected, and a full-thickness block of iliac crest fitted to the defect and secured with metallic internal fixation.

Fig. 5 (right).—Giant cell tumor of femoral head and neck eradicated by resection. Reconstruction was accomplished by insertion of an endoprosthesis.

graft material. Locally aggressive or recurrent lesions of the femoral head and neck are in this category (Fig. 5).

Next are the lesions that require supplementation with allograft or autograft to support the prosthesis secured by methylmethacrylate. Trochanteric and proximal shaft lesions are examples of this category (Fig. 6).

Lesions whose anatomical site and/or size jeopardize joint function by involving the joint surface, because of the need for major resection involving the joints, are the ones in which reconstruction presents the greatest problem. These lesions are also those in which the most disagreement exists among surgeons regarding reconstruction. Classically, distal femoral and proximal tibial giant cell tumors fit this category (Fig. 7). It is our feeling that lesions in this region, which require partial resection of a joint surface, can quite satisfactorily, and rather consistently, be managed by radical excision and allograft transplant involving a partial joint surface, with good functional result. Lesions that require the resection of one complete joint surface, such as the distal femur, can also be managed by allograft transplant; however, it is important to consider the significance and severity of complications associated with whole-joint surface transplants by massive allografts. Amputation may be necessary to manage complications in this procedure.

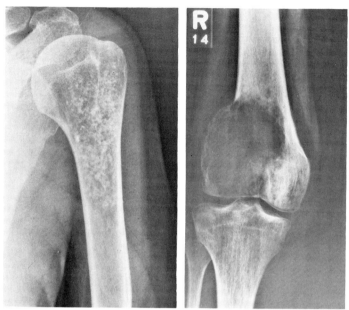

Fig. 6 (left).—Chondrosarcoma of the proximal humerus eradicated by resection. Reconstruction was carried out utilizing a segment of allograft and a Neer prosthesis.

Fig. 7 (right).—Giant cell tumor of the distal femur requiring resection of the entire distal femur. Reconstruction by allograft transplant was tailored to match the surgical defect.

These comments are not meant to answer specific problems, but are presented for consideration as a basic concept. Again, the single mandatory function of the surgeon in the approach to the surgical management of neoplasia of bone is to eradicate the neoplasia.

REFERENCES

Dahlin, D. C.: *Bone Tumors.* 2nd edition. Springfield, Illinois, Charles C Thomas, 1967, 285 pp.

Dahlin, D. C., and Coventry, M. B.: Osteogenic sarcoma. The Journal of Bone and Joint Surgery, 49A:101–110, January–June 1967.

Enneking, W. F.: Personal communication.

Fernandez, C. H., Lindberg, R. D., Sutow, W. W., and Samuels, M. L.: Localized Ewing's sarcoma. Cancer, 34:143–148, July 1974.

Spjut, H. J., Dorfman, H. D., Fechner, R. E., and Ackerman, L. V.: *Tumors of Bone and Cartilage.* 2nd series. Washington, D.C., Armed Forces Institute of Pathology, Fascicle #5, 1971.

Total Resection of Giant Cell Tumors of the Extremities

FRANK F. PARRISH, M.D.

Clinical Associate Orthopedist,
The University of Texas System Cancer Center
M. D. Anderson Hospital and Tumor Institute,
Houston, Texas

GIANT CELL TUMOR of bone more commonly affects the ends of long bones of young and middle-aged adults. This neoplasm produces marked lysis of bone and generally appears only after the epiphyseal plate has closed. One of the principal characteristics is its extension across the epiphyseal line to involve subchondral bone. While its origin is usually eccentric, as opposed to central, its growth may progress to involve the entire end of the long bone. Microscopically, it is an enigma to the pathologist because, in many instances, while its histological characteristics are benign, clinically, it is highly aggressive and may even metastasize to the lung, without the characteristic microscopic evidence of malignancy.

The tumor lends itself to surgical treatment in the extremities much more readily than in the axial skeleton. In the latter instance, total excision frequently is not feasible. The common treatment upon initial presentation of a giant cell tumor of the extremities thus far has been basically curettage of all possible tumor, followed by packing of the residual cavity with bone chips. In many series, this form of management resulted in 40%–60% recurrence, which must be considered an inadequate surgical procedure by most surgical standards. Furthermore, the longer a series of giant cell tumors is studied after such an initial procedure, the more likely it is to recur after a long period of time, and the more amputations must be done; occasionally, the lesion is found in the lung.

With these facts in mind, it must become apparent that the generally accepted treatment of an initial giant cell tumor of bone, as judged by current standards, is inadequate. Combinations of surgery, radiotherapy, chemotherapy and immunology are not the answer to treatment of this tumor in light of current scientific advances. Therefore, a more radical surgical treatment appears to be indicated. The philosophy of total excision of the tumor at the time of initial presentation, excising a margin of normal bone beyond the tumor borders, appears to be the treatment of choice. This is best effected when the tumor involves a bone in 1 of the extremities, rather than in the axial skeleton where total excision is most difficult. If we follow this dictum in the surgical management of giant cell tumors of bone, procedures must be devised in which the tumor can be totally excised, amputation avoided, and, it is hoped, the patient, through reconstructive measures, left with the least possible functional disability.

Following radical excision of a giant cell tumor in the extremity, the orthopedic surgeon has at his disposal for the reconstruction of the extremity autographs, allografts (which in some cases would involve osteocartilaginous graft to replace the entire end of long bone), nu-

Fig. 1.—Major distal femoral resection with allograft replacement. (Adapted from Parrish, 1973.)

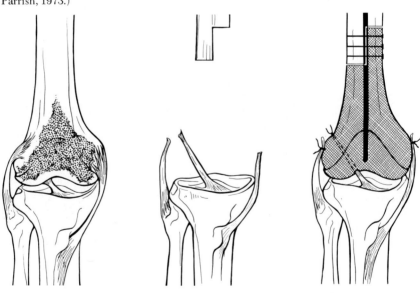

merous prosthetic appliances for total or partial joint surface replacement, bone cement, and certain synthetic materials which may be employed to reconstruct the joint capsule, a wide fascial defect, and major joint ligaments. Some of the methods of total excision and replacement of the residual defect with an allograft are graphically illustrated in Figures 1–5.

In the past 20 years, 47 cases of giant cell tumor involving extremi-

Fig. 2.—Techniques of partial distal femoral resection.

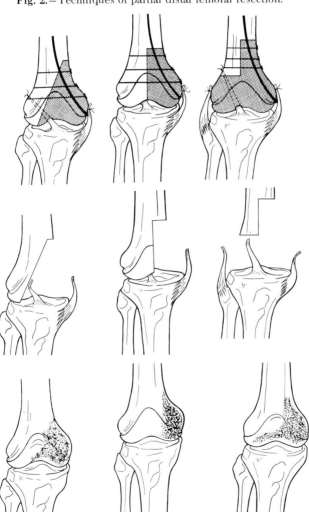

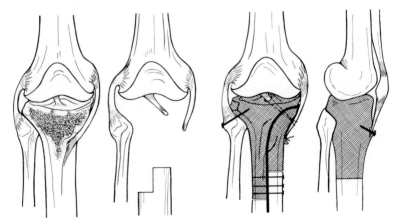

Fig. 3.—Total proximal tibial resection with allograft replacement. (Adapted from Parrish, 1973.)

ties have been treated by total surgical excision at the time of initial presentation. Of this number, 26 patients had primary tumors with no previous definitive surgery, and 21 presented with 1 or more recurrences. Of the group so treated, only 1 patient in the series has had a local recurrence in bone at the site of the original tumor. This recurrence proved to be a malignant fibrohistiocytic tumor, and the patient's extremity was sacrificed. Two patients required amputation because of failure of the graft in total distal femoral transplant. Both had had multiple previous operative procedures. One patient with 3 previous procedures developed infection after a secondary procedure following a distal femoral transplant and required amputation. A fifth

Fig. 4.—Partial proximal tibial resection with allograft replacement.

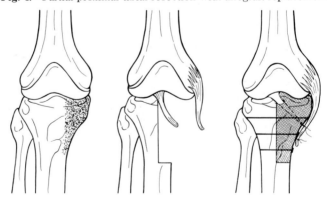

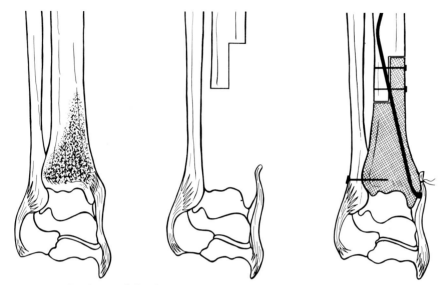

Fig. 5.—Total distal tibial resection. (Adapted from Parrish, 1973.)

patient died of pulmonary embolism 6 weeks after distal femoral transplant. Only 1 tumor, in fact, recurred in the entire series. Local soft tissue recurrences occurred in 2 patients, both of whom had had 2 previous procedures elsewhere. These 2 patients presented no problems after local excision of the soft tissue tumor. The patient with local recurrence at the site of a total excision in the distal femur which had progressed to malignant fibrohistiocytic tumor of bone developed a lesion in his lung. One patient with a primary excision in the 2nd metacarpal bone has now developed metastatic disease in the lung. The chest is clear in all remaining patients.

REFERENCES

Parrish, F. F.: Allograft replacement of all or part of the end of a long bone following excision of a tumor. Report of 21 cases. The Journal of Bone and Joint Surgery, 55A:1–22, January 1973.

Parrish, F. F.: Treatment of bone tumors by total excision and replacement with massive autologous and homologous grafts. Journal of Bone and Joint Surgery, 48A:968–990, July 1966.

Biopsy of Bone Lesions

RICHARD G. MARTIN, M.D.

Professor of Surgery, Chief, Section of General Surgery,
Department of Surgery, The University of Texas System
Cancer Center M. D. Anderson Hospital and Tumor
Institute, Houston, Texas

A BONE BIOPSY IS PERFORMED for 2 main reasons: (1) diagnosis, and (2) determination of the type of treatment best suited for the particular lesion. It is essential to obtain enough tissue from a bone biopsy for histological diagnosis and to determine whether the tissue is malignant or benign, primary or metastatic, and whether it is radiosensitive, e.g. Ewing's sarcoma or lymphoma.

Because of the biopsy's use in determining the type of treatment used for a lesion we strongly believe that, whenever possible, the biopsy should be performed by the surgeon or team responsible for the definitive treatment of the patient. We believe that this individual or team will have the best knowledge of how and where the biopsy incision should be made. In the performance of a biopsy, the radiologist and the pathologist should be consulted so that adequate and representative tissue will be obtained. It is because of these beliefs that all patients with primary bone lesions referred to M. D. Anderson Hospital are seen by a group consisting of an orthopedist, general surgeon, pathologist, radiologist, radiotherapist, and chemotherapist. Pediatric patients are seen by a pediatrician as well.

Types of Biopsies

The three types of biopsies are: excisional, incisional, and needle. An excisional biopsy is rarely performed because of the location and magnitude of the lesions of bone; an incisional biopsy is the most common type used for lesions of bone. This usually requires a general anesthesia, with the incision then made over the tumor mass and down through to the soft tissue. Whenever possible, soft tissue tumor as well as some bone should be obtained. Frequently, these biopsy sites bleed quite profusely and may require packing.

Needle biopsies are especially appropriate for lesions that are difficult to reach surgically, and their use eliminates the need of a difficult surgical procedure. If the lesion is soft, a True Cut or disposable Vim Silverman Needle (or a similar type needle) is used. In the case of blastic or hard lesions, a needle similar to the Ackerman or one with a serrated tip is used in order to permit cutting a core for sample. The chief criticism of this method is, of course, the amount of tissue obtained for histologic study. The needle biopsy may also be of value in preclinical areas that are positive on bone scans. Frequently, a negative biopsy is not significant. These procedures may be done under local anesthesia using either ultrasound or fluoroscopic control. General anesthesia, however, is necessary in cases involving the vertebra.

Frozen Sections

Frozen sections are obtained in those cases where a diagnosis of osteogenic sarcoma, fibrosarcoma, or chondrosarcoma is most likely and where the intention is to perform immediate definitive surgery under the same anesthetic. In cases such as lymphoma and Ewing's sarcoma, the incision is closed and treatment is primarily radiotherapy and/or chemotherapy. Metastatic lesions are also usually treated by radiotherapy, but at times, definitive surgical resection at the time of initial anesthesia may be necessary. If frozen section diagnosis is impossible, as in trauma or myocytis ossificans, therapy may be postponed until results of permanent section studies are known. Frozen sections are always done to be sure that adequate and representative material has been obtained, even though further definitive treatment is not contemplated at that time. This is especially true in the case of large tumors, in which much of the tumor material may be necrotic and therefore not suitable for histologic study. For this reason, it is best to try to obtain tissue from the margins of the lesion where normal tissue and tumor may be seen in the same field and where necrotic tissue is least likely to be seen. In some bone lesions, decalcification is necessary, and when this is true, the surgeon must wait for a permanent section study. In lesions where purulent material is noted, cultures and sensitivity tests, as well as studies for fungus and tuberculosis, must be made.

Location of Biopsy Site

The location and size of the biopsy scar are most important; in fact, just as important to the surgeon, orthopedist, and radiologist as is the need for adequate biopsy material to the pathologist. Incisions must be planned, so that the biopsy scar can be removed with the surgical procedure. It also must not compromise the skin flap, especially in patients undergoing fore- and hindquarter amputations. The scar must be well-healed for the radiotherapist. The placement of the scar may also have much to do with the patient's ability to be mobile; this is especially true with lesions in the calf and around the Achilles tendon, foot, and hand. Care must be taken at the time of biopsy to prevent fracture; it may be necessary to immobilize the bone by the use of splints.

When possible, the biopsy site should be over the area of soft tissue swelling, often the maximum point of tenderness. Frequently, it is necessary that X-ray films be obtained at the time of biopsy of bone lesions with markers in place to be sure that the area desired is the one biopsied.

Often, in obtaining a biopsy specimen of bone lesions, bleeding is profuse, requiring gel foam, or a similar substance, packed into the wound to control the bleeding. These lesions are apt to develop hematomas, and to break down and become infected, causing sinus tracts. Radiotherapy in such cases must be delayed; therefore, the smaller the incision and the more meticulous and proper the closure of the skin edges, the better the healing.

Summary

A biopsy is important not only for diagnostic purposes but also to determine the type of treatment procedure best suited for the particular lesion. The method and location of the biopsy are of utmost importance for diagnostic purposes and for producing the best skin flaps for amputations, especially for hind- and forequarter procedures. Also, well-healed, well-placed small scars are essential for further use of radiotherapy and chemotherapy in cases of lymphoma and Ewing's sarcoma. It is our belief, therefore, that the surgeon or team that is to give the definitive treatment for a primary bone lesion should have the privilege of performing the biopsy.

Surgical Treatment of Chondrosarcoma

MARVIN M. ROMSDAHL, M.D., Ph.D., HARRY L.
EVANS, M.D., and ALBERTO G. AYALA, M.D.

*Departments of Surgery and Pathology, The University
of Texas System Cancer Center
M.D. Anderson Hospital and Tumor Institute,
Houston, Texas*

THE CLINICAL BEHAVIOR of chondrosarcomas is highly variable compared to that of the majority of other solid tumors found in man. In particular, it differs from the more predictable pattern of osteosarcoma or Ewing's sarcoma, both common primary tumors of bone. Chondrosarcomas which remain localized may grow either slowly or very rapidly; however, local growth features do not usually allow one to predict which tumors will metastasize. These, as well as other features, have served to complicate the management of chondrosarcomas. Consequently, many patients are subjected to repetitive surgical procedures in attempts to control local disease. In addition, criteria for identifying patients whose tumors are likely to spread, and who thereby are candidates for early systemic treatment, have not been established for use by the medical community.

It is not appropriate to suggest that complete answers to these considerations are now available. Nevertheless, attempts to utilize histopathological criteria and clinical information pertinent to patients with chondrosarcoma have led to concepts which appear noteworthy and practical in the treatment of individuals with this disease (Barnes and Catto, 1966). In this regard, patients with chondrosarcoma treated at M. D. Anderson Hospital over a period of 26 years, ending in 1974, were examined in a retrospective manner (Evans, Ayala, and Romsdahl, in press). Only those individuals for whom histological slides were obtainable and for whom a reliable evaluation of the clinical course could be ascertained were included for review. The histopathological aspects of this subject material indicate that chondrosarcomas can be appropriately graded in a manner which usually correlates with clinical behavior and survival. Basically, such grading considers the number of mitoses in representative microscopic fields as well as the staining and morphological characteristics of cell nuclei.

Eighty-one patients with chondrosarcoma (53 men and 28 women) were evaluable for review. Individuals ranged from 16 to 81 years of age, with the greatest number in the sixth and seventh decades. Pain and/or a noticeable mass were the most common presenting symptoms. A survey of the location of these neoplasms indicates a wide distribution and a propensity for involvement of the pelvis and femur (Fig. 1).

The anatomical distribution of chondrosarcoma for both sexes suggests that the male-female ratio of 2:1 generally applies to every anatomical region (Table 1). Certain bones appearing to deviate from this ratio, such as those of the face, scapula, and humerus, are not involved

Fig. 1.— The anatomical distribution of documented chondrosarcoma in 81 M. D. Anderson Hospital registered patients indicates that numerous sites may be involved, with a large proportion being in the pelvis and proximal long bones.

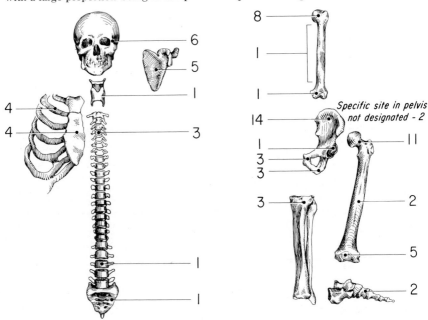

TABLE 1.—ANATOMICAL DISTRIBUTION OF
CHONDROSARCOMAS IN RELATION TO SEX AND AGE

ANATOMICAL REGION	NUMBER OF MALES	DECADE	NUMBER OF FEMALES	DECADE
Facial bones	2	4,6	4	2,5,6,8
Larynx	1	8		
Spine:				
Cervical	3	4,5,7		
Lumbar	1	6		
Sacrum			1	4
Sternum	2	7,8	2	2,8
Scapula	5	2,5,6,6,7		
Ribs	3	5,8,9	1	7
Humerus:				
Proximal	3	3,6,7	5	3,4,5,6,7
Distal	1	5		
Entire Bone	1	8		
Pelvis:				
Ilium	10	3,4,4,4,5,5,5,5,6,7	4	3,4,5,6
Pubis	2	3,4	1	2
Ischium	2	3,6	1	3
Acetabulum	1	7		
Not designated	2	3,4		
Femur:				
Proximal	7	6,7,7,7,7,7,7,	4	3,4,6,7
Mid			2	6,8
Distal	3	4,6,6	2	3,5
Tibia	3	4,6,7		
Foot	2	5,8		
Totals	54	Medium 6th decade	27	Medium 5th decade

frequently enough to indicate a sexual influence in distribution. The median age at diagnosis of chondrosarcoma is less for females than for males.

Histological grades of chondrosarcoma were tabulated for the different anatomical regions of involvement (Table 2). While most sites were represented by tumors of different grades, a predominance of a certain grade appeared evident in some bones; for example, 11 of 14 tumors originating in the ilium were of Grade 1 histological type. Contrary to this finding was that concerning the proximal femur, where 8 of 11 lesions were classified as Grade 3. The proximal humerus appeared to favor a low-grade histology, with 6 of 8 chondrosarcomas at this site being Grade 1. Overall, there were 35 (43%) lesions designated Grade 1, 26 (32%) designated Grade 2, and 20 (25%) designated Grade 3. The survival of patients for the respective grades for chondrosarcomas is as follows: Grade 1, 90% at 5 years and 87% at 10

TABLE 2.—HISTOLOGICAL GRADES OF
CHONDROSARCOMAS IN RELATION TO
ANATOMICAL REGION

ANATOMICAL REGION	TOTAL NUMBER OF PATIENTS	HISTOLOGICAL GRADE		
		1	2	3
Facial bones	6	2	3	1
Larynx	1		1	
Spine:				
Cervical	3	1	2	
Lumbar	1	1		
Sacrum	1			1
Sternum	4	3	1	
Scapula	5	1	1	3
Ribs	4		2	2
Humerus:				
Proximal	8	6	2	
Distal	1		1	
Entire Bone	1			1
Pelvis:				
Ilium	14	11	1	2
Pubis	3	2	1	
Ischium	3	1	2	
Acetabulum	1			1
Not designated	2	2		
Femur:				
Proximal	11	1	2	8
Mid	2	1	1	
Distal	5		5	
Tibia	3	2	1	
Foot	2	1		1
Totals	81	35	26	20

years; Grade 2, 81% at 5 years and 64% at 10 years; and Grade 3, 43% at 5 years and 29% at 10 years (Evans, Ayala, and Romsdahl, in press).

Patients treated at M. D. Anderson Hospital during the 25-year period prior to this report included many having biopsies, surgical excisions, and partial excisions of their tumors. This hetergenous approach to initial management precludes an accurate assessment of a relationship of histological grade to recurrence rates. However, it was feasible to establish a relationship between the occurrence of metastatic disease and the histological grade. In this regard, no metastases were observed in patients with Grade 1 chondrosarcomas. Patients with Grade 2 tumors had a 10% incidence of metastatic spread. In contrast, 71% of patients with histological Grade 3 chondrosarcomas eventually developed metastases. Consequently, analysis of the information available for this large group of patients indicates a correlation between histological grade and development of metastases, but not a reliable correlation with local recurrence of tumor.

In spite of these limitations, an attempt was made to relate wound recurrence to the type of surgical procedure initially performed. Patients initially treated by curettage or limited local excisions without a substantial margin had a local wound recurrence of 92%. Uncontrolled recurrence, in which further surgery either was not feasible or, if done, was unable to control the local tumor, occurred in 46% of these patients; however, it is acknowledged that referral of individuals to this institution is often for management of recurrent disease.

When (1) amputation or (2) resection of all or a part of an involved bone was done as the initial procedure for this tumor, the local wound recurrence rate was 19% and uncontrolled recurrences were reduced to 9.5%. In spite of the limitations inherent in this type of clinical assessment, it appears reasonable that patients are best treated by wide surgical resection, including amputation where indicated, instead of by local or restricted excision of the primary chondrosarcoma. Individuals with local recurrence of tumor, however, usually benefit by subsequent surgical procedures. In the event that such patients have a histological Grade 1 or Grade 2 lesion, an appropriate second or third operation can result in favorable expectations of long-term survival.

The principal consideration in the surgical management of chondrosarcoma is that the primary lesion be widely excised, regardless of its site of presentation. Enucleations, limited or marginal excision, or removal of lesions in fragments are ill-advised procedures. Preferably, the mass should be removed en bloc, with a margin of normal bone encompassing the entire biopsy tract with a modest but definite amount of contiguous soft tissue. For this reason, those who perform the initial biopsies should consider tactical approaches to definitive surgical management at a later time. The specific resection will depend on the bone of involvement, the extent of the disease process, and the anticipated behavior based on X-ray interpretations and histological grade. Consequently, it becomes apparent that the treatment of patients must indeed be individualized. The rationale for this treatment concept, as well as for the restricted use of adjunctive systemic measures, is supported by an analysis of treated chondrosarcoma patients referred to our institution.

While 81 patients were treated at M. D. Anderson Hospital in the period covered by this report, a subset of 53 patients received their initial treatment at this institution. This group permits an objective assessment of clinical and pathological parameters as well as the natural history of this disease as encountered in a single referral center. The anatomical distribution of primary chondrosarcoma, as well as the age of subjects, was not different from that observed for the comprehensive group of 81 patients.

Of 53 patients, 3 operative deaths occurred (6%) and 4 patients underwent only a biopsy or partial excision (8%) because of circumstances relating to their clinical presentation (Table 3). Consequently, 46 patients were evaluable for assessment of clinical management, histological grading, and survival. While 34 (74%) patients are considered survivors without evidence of disease, there are 2 patients alive with disease and 10 dead due to disease.

The surgical management of chondrosarcoma is currently based on a policy recommending wide surgical excision, partial or total excision of the bone of involvement, or amputation according to extent or character of the tumor. It is our practice to perform wide exicision for chondrosarcoma arising in the axial skeleton for tumors of Grade 1 and Grade 2, although more radical procedures have been done in past years for scapular and pelvic tumors. Grade 3 lesions are treated similarly, except for those presenting in the scapula and pelvis, which are managed by standard or modified hemipelvectomy or thoracoscapular amputation. Grade 1 and Grade 2 chondrosarcomas of the extremities, particularly the humerus, femur, and tibia, are usually resected and the bone segment is replaced with an allograft (Parrish, 1973) or, where applicable, with an internal prosthesis. Grade 3 tumors are usually treated by amputation to include the entire affected bone. Since 1973 we have treated patients with Grade 3 chondrosarcomas with systemic chemotherapy after wide surgical extirpation, using a combination drug program.

Surgical management of chondrosarcoma according to our guidelines has resulted in 7 (15%) of the 46 evaluable patients developing local wound recurrence (Fig. 2). Of these, there were 5 whose disease was not subsequently controlled, resulting in an uncontrolled recurrence rate of 11%. Nine (20%) patients developed metastatic disease. Histological grading of this patient population revealed 21 (46%) patients with Grade 1, 11 (24%) with Grade 2, and 14 (30%) with Grade 3 chondrosarcomas.

TABLE 3.—CHONDROSARCOMA OF BONE
MDA SERIES

	Total Number Patients	53	
	Operative Deaths	3 (6%)	
	Biopsy Only/Partial Excision	4 (8%)	
	Evaluable Patients	46	
Recurrence:	7 (15%)	Grade I:	21 (46%)
Uncontrolled Recurrence:	5(11%)	Grade II:	11 (24%)
Metastasis:	9 (20%)	Grade III:	14 (30%)
	Survivors Without Disease: 34 (74%)		

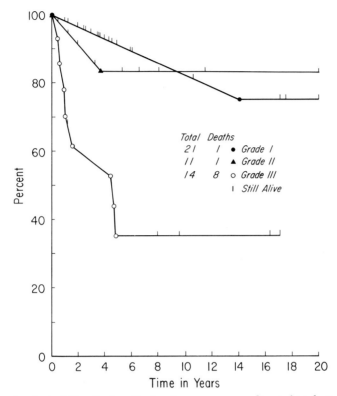

Fig. 2.—Survival of 46 patients with chondrosarcoma according to histological grade (Kaplan-Meier method).

Since local wound recurrence, uncontrolled wound recurrence, and development of metastasis are of primary importance and may be influenced by surgical management, a detailed evaluation of clinical and pathological features and outcome was done. An analysis of individuals developing local wound recurrence is indicated in Table 4. Three recurrences occurred in the pelvis, 2 in the ribs, and 1 each in the scapula and humerus. Four of the 7 patients had Grade 3 chondrosarcomas, and 3 eventually developed metastatic disease. Recurrence was detected within 10 months in those individuals with Grade 3 chondrosarcomas, while patients with Grade 1 and Grade 2 tumors developed local recurrence between 2 and 9 years following their initial surgery. Five of these 7 patients subsequently developed uncontrolled local recurrence (Table 5). Individuals with Grade 3 chondrosarcomas died within 1 year, while those with Grade 1 and Grade 2 sarcomas died after 14 and 4 years, respectively.

TABLE 4.—CHONDROSARCOMA CHARACTERISTICS OF
MDA PATIENTS DEVELOPING LOCAL RECURRENCE

PATIENT	SITE	HISTOLOGICAL GRADE	METASTASIS	SURVIVAL (YRS.)	DIED (YRS.)
1	Ischium	1	—	21	—
2	Ilium	1	—	—	14
3	Rib	2	—	—	4
4	Rib	3	—	—	1
5	Scapula	3	+	—	1
6	Ilium	3	+	—	1
7	Humerus	3	+	—	1

These observations indicate that local recurrence, as well as uncontrolled local recurrence, is not strictly correlated with histological grade, since 3 of 7 local recurrences were either Grade 1 or Grade 2 chondrosarcomas. This lack of correlation between grade and local recurrence was also observed in an analysis of the larger group of 81 patients (Evans, Ayala, and Romsdahl, in press).

The clinical characteristics of those individuals developing metastatic chondrosarcoma are indicated in Table 6. The most pertinent finding was that all 9 patients with metastases had Grade 3 chondrosarcomas on histological examination. Three of these 9 also had uncontrolled local wound recurrence. The interval from primary treatment to the detection of metastatic disease was between 2 and 74 months. Five of the 9 patients, however, developed metastatic disease within 1 year. Two individuals are alive with disease, 1 for 8 years after the initial surgical treatment. This exceptional circumstance illustrates the indolent course this disease may take when primary surgical treatment has not been curative. Patients developing metastatic disease within 1 year following surgical treatment have usually died within a short time.

Survival of patients with chondrosarcoma has correlated well with the designated histological grade (Fig. 2), as determined for this group

TABLE 5.—CHONDROSARCOMA CHARACTERISTICS OF MDA
PATIENTS DEVELOPING UNCONTROLLED LOCAL RECURRENCE

PATIENT	SITE	HISTOLOGICAL GRADE	METASTASIS	SURVIVAL (YRS.)	DIED (YRS.)
1	Ilium	1	—	—	14
2	Rib	2	—	—	4
3	Rib	3	—	—	1
4	Scapula	3	+	—	1
5	Ilium	3	+	—	1

TABLE 6.—CHONDROSARCOMA CHARACTERISTICS OF MDA
PATIENTS DEVELOPING METASTATIC DISEASE

PATIENT	AGE	SEX	SITE	HISTOLOGICAL GRADE	SURVIVAL (YRS.)	DIED (YRS.)
1	63	M	Proximal femur	3	8	—
2	28	F	Ilium	3	1	—
3	65	M	Acetabulum	3	—	5
4	61	M	Proximal femur	3	—	5
5	68	M	Proximal femur	3	—	1
6	50	M	Scapula	3	—	5
7	68	M	Scapula	3	—	1
8	53	F	Ilium	3	—	1
9	75	M	Humerus	3	—	1

of 46 individuals. The estimated 10-year survival of patients with
Grade 1 and Grade 2 tumors is approximately 83%; this is substantially greater than the 35% survival observed for individuals with Grade 3
chondrosarcoma, as determined by the method of Kaplan and Meier
(1958). Using a generalized Wilcoxon test (Gehan, 1965), the difference in survival between individuals with Grade 2 and Grade 3 chondrosarcoma is significant (P =0.03). Overall survival for this group of
46 patients at 10 years is estimated at 67% (Fig. 3). These statistics
serve to indicate that histological grading of primary chondrosarcomas
can reflect, to a reasonable extent, the eventual clinical behavior and
outcome.

The practice of wide surgical resection, or amputation where indicated, has served to reduce the local wound recurrence rate. In fact,
appraisal of clinicopathological information strongly suggests that local recurrence of chondrosarcoma is much more closely dependent on
the extent of surgical excision than on the histological grade. Thus, it
is prudent to excise all tumors, regardless of anticipated histological
grade, with adequate margins of normal bone and adjacent soft tissues. It is important, therefore, to plan the initial biopsy approach to
facilitate excision of the entire biopsy wound in the event a subsequent and definitive surgical procedure is necessary.

Depending on the management team, certain circumstances may
call for complete excisional biopsy rather than incisional biopsy.
While incisional biopsy will usually confirm whether a lesion is malignant, complete excision will permit more extensive pathological
examination and more accurate histological grading. This latter con-

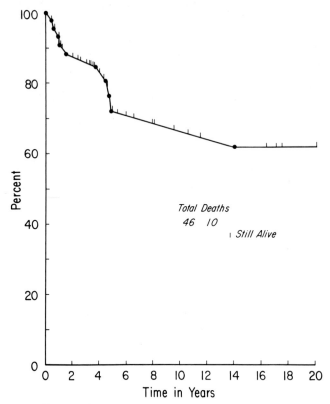

Fig. 3.—Overall survival of 46 patients with chondrosarcoma, as estimated by the Kaplan-Meier method.

sideration assumes greater relevance as management programs for Grade 3 chondrosarcomas are developed.

The management policy of wide surgical excision, or amputation where indicated, has also contributed to our overall survival rate, which is 77% at 5 years and 67% at 10 years (Evans, Ayala, and Romsdahl, in press). The contribution of aggressive surgical treatment has also improved survival in other centers (Barnes and Catto, 1966; Marcove *et al.*, 1972; Dahlin and Henderson, 1956; and Lindbom, Soderberg, and Spjut, 1961). Consequently, the practice of restricted excisions, enucleations, removal of lesions in fragments, and curettage will both increase the incidence of local recurrence and adversely affect survival.

Histological grading of chondrosarcoma has been examined for potential correlation with the clinical course of disease ever since the distinctive features of benign and malignant cartilage tumors were defined by Lichtenstein and Jaffe (1943) as well as Copeland and Geschicter (1949). In general, the features of pleomorphism, degree of nuclear hyperchromatism, and proportion of multinucleated tumor cells have been used as criteria for this purpose (Marcove *et al.*, 1972; Dahlin and Henderson, 1956; and Lindbom, Soderberg, and Spjut, 1961). In most of these studies, the histological grade generally appeared to correlate with prognosis and frequency of metastasis. Histological grading of chondrosarocma at M. D. Anderson Hospital, including those patients in this report, has emphasized the criteria of mitotic rate and cellularity in preference to other microscopic features. It appears at this time that these criteria offer the best means of identifying metastatic potential and survival.

Using the system of histological grading, we can predict a 5-year survival of 43% and a 10-year survival of 29% for patients with Grade 3 chondrosarcoma. When considering only those patients receiving their initial treatment for chondrosarcoma at our institution, all of the 9 individuals who eventually developed metastatic disease had Grade 3 lesions. It therefore seems plausible to use these criteria to identify patients who, because of the threat of metastatic disease, may benefit from systemic cancer chemotherapy as an adjunct to their surgical treatment.

Acknowledgments

The authors acknowledge Mrs. Terry L. Smith for statistical analyses and Mr. John Kuyendall for photography.

This study was supported in part by American Cancer Society Clinical Fellowship No. 3588, and funds from various donors for surgical research on sarcomas.

REFERENCES

Barnes, B., and Catto, M.: Chondrosarcoma of bone. The Journal of Bone and Joint Surgery, 48B:729–764, November 1966.

Copeland, M. M., and Geschicter, C. F.: Chondrosarcoma tumors of bone: Benign and malignant. Annals of Surgery, 129:724–735, May 1949.

Dahlin, D. C., and Henderson, E. D.: Chondrosarcoma, a surgical and pathological problem. The Journal of Bone and Joint Surgery, 38A:1025–1038, October 1956.

Evans, H. L., Ayala, A. G., and Romsdahl, M. M.: Prognostic factors in chondrosarcoma of bone: A clinicopathological analysis with emphasis on histological grading. Cancer. (In press.)

Gehan, E.: A generalized Wilcoxon test for comparing arbitrarily singly-censored samples. Biometrika, 52:203–223, June 1965.

Kaplan, E. L., and Meier, P.: Nonparametric estimation from incomplete observations. Journal of the American Statistical Association, 53:457, 1958.

Lichtenstein, L., and Jaffe, H. L.: Chondrosarcoma of bone. American Journal of Pathology, 19:553–574, 1943.

Lindbom, A., Soderberg, G., and Spjut, H. J.: Primary chondrosarcoma of bone. Acta Radiologica, 55:81, 1961.

Marcove, R. C., Miké, V., Hutter, R. V. P., Huvos, A. G., Shoji, H., Miller, T. R., and Kosloff, R.: Chondrosarcoma of the pelvis and upper end of the femur. The Journal of Bone and Joint Surgery, 54A:561–572, April 1972.

Parrish, F. F.: Allograft replacement of all or part of the end of a long bone following excision of a tumor. The Journal of Bone and Joint Surgery, 55A: 1–22, January 1973.

Surgical Management of Osteosarcoma

MARVIN M. ROMSDAHL, M.D., Ph.D., and ALBERTO
G. AYALA, M.D.
*Departments of Surgery and Pathology, The University
of Texas System Cancer Center
M. D. Anderson Hospital and Tumor Institute,
Houston, Texas*

THE SURGICAL TREATMENT of primary osteosarcoma, namely amputation of the affected extremity, appears at this time to offer the only chance for local tumor control and possible cure for most patients. A search for other approaches to management, as a means of preserving the affected extremity, has not been successful. Currently, there is substantial interest in limb-saving measures which entail resection of all or part of the affected bone, with insertion of a bone allograft or other suitable internal prosthesis.

Measures in addition to surgical treatment have been tried in an attempt to increase the number of survivors, but without convincing success. Preoperative radiotherapy followed by amputation after an intervening period of up to 6 months has not proven helpful (Lee and MacKenzie, 1964; Poppe, Liverund, and Efsking, 1968). Preoperative radiotherapy followed by immediate amputation has been carried out presumably to decrease the number of viable tumor cells that gain entrance to the systemic circulation during the operation (Farrell and Raventos, 1964; Caceres, Zaharia, and Tantalean, 1969).

Prophylactic irradiation of lung fields has been considered as an adjunct to surgical management, but is not favored because of the threat of diffuse pulmonary fibrosis and respiratory insufficiency. Extracorporeal supervoltage irradiation, even up to 20,000 rads, has been attempted without success (Spiro and Lubin, 1968). Isolation perfusion and intra-arterial irradiation with microspheres have not been shown to alter survival (Rocklin, 1963; Simon *et al.*, 1968).

Five-year survival rates have at best only approximated 20% in the past, principally because of pulmonary metastases which, if not detected at the time of diagnosis, develop soon in the course of the disease. It is assumed that most pulmonary metastases are occult when the disease is discovered. For this reason, it has seemed appropriate to implement adjunctive chemotherapy immediately after surgical amputation—before clinical or roentgenological evidence of metastasis is apparent. Early attempts using a single agent as adjuvant chemotherapy for nonmetastatic osteosarcoma following surgery were not considered successful (Sutow *et al.*, 1971). However, the development of treatment regimens utilizing multiple drugs, with each agent having shown some indication of therapeutic efficacy against osteosarcoma, appears promising in clinical trials of adjunctive chemotherapy in children (Sutow, Sullivan, Wilbur, and Cangir, 1975; Sutow *et al.*, 1975b).

Surgical Management

In the surgical management of osteosarcoma at M. D. Anderson Hospital, it has been our practice to resect the entire bone of involvement, principally to reduce or eliminate the prospects for recurrence of disease at the surgical margin of amputation (Francis, Hutter, and Coley, 1964).

Therefore, hip disarticulation is carried out for lesions of the distal femur, while hemipelvectomy is performed for tumors arising in the proximal femur and the pelvis. Smaller tumors of the proximal femur and those arising anterior to the region of the acetabulum are often treated by a modification of the standard hemipelvectomy, transecting the ilium lateral to the greater sciatic notch. This permits preservation of the wing of ilium, thereby facilitating, to some extent, the wearing of certain apparel and weight bearing, as well as the fitting of a prosthesis. Low midthigh or midthigh amputation is done for osteosarcoma of the proximal tibia. Tumors developing in the proximal humerus are treated by interscapulothoracic amputation, or a modification of this procedure, preserving the medial aspect of the clavicle and both the anterior and posterior shoulder muscle groups.

Surgical procedures for osteosarcoma are done with careful consideration with regard to skin flaps. Biopsy and histological verifications are mandatory prior to any amputation. When subsequent amputation is contemplated, these are done so that the biopsy track is remote from the skin flaps. Prior to primary wound closure following either amputation, hemipelvectomy, or interscapulothoracic amputation, strict hemostasis is secured and 2 wound suction catheters are inserted for drainage. A modest pressure dressing is applied only as an aid to immobilizing the large operative wound. Surprisingly, wound drainage is usually slight, and wound catheters are usually removed on the third to fifth postoperative day when drainage is below 15 cc for a 24-hour period. Patients are mobilized to bedside on the second postoperative day and ambulation is increased substantially on removal of the wound catheters.

Narcotics are used quite liberally during the 48 hours following surgery for relief of pain, and to reduce the severe anxiety and fear during this important period of adjustment to the surgical procedure. The narcotics are then progressively decreased according to the individual patient's needs. During this time, the patient requires substantial support from the professional staff as well as from members of his family. The phantom limb syndrome is managed by a careful explanation of its cause early in the postoperative period and by the combined use of a narcotic or narcotic substitute combined with an antidepressant, usually Valium. These agents, when used in combination, are considerably more effective that when used alone. As the phantom limb syndrome subsides, narcotics are reduced or eliminated, with Valium being used alone for relief of sporadic phantom symptoms.

Implementation of rehabilitation measures are included among the responsibilities of the surgeon and should reach an acceptable level before the patient is discharged from the hospital. At this time, the patient should be able to ascend and descend stairs, walk outdoors, and independently erect himself from a flat position on the floor with the aid of crutches. These measures, when appropriately taught and learned, represent a substantial aspect in the treatment of these individuals and prepare the patients for subsequent rehabilitation measures to improve their quality of life.

Results of Surgical Treatment

The surgical management of primary osteosarcoma at M. D. Anderson Hospital for a 24-year period extending from 1950 to 1974 was recently reviewed (Uribe-Botera, Russell, Sutow, and Martin, in press). An attempt was made to carefully exclude postirradiation sarcoma, extraskeletal osteosarcoma (Wurlitzer, Ayala, and Romsdahl, 1972), parosteal osteosarcoma, Ewing's sarcoma, chondrosarcoma, fibrosarcoma, and histiocytic lymphoma. In addition, patients treated with the Conpadri I adjunctive chemotherapy program were excluded from surgical analysis since examination confirms an improvement in both the percentage of patients disease-free at 2 years (54%) and the percentage surviving at 2 years (79%) for this group (Gehan *et al.*, in press). This compares favorably with patients treated by surgery alone, of whom only 18% were disease-free and 34% were surviving at 2 years following surgical management.

Of the 243 patients with osteosarcoma treated at M. D. Anderson Hospital over a 24-year period, 121 (49.8%) had lesions in the femur, 47 (19.3%) in the tibia, and 26 (11%) in the humerus. There was a concentration of tumors near the knee, with 101 (41.6%) involving the distal femur, 46 (18.9%) involving the proximal tibia, and 9 (3.7%) arising in the proximal fibula, for a total of 156 (64.2%) at this location (Fig. 1).

Lung metastases were observed in all but 1 of 54 subjects having complete postmortem examinations, while lymph node metastases were found in only 3 instances. The 3-year survival for the entire series was 21.7%, and the 5-year survival only 12.6%. Histologically, patients with osteoblastic tumors had the poorest survival, followed by those whose tumors exhibited predominantly chondroblastic features. Individuals with a fibroblastic pattern of osteosarcoma survived for the longest period of time.

Fig. 1.—Osteosarcoma of the lower extremity is found most frequently in the region of the knee. The distal femur, with proximal tibia and fibula, accounts for 64.2% of all osteosarcomas treated at M. D. Anderson Hospital.

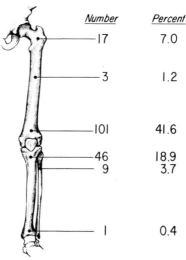

	Number	Percent
	17	7.0
	3	1.2
	101	41.6
	46	18.9
	9	3.7
	1	0.4

Level of Surgical Amputation

Since 41.6% of osteosarcomas seen at this institution occurred at the distal femur, serious consideration regarding the level of amputation seems appropriate. In principal, amputation proximal to the bone involved, rather than amputation through the bone or transmedullary amputation, has been advocated. There is, however, little objective evidence indicating that disarticulation of the hip results in more effective management than midthigh or upper-thigh amputation. Reviews dealing with the management of osteosarcoma rarely document the incidence of local recurrence, probably mainly because of the rapid death of most patients as a result of pulmonary metastasis. Whether this pattern will change in the future, with an anticipated increase in survival because of adjunctive chemotherapy, remains to be seen. Lichtenstein, in his monograph entitled *Bone Tumors*, states that the infrequent recurrence of osteosarcoma at the amputation site does not justify routine disarticulation of tumors of the lower femur (Lichtenstein, 1972). A recent study conducted to elucidate this problem included careful pathological examination of 20 long bones affected with osteosarcoma (Lewis and Lotz, 1974). In none of these instances was unappreciated intramedullary extension, or "skip areas," observed. Microscopic medullary extension, when observed, was within 1.0 cm of the gross intramedullary extent of tumor. In 2 series from a center performing transmedullary amputation for osteosarcoma, 5-year survival rates are equal to or better than those for centers performing radical amputations (Hayles, Dahlin, and Coventry, 1960; Dahlin and Coventry, 1967). While Dahlin and Coventry report a recurrence incidence of approximately 2% with transmedullary amputation, 2 other studies show recurrence rates of 14% and 16% with this procedure (Marcove *et al.*, 1970; McKenna, Schwinn, Soong, and Higenbotham, 1966). However, with only 1 exception, local recurrence occurred as a preterminal event associated with widespread bone metastases.

Contrary to these observations, Enneking has described "skip" lesions in 10 of 40 patients by conducting a careful, prospective research for small metastatic foci of osteosarcoma (Enneking and Kagan, 1975). Five of these 10 "skip" tumors were transarticular and 5 were intraosseus. His study utilized tetracycline-positive flourescence, which played an important role in detection of 6 "skip" areas. Four "skip" lesions were grossly evident by inspection. Consequently, it appears that excision of osteosarcoma through the bone of involvement, as opposed to total bone removal, carries with it some risk of leaving microscopic foci of tumor.

Since 1974, an attempt has been made at M. D. Anderson Hospital to determine whether intramedullary spread of osteosarcoma could be demonstrated in completely excised bones. In the immediate preoperative period, patients are given tetracycline, which has the properties of binding to osteoid and of being fluorescent in the presence of ultraviolet light. Following amputation, the affected bone is cut longitudinally with a band saw, thereby exposing the entire length of the

Fig. 2.—**A,** osteosarcoma of distal femur showing a permeative pattern in the metaphyseal area and mineralized osteoid extending through the cortex. **B,** an X-ray film of the femur above the level of the primary osteosarcoma does not show evidence of intramedullary disease suggestive of tumor "skip" areas.

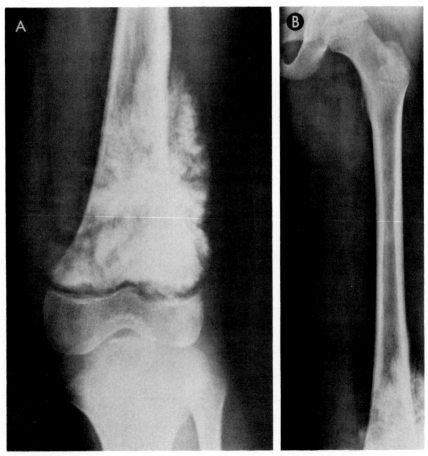

medullary cavity. The length of the marrow cavity is then inspected under ultraviolet light for areas of fluorescence. In addition, areas remote from as well as contiguous to the primary tumor are inspected for gross evidence of intramedullary spread. All regions of suspicion, as well as random areas of the marrow, are examined for histological evidence of osteosarcoma.

Of 48 separate surgical specimens examined, 3 have satisfied the criteria of noncontiguous spread in the affected bone. Clinical and pathological findings concerning these 3 patients have been analyzed.

One patient, an 11-year-old boy with a large osteosarcoma of the distal femur, had a hip disarticulation. The preoperative X-ray film of the involved femur did not show evidence of any abnormality remote from the primary tumor (Fig. 2A and B). Full chest tomograms taken prior to amputation showed metastatic disease to both lungs. Following surgery and longitudinal transection of the femur, 2 areas of interosseous tumor were observed, one being as far as the mid-diaphysis (Fig. 3A and B). These areas were visualized grossly and without the aid of fluorescence techniques. However, in the presence of ultraviolet light, these 2 areas, as well as the primary tumor, were highly fluorescent. Metastatic osteosarcoma was found in both of 2 popliteal lymph nodes and in 2 of 15 regional lymph nodes removed with the extremity. This patient was placed on high-dose methotrexate with citrovorum factor and vincristine, in combination with radiotherapy to the lungs. He died of extensive pulmonary metastases 9 months following surgical amputation.

The second patient, a 13-year-old girl, presented with a painful, progressively enlarging mass of the distal femur measuring 10 cm × 15 cm in transverse dimensions. X-ray examinations confirmed the soft tissue extension, showing a mineralized osteoid pattern which also involved the shaft. A large "skip" area was seen roentgenographically, as was some abnormal mineralization near the midshaft level. Hip disarticulation was performed. Although 10 femoral lymph nodes showed no evidence of tumor, there was intramedullary spread extending to the upper one third of the femur. Two "skip" areas of tumors were observed, one 0.5 cm in diameter and in the femoral neck, and another 0.3 cm in diameter in the head of the femur. The "skip" area in the femoral head showed flourescence, while the femoral neck lesion did not. Several areas of fluorescence were observed along the course of the medullary cavity and in the large tumor mass extending into the soft tissues of the lower thigh. This individual demonstrated no evidence of distant metastases and was placed on an adjunctive chemotherapy program.

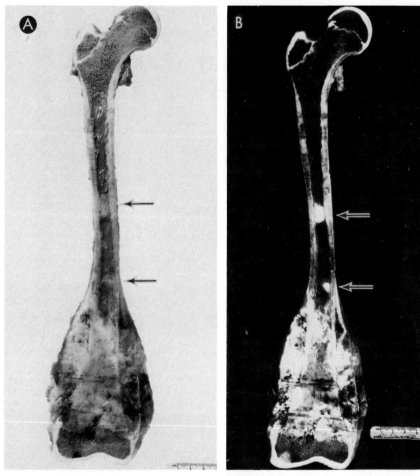

Fig. 3.—A, longitudinal section through entire femur represented in Fig. 2. In addition to the large primary osteosarcoma in the distal femur, 2 separate foci of intramedullary spread are grossly evident *(arrows)*. **B,** examination with ultraviolet light shows brilliant fluorescence of osteoid in primary tumor as well as in the 2 areas of "skip" metastases *(arrows)*.

The third patient demonstrating "skip" metastases also presented with a large primary tumor of the distal femur at our institution. A transmedullary amputation was performed as a palliative measure because multiple pulmonary metastases were evident on initial studies. A single focus of interosseous osteosarcoma was evident in the mid-diaphysis, close to the level of amputation. This lesion was also visible grossly without the aid of tetracycline-positive fluorescence.

The finding of "skip" areas in 3 of 48 bones examined for remote spread of osteosarcoma is less than that reported by Enneking (Enneking and Kagan, 1975), who found 5 interosseous "skip" tumors in 40 bones examined. His report, however, also describes 5 transarticular "skip" tumors. We did not observe transarticular metastasis in this series of patients, although this phenomenon has been noted at this institution. It appears, seemingly, that transarticular deposits of osteosarcoma represent a late stage in the blood-borne metastatic process. They may, however, be due to an increased propensity for tumor cells in venous tributaries leading from the primary tumor to arrest in or near the affected limb. The former explanation would not, in a strict pathophysiological sense, be consistent with the concept of ascending tumor spread with intervening "normal" tissue. The latter explanation, if true, would denote a lesion consistent with the definition of "skip" metastases.

Interosseous metastatic deposits seemingly represent a strictly regional event; however, the possibility that such lesions may actually represent another manifestation of arterial blood-borne tumor cells cannot be excluded. The finding of metastatic pulmonary disease in 2 of our 3 patients showing interosseous "skip" lesions, and involved regional nodes in 1 of those 3 subjects, suggests, but does not clearly document, a relationship of this finding to exceptionally advanced disease. Clearly, further studies are needed to elucidate the complex mechanisms and factors responsible for these remote foci of metastatic osteosarcoma.

Surgery in the Management of Metastatic Osteosarcoma

In the past, the role of surgery for metastatic osteosarcoma has been limited to an occasional resection of a single (or at most only several) pulmonary nodule and, rarely, palliative management of other problems. Usually, pulmonary metastases were so numerous that surgical intervention was unwarranted. Adjunctive chemotherapy programs following potentially curative surgery, however, have resulted in a certain number of patients who develop restricted metastatic disease to the lung — often only a single lesion. Under these circumstances, an intensive multimodal regimen utilizing pulmonary resection, irradiation, and chemotherapy is implemented (Sutow *et al.*, 1975A). The adjunctive chemotherapy program instituted initially following primary surgery is discontinued. The metastatic nodule(s) is resected surgically. High-dose methotrexate with citrovorum factor is then administered in conjunction with whole-lung irradiation. Treatment of patients in this manner has resulted in some patients remaining free of disease for as long as 2 years.

A certain number of patients will have a limited number of pulmonary metastatic nodules when initially presenting for management of primary osteosarcoma. Full chest tomography is routinely done to verify whether additional lesions undisclosed by a routine chest X-ray examination are present. Surgical management of the primary tumor receives the greatest priority, and resection or amputation is carried out immediately. In some patients, the primary tumor is large, painful, or otherwise disabling, and removal affords both local relief and systemic improvement (Fig. 4). Such patients are then placed on an intense systemic chemotherapy regimen and observed several months later for evidence of progression of metastatic disease. In the event that pulmonary disease is static or decreasing, pulmonary resection is seriously considered if it appears possible to extirpate all evident disease. Subsequently, systemic chemotherapy is continued, as in adju-

Fig. 4.—This extensive osteosarcoma of the proximal humerus was responsible for considerable disability. Interscapulothoracic amputation permitted local control, while systemic chemotherapy was utilized as the initial measure to treat 2 pulmonary nodules and prevent further development of metastases.

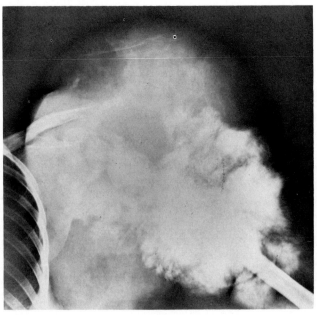

vant therapy, to attempt to destroy potential microscopic foci of metastatic osteogenic sarcoma which are not evident by usual clinical examination.

Conservative Surgery with Internal Prosthesis

Selected patients with osteogenic sarcoma of the extremities are currently being evaluated for resection of the segment of bone containing the involved primary tumor and are being fitted with an internal prosthesis. This approach is considered to be feasible in view of the potential therapeutic effectiveness of adjunctive chemotherapy programs now developed for osteosarcoma. Candidates for this method of management have been restricted to adults or younger patients in whom bone growth is almost complete and to patients with confined lesions without extensive soft tissue extension. While this approach is now considered preliminary, it has the potential of permitting control of disease with preservation of the affected limb.

Discussion

The successful management of osteosarcoma requires surgical excision, since radiotherapy and chemotherapy are not capable of offering permanent control. The principal goal of surgical treatment is to cure the patient, even with amputation. The secondary goal is to accomplish this cure with the least amount of physical disability. Consequently, it appears noteworthy to consider transmedullary amputation whenever it seems reasonable to the surgical oncologist. Obviously, certain massive tumors of the distal femur with proximal extension and soft tissue involvement will not be candidates for such a procedure, and in these cases immediate amputation at the hip should be done. The prudent use of conservative surgical excision of confined lesions, combined with intensive and effective systemic chemotherapy as a means of preserving an extremity, appears to have merit. It is hoped that future progress will allow this approach to be utilized for more patients. These and additional innovative measures should eventually result in improved survival as well as less disability for the patient with osteosarcoma.

Acknowledgments

This study was supported in part by funds from various donors for surgical research on sarcomas.

REFERENCES

Caceres, E., Zaharia, M., and Tantalean, E.: Lymph node metastases in osteogenic sarcoma. Surgery, 65:421–422, 1969.

Dahlin, D. C., and Coventry, M. B.: Osteogenic sarcoma—A study of 600 cases. Journal of Bone and Joint Surgery, 49A:101–110, 1967.

Enneking, W. F., and Kagan, A.: "Skip" metastases in osteosarcoma. Cancer, 36:2192–2205, 1975.

Farrell, C., and Raventos, A.: Experiences in treating osteosarcomas at the hospital of the University of Pennsylvania. Radiology, 83:1080–1083, 1964.

Francis, K. C., Hutter, R. V. P., and Coley, B. C.: Treatment of osteogenic sarcoma. In Pack, G. T., and Ariel, I. M., Eds.: *Treatment of Cancer and Allied Diseases*. New York, New York, Harper and Row, 1964, pp. 374–399.

Gehan, E. A., Sutow, W. W., Uribe-Botero, G., Romsdahl, M. M., and Smith, T. L.: Osteosarcoma: The M. D. Anderson Experience, 1950–1974. In *Immunotherapy of Cancer*, Raven Press. (In press.)

Hayles, A. B., Dahlin, D. C., and Coventry, M. B.: Osteogenic sarcoma in children. Journal of the American Medical Association, 174:1174–1177, 1960.

Lee, E. S., and MacKenzie, D. H.: Osteosarcoma, a study of the value of preoperative megavoltage radiotherapy. British Journal of Surgery, 51: 252–274, 1964.

Lewis, R. J., and Lotz, M. J.: Medullary extension of osteosarcoma—implications for rational therapy. Cancer, 33:371–375, 1974.

Lichtenstein, L.: *Bone Tumors*. 4th edition. St. Louis, Missouri, The C. V. Mosby Company, 1972, p. 235.

Marcove, R. C., Miké, V., Hajek, J. V., Levin, A. G., and Hutter, R. V. P.: Osteogenic sarcomas under the age of twenty-one. Journal of Bone and Joint Surgery, 52A:411–423, 1970.

McKenna, R. J., Schwinn, C. P., Soong, K. Y., and Higenbotham, N. L.: Sarcomata of the osteogenic series. Journal of Bone and Joint Surgery, 48A: 1–26, 1966.

Poppe, E., Liverund, K., and Efsking, J.: Osteosarcoma. Acta Chirurgica Scaninavica, 134:549–556, 1968.

Rocklin, D. B.: The therapy of sarcomas by isolation perfusion. American Journal of Surgery, 105:615–618, 1963.

Simon, N., Siffert, S., Baron, M. G., Mitty, H. A., and Rudavsky, A.: Preoperative irradiation of osteogenic sarcoma with intra-arterially injected Yttrium 90 microspheres. Cancer, 21:453–455, 1968.

Spiro, E., and Lubin, E.: Extracorporeal irradiation of bone tumors. Israel Journal of Medical Science, 4:1015–1019, 1968.

Sutow, W. W., Fernandez, C. H., Mountain, C. F., King, O. Y., Rivera, R. L., and Mumford, D. M.: Multimodal treatment of pulmonary metastases in osteogenic sarcoma. (Abstract) Proceedings of the American Association for Cancer Research and American Society for Clinical Oncology, 16:39, March 1975a.

Sutow, W. W., Sullivan, M. P., Fernbach, D. J., Cangir, A., and George, S. L.: Adjuvant chemotherapy in primary treatment of osteogenic sarcoma. Cancer, 36:1598–1602, 1975b.

Sutow, W. W., Sullivan, M. P., Wilbur, J. R., and Cangir, A.: Study of adjuvant chemotherapy in osteogenic sarcoma. Journal of Clinical Pharmacology, 15(7):530–533, 1975.

Sutow, W. W., Sullivan, M. P., Wilbur, J. R., Vietti, T. J., Kaizer, H., and Naga-moto, A.: L-phenylalanine mustard (NSC-8806) administration in osteogenic sarcoma: An evaluation of dosage schedules. Cancer Chemotherapy Reports, 55:151–157, 1971.

Uribe-Botero, G., Russell, W. O., Sutow, W. W., and Martin, R. G.: Primary osteosarcoma of bone: A clinicopathologic investigation of 243 cases with necropsy studies in 54. (In press.)

Wurlitzer, F., Ayala, A., and Romsdahl, M. M.: Extraosseous osteogenic sarcoma. Archives of Surgery, 105:691–695, 1972.

The Treatment of Osteosarcoma with Radiation: Current Indications

R. DEREK T. JENKIN, M.B.

Department of Radiation Oncology, The Princess
Margaret Hospital, and Department of Pediatrics,
The Hospital for Sick Children,
Toronto, Ontario, Canada

A REVIEW OF PATIENTS with osteosarcoma treated from 1958 – 1970 at The Princess Margaret Hospital, Toronto, demonstrated that for those younger than 30 years at diagnosis, the 5-year survival rate was only about 10%. Eighteen months after diagnosis only 2 of 33 patients were without metastatic disease. During these years, we had hoped that initial high-dose irradiation of the primary tumor followed by amputation at about 6 months, in the absence of pulmonary metastases, would offer the best available palliation for the majority of patients without jeopardizing the small chance for cure. However, the response of the primary tumor was inadequate to provide this palliation: In 27 patients less than 30 years of age, the response to irradiation was complete in 3, partial in 17, and absent in 7. The primary tumor relapsed in all 27 patients, with a median time of only 3.6 months; this was shorter than the median time of 4.5 months to the development of metastases (Jenkin, Allt, and Fitzpatrick, 1972). Since that time, preoperative irradiation has not been practiced in Toronto. When feasible, all patients undergo prompt resection as the first treatment. A similar unsatisfactory experience with radiation and selective delayed amputation in North America has been reported (Beck, Wara, Bovell, and Phillips, 1976).

151

Massive preoperative irradiation of the primary tumor prior to prompt amputation has been advocated by some on the grounds that viable tumor cells will not be liberated into circulation at the time of amputation and with the speculation that this might be a beneficial tumor-specific immunological stimulant. An unequivocally negative result was obtained when 8,000–12,000 rads in 8–12 days in 1,000–1,200 rads dose fractions was given preoperatively (Fig. 1) (Caceres and Zaharia, 1972).

A compilation of data from the literature of 1953–1971 for the treatment of osteosarcoma by radiation alone indicated that 18 of 143 patients (12.5%) were alive at 5 years (Friedman and Carter, 1972). However, the evolution of the histopathology of osteosarcoma during these years and the absence from the literature of single institution reports of series of young patients with classical osteosarcoma cured by radiation alone suggest that, at least in classical osteosarcoma, the prospect of cure by radiation alone is very small indeed.

Two notable advances in the treatment of osteosarcoma have been made very recently. On the one hand, it has been demonstrated that a proportion of patients with lung metastases have only a small finite number which may be eradicated by repeated resections (Martini *et al.*, 1971; Beattie, Martini, and Rosen, 1975), and on the other hand, effective adjuvant therapy with either Adriamycin or high dose methotrexate with citrovorum rescue has been described (Cortes *et al.*, 1974; Jaffe, Frei, Traggis, and Bishop, 1974). The combination of these 2 treatment modalities, if necessary, after resection of the primary tumor has significantly improved the prospect for survival, at

Fig. 1.—Survival after local irradiation of the primary tumor to 8,000–12,000 rads and prompt amputation, compared with amputation alone. (Courtesy of Caceres and Zaharia, 1972.)

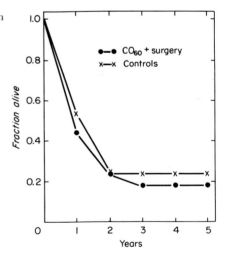

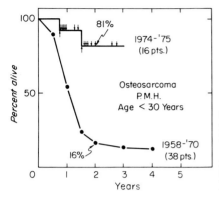

Fig. 2.—The survival of 16 consecutive patients less than 30 years of age referred postoperatively to The Princess Margaret Hospital during 1974–1975 for elective systemic therapy is compared with historical controls treated during 1958–1970 at The Princess Margaret Hospital.

least for young patients with osteosarcoma. For example, the 2-year survival rate at The Princess Margaret Hospital has increased from 16% to 81% (Fig. 2). Since this major change in the prospect for survival coincided with the introduction of 2 new effective treatments, it is assumed to be causally related.

The present treatment policy at The Princess Margaret Hospital is that both primary and secondary osteosarcoma should be resected whenever this is feasible. Radiation treatment of the primary tumor is employed only when the primary tumor is not resectable, or when the price of resection would be prohibitive; that is, in less than 10% of patients less than 30 years of age. No patient treated at The Princess Margaret Hospital with radiation alone prior to 1970 survived. Our recent experience is different.

Case Histories

CASE 1.—This 12-year-old girl presented in January, 1974, with a 4-month history of progressive right hip and buttock pain, and with a limp. On admission, she was in severe pain, unable to walk or stand, and could only lie prone in bed. There was a large diffuse mass in the right buttock and radiological evidence of a bone lesion in the right sacroiliac region, with gross destruction of the right sacrum and ilium (Fig. 3). Osteosarcoma was confirmed histologically. The right os calcis was considered to be a second site of osteosarcoma on the basis of a markedly abnormal bone scan, local pain, and tenderness, but with equivocal X-ray abnormalities.

The primary site was irradiated, utilizing ^{60}Co gamma rays by means of 18 × 18 cm parallel opposed fields. A midline dose of 6,000 rads was given in 30 fractions over 42 days. The field size was reduced to 15 ×

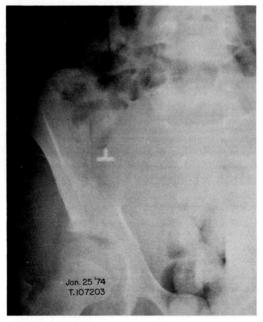

Jan. 25 '74
T.107203

Fig. 3.—Case 1. Extensive destruction of the right sacrum and adjacent ilium by primary osteosarcoma. Appearance at diagnosis. The volume irradiated is indicated.

15 cm at 5,600 rads. The right os calcis was given a midline dose of 2,500 rads in 5 fractions over 7 days with parallel opposed fields. One to 2 hours prior to each radiation treatment, metronidazole 1–2 gm was given by mouth. Two weeks after completing irradiation, she began Adriamycin treatment. Eleven single injections were given to a cumulative dose of 540 mg/m² over 8 months. She then started methotrexate, which was escalated to 250 mg/kg, given as a 6-hour infusion with folinic acid, 15 mg i.v., every 3 hours for 72 hours, commencing 2 hours after completion of the methotrexate infusion. Methotrexate was given every 21 days for 6 months, every 28 days for 7 months, and then every 3 months as illustrated in Figure 4.

Approximately 3 months after completing Adriamycin treatment, the patient developed an episode of cardiac dysfunction, characterized by cardiomegaly, tachycardia, and gallop rhythm, which responded to digitalis, diuretics, and rest, and which was attributed to Adriamycin cardiotoxicity. A complete tumor response was obtained and continues 33+ months from diagnosis. For 5 months, she required canes for walking, with the pain in the right foot being the slowest symptom to resolve. Within 2 months of completing irradiation, near

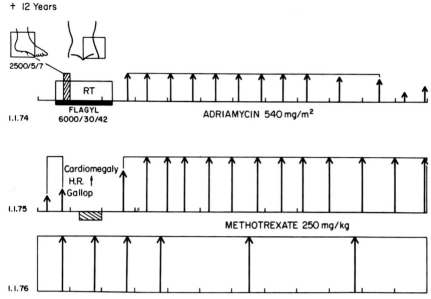

Fig. 4.—Case 1. Sequencing of radiation, Adriamycin, and methotrexate, January 1, 1974 through December 31, 1976.

total collapse of the bony framework at the primary site occurred (Fig. 5). Subsequently, progressive degenerative changes within the irradiated volume appeared (Fig. 6). Despite the radiological appearance, she has a functioning limb and walks reasonably well with a 5 cm lift in the right shoe.

CASE 2.—This 16-year-old girl presented with intermittent but progressive left sciatic pain of 7 months duration and a limp which had been present for 1 month. On X-ray examination, a bone lesion was seen on both sides of the left sacroiliac joint. A diagnosis of osteosarcoma was confirmed. A small lesion in the left lower lung was possibly a metastasis. A poorly defined buttock mass was present over the sacroiliac joint.

Treatment was by local irradiation of the primary site, 5,000 rads in 25 fractions over 39 days, using 16 × 16 cm opposed ⁶⁰Co fields. A first dose of Adriamycin, 75 mg/m², was given during irradiation at 4,200 rads tumor dose. A severe episode of diarrhea with some vomiting was precipitated which required hospitalization, parenteral fluids, and interruption of irradiation for 7 days. The patient commenced high-dose methotrexate therapy 14 days after completion of irradiation without unusual toxicity. She is now maintained on a 28-day cycle

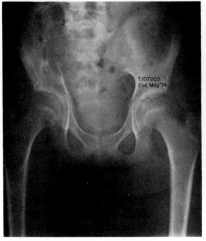 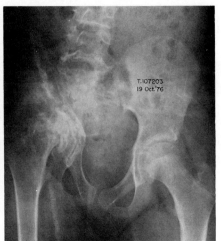

Fig. 5 (left).—Case 1. Two months after completion of irradiation, gross collapse of bone has occurred at the primary tumor site.

Fig. 6 (right).—Case 1. Thirty-five months after diagnosis, additional gross degenerative changes may be seen.

with methotrexate, 250 mg/kg, on day 1 and Adriamycin, 60–75 mg/m², on day 8. She continues in complete remission 6+ months from diagnosis.

Primary Tumor Control

Radiation, Adriamycin, and methotrexate together appear more effective than radiation alone in control of the primary tumor. In the only 2 patients treated in this manner, complete remission has been achieved for 6+ and 33+ months. This compares with our former experience of complete remission of 3–6 months duration in 3 of 27 patients less than 30 years of age and complete remission in 4 of 9 patients older than 30 years with a duration of 6, 6, 15, and 18 months, using radiation alone.

It may be anticipated that the radiation dose-response curve for tumor control will be favorably modified by concurrent exposure to effective systemic agents. Analogy may be made with tumor control by radiation and MOPP in Hodgkin's disease; radiation and Adriamycin, cyclophosphamide, vincristine, and actinomycin D in embryonal rhabdomyosarcoma; and radiation, actinomycin D, and vincristine in Wilms' tumor. In none of these circumstances is the shape of the dose-response curve for combined treatment established, although a change favoring increased tumor control for a given radiation dose may well exist. A current important question in the treatment of osteosarcoma is, therefore: Does combined treatment with radiation, Adriamycin, and methotrexate offer any reasonable chance for eradication of the tumor at the primary site? Observation of quite a small number of unresected primary tumors will provide an answer, due to the previous very poor results with irradiation alone. A definite positive answer in this restricted group is required before this treatment can be properly explored as a medical alternative for the peripheral primary.

Combined Modality Toxicity

In Case 1, degenerative change in the irradiated bone has been excessive and greater than might be expected with 6,000 rads alone. This can be explained only in part by the direct and delayed consequences

Fig. 7. – Sequencing of administration of radiation (RT), Adriamycin (A), and methotrexate (MTX) in the treatment of primary unresected osteosarcoma for 2 current cooperative clinical trials: **A,** C C G – 741, **B,** N C I (Canada).

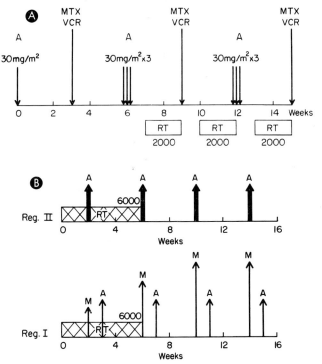

of collapse of that part of the bone initially destroyed by osteosarcoma. Moderate to marked subcutaneous fibrosis is also present in irradiated skin. Augmentation of the late effects of irradiation by Adriamycin and/or methotrexate is, as yet, a poorly defined area of toxicity. Because of this complication, the tumor dose was reduced to 5,000 rads in the second patient. No acute toxicity was seen in Case 1 when Adriamycin was commenced 2 weeks after 6,000 rads to a wide pelvic field, whereas in Case 2, acute enteritis occurred when Adriamycin 75 mg/m² was given concurrently with radiation at 4,200 rads tumor dose. Only mild-to-moderate erythemia was seen in the irradiated skin without moist desquamation.

Optimal timing of administration of radiation, Adriamycin, and methotrexate is not known, but may be expected to be determined by the degree of acute combined treatment toxicity (Cassady, Richter, Piro, and Jaffe, 1975; Phillips and Fu, 1976; Tefft et al., 1976). The sequencing utilized in 2 cooperative group protocols, from the Children's Cancer Study Group (CCG-741) and the National Cancer Institute of Canada, is illustrated in Figure 7.

Radiation Modulators

METRONIDAZOLE

The patient in Case 1 received metronidazole (flagyl) 1–2 gm prior to each radiation treatment during establishment of tolerance to and pharmacokinetics of this drug, which at that time was known to be (in the laboratory, both in vitro and in vivo) an hypoxic cell sensitizer to irradiation (Adams, Dische, Fowler, and Thomlinson, 1976). Subsequently, this agent was shown, in addition, to be selectively toxic to hypoxic cells (Sutherland, 1974; Mohindra and Rauth, 1976). The serum levels, up to 0.5 mM, obtained in this patient would be low to obtain hypoxic cell sensitization. At present there is only weak evidence that metronidazole is of value in clinical practice (Urtasun et al., 1976). Its use in this patient is not evaluable.

HYPOXIC IRRADIATION

To eliminate the differential in radiosensitivity between hypoxic and well-oxygenated cells in a limb tumor, all tissues may be made equally hypoxic by tourniquet isolation of the limb, and the radiation dose may be appropriately increased. This technique has been evaluated in osteosarcoma (Suit, 1963; Jenkin, Allt, and Fitzpatrick, 1972);

however, the results have not improved upon classically delivered radiation, and the technique has been abandoned.

RADIOSENSITIZERS

Local control of the primary tumor has been reported in 3 children treated by combined intraarterial 5′ bromodeoxyuridine infusion and high-dose-per-fraction (600 rads) megavoltage irradiation (Goffinet *et al.*, 1975). Large dose fractions were chosen in the hope of overcoming the unusually broad shoulder seen, in vitro, in cell survival curves due, at least in part, to efficient repair of radiation damage in human osteosarcoma cells (Weichselbaum and Little, 1976). Systemic therapy with methotrexate, Adriamycin, cyclophosphamide, and vincristine was added.

Subsequent data indicated that 6 of 7 patients achieved local control. However, the initial dose of eight 600-rad fractions produced excessive soft tissue damage. It is noteworthy that it was possible to give high-dose methotrexate concurrently with irradiation (Donaldson, personal communication).

Elective Lung Irradiation

Prior to the development of effective systemic treatment, elective whole lung irradiation was undertaken at a number of institutions in the hope of eradicating pulmonary metastases when the foci were undetectable and the total tumor cell number small. The results were difficult to evaluate. Recently, 2 prospective randomized clinical trials have been undertaken to settle the point. At the Mayo Clinic, 53 patients without clinical evidence of pulmonary metastases after resection of the primary tumor were randomized to receive whole lung irradiation (1,500 rads ^{60}Co in 14 days) or no further treatment. All were less than 40 years of age. Parosteal osteosarcoma and tumors occuring in Paget's disease or in the jaw were excluded. No difference was found in the subsequent incidence of pulmonary metastases (Fig. 8) (Rab *et al.*, 1976).

A dissimilar result has emerged from an E.O.R.T.C. (European Organization for the Treatment of Cancer) prospective randomized cooperative clinical trial. Elective whole lung irradiation (1,750 rads in 10 fractions in 12 days with megavoltage irradiation) was compared with no additional treatment in patients with osteosarcoma of the extremities after treatment of the primary tumor by resection or irradiation. Patients were less than 50 years old. At present, with 82 patients

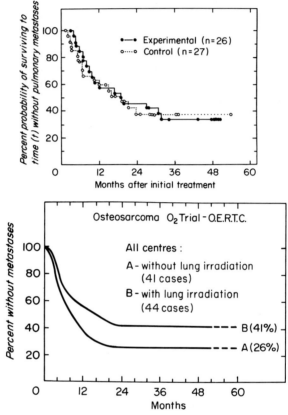

Fig. 8 (top).—Results of the Mayo Clinic trial of adjuvant lung irradiation in osteosarcoma. Patients in the experimental group received 1,500 rads whole lung irradiation in 14 days. (Courtesy of Rab *et al.*, 1976.)

Fig. 9 (bottom).—The overall interim results of the E.O.R.T.C. trial of adjuvant lung irradiation in osteosarcoma. (Courtesy of Breuer, in press.)

in the trial and after 4 years of follow-up, 41% of the electively irradiated patients are without metastases, compared to 26% of those with no further treatment (P = 0.08). This is illustrated graphically in Figure 9 (Breur and Cohen, 1975; Breur *et al.*, in press).

Since these results conflict, it seems necessary to conclude that the value of adjuvant lung irradiation alone in eradicating micrometastases remains unproven, but it is possible that a small positive effect exists. In this situation, it might be best to be cautious in introducing lung irradiation into adjuvant systemic therapy until the magnitude of the effect of Adriamycin and high-dose methotrexate, combined with resection of focal deposits, is evident.

Conclusions

(1) The current treatment of choice for primary and metastatic osteosarcoma is resection.

(2) Combined treatment with radiation and systemic therapy, including at least high-dose methotrexate and Adriamycin, may increase the chance of local control of the primary tumor, compared with radiation alone. Time-dose parameters and the tolerance of concurrent or sequential radiation and systemic therapy are under active study.

(3) The value of adjuvant pulmonary irradiation remains equivocal.

REFERENCES

Adams, G. E., Dische, S., Fowler, J. F., and Thomlinson, R. H.: Hypoxic cell sensitisors in radiotherapy. Lancet, 1:186–188, January 24, 1976.

Beattie, E. J., Jr., Martini, N., and Rosen, G.: The management of pulmonary metastases in children with osteogenic sarcoma with surgical resection combined with chemotherapy. Cancer, 35:618–621, March 1975.

Beck, J. C., Wara, W. M., Bovell, E. G., and Phillips, T. L.: The role of radiation therapy in the treatment of osteosarcoma. Radiology, 120:163–165, July 1976.

Breur, K., *et al.*: Adjuvant lung irradiation in the treatment of osteosarcoma. European Journal of Cancer. (In press.)

Breur, K., and Cohen, P.: Prophylactic irradiation of the lungs in patients with osteosarcoma. Data presented at the VIIIth Meeting International Society Paediatric Oncology, Stockholm, September 1975.

Caceres, E., and Zaharia, M.: Massive preoperative radiation therapy in the treatment of osteogenic sarcoma. Cancer, 30:634–638, September 1972.

Cassady, J. R., Richter, M. P., Piro, A. J., and Jaffe, N.: Radiation-Adriamycin interactions: Preliminary clinical observations. Cancer, 36:946–949, September 1975.

Cortes, E. P., Holland, J. F., Wang, J. J., Sinks, L. F., Blom, J., Senn, H., Bank, A., and Glidewell, O.: Amputation and Adriamycin in primary osteosarcoma. The New England Journal of Medicine, 291:998–1000, November 7, 1974.

Donaldson, S. S.: Personal communication.

Friedman, M. A., and Carter, S. K.: The therapy of osteogenic sarcoma: Current status and thoughts for the future. Journal of Surgical Oncology, 4:482–510, 1972.

Goffinet, D. R., Kaplan, H. S., Donaldson, S. S., Bagshaw, M. A., and Wilbur, J. R.: Combined radiosensitizer infusion and irradiation of osteogenic sarcomas. Radiology, 117:211–214, October 1975.

Jaffe, N., Frei, E., III, Traggis, D., and Bishop, Y.: Adjuvant methotrexate and citrovorum-factor treatment of osteogenic sarcoma. The New England Journal of Medicine, 291:994–997, November 7, 1974.

Jenkin, R. D. T., Allt, W. E. C., and Fitzpatrick, P. J.: Osteosarcoma: an assessment of management with particular reference to primary irradiation and selective delayed amputation. Cancer, 30:393–400, August 1972.

Martini, N., Huvos, A. G., Miké, V., Marcove, R. C., and Beattie, E. J., Jr.:

Multiple pulmonary resections in the treatment of osteogenic sarcoma. Annals of Thoracic Surgery, 12:271–297, September 1971.

Mohindra, J. K., and Rauth, A. M.: Increased cell killing by metronidazole and nitrofurazone of hypoxic compared to aerobic mammalian cells. Cancer Research, 36:930–936, March 1976.

Phillips, T. L., and Fu, K. K.: Quantification of combined radiation therapy and chemotherapy effects on critical normal tissues. Cancer, 37 (Suppl.): 1186–1200, February 1976.

Rab, G. T., Ivins, J. C., Childs, D. S., Jr., Cupps, R. E., and Pritchard, D. J.: Elective whole lung irradiation in the treatment of osteogenic sarcoma. Cancer, 38:939–942, August 1976.

Suit, H. D.: Radiation therapy given under conditions of local tissue hypoxia for bone and soft tissue sarcoma. In *Tumors of Bone and Soft Tissue* (The University of Texas M. D. Anderson Hospital and Tumor Institute, 8th Annual Clinical Conference on Cancer). Chicago, Illinois, Year Book Medical Publishers, Inc., 1963, pp. 143–169.

Sutherland, R. M.: Selective chemotherapy of noncycling cells in an in vitro tumor model. Cancer Research, 34:3501–3503, December 1974.

Tefft, M., Lattin, P. B., Jereb, B., Cham, W., et al.: Acute and late effects on normal tissues following combined chemo- and radiotherapy for childhood rhabdomyosarcoma and Ewing's sarcoma. Cancer, 37 (Suppl.): 1201–1217, February 1976.

Urtasun, R., Band, P., Chapman, J. D., Feldstein, M. L., Meilke, B., and Fryer, C.: Radiation and high-dose metronidazole in supratentorial glioblastomas. The New England Journal of Medicine, 294:1364–1367, June 17, 1976.

Weichselbaum, R. R., and Little, J. B.: Efficient repair of radiation damage in human osteosarcoma cells. (Abstract) Proceedings of the American Association for Cancer Research, 17:17, March 1976.

Chemotherapy in the Management of Osteosarcoma

WATARU W. SUTOW, M.D.

Department of Pediatrics, The University of Texas
System Cancer Center M. D. Anderson Hospital
and Tumor Institute, Houston, Texas

OSTEOSARCOMA is a malignant bone tumor of considerable importance to the pediatric oncologist. The age distribution of the tumor shows a peak incidence during the second decade of life, in individuals from 10 to 20 years of age, when approximately 80% of all cases are seen (Uribe-Botero, Russell, Sutow, and Martin, 1976).

It had been presumed, with good clinical evidence, that osteosarcoma was unresponsive to drugs (Friedman and Carter, 1972; Livingston and Carter, 1970; Sutow, 1975a,b; Sutow *et al.*, 1971). Regardless of treatment modality used, the long-term survival rate had remained at less than 20% (Friedman and Carter, 1972). In the past 6 years, however, the development of effective chemotherapy has brought about exciting and dramatic changes in the concepts of treatment of osteosarcoma.

This review will outline briefly the adjuvant chemotherapy programs that have been investigated since 1962 by the Department of Pediatrics at M. D. Anderson Hospital. In particular, the basic principles incorporated in the various regimens and the evolution of the guidelines for the strategy of therapy will be examined. Several of these regimens have been utilized as Southwest Oncology Group studies.

In 1962, significant regression of large pulmonary metastases in a 12-year-old girl was noted following treatment with phenylalanine mustard (PAM). Following 2 subsequent thoracotomies, the patient is

163

living without evidence of disease, 15 years later (Sullivan, Sutow, and Taylor, 1963).

The prerequisites for adjuvant chemotherapy in osteosarcoma established at that time are still being observed: (a) surgical extirpation of the primary lesion (amputation) is considered necessary, and (b) the patient must be free of demonstrable metastases (Sutow, 1975a,b).

PAM was utilized as single-agent adjuvant chemotherapy following

Fig. 1.—Disease-free survival curves in osteosarcoma with adjuvant chemotherapy. PAM series received phenylalanine mustard (PAM) as single-drug therapy. VAC-pulse series represent those treated with vincristine, actinomycin D, and cyclophosphamide pulses. The surviving patients are still living with no evidence of disease more than 8 years from diagnosis. The comparison series included children with osteosarcoma treated without adjuvant chemotherapy. (Courtesy of Sutow, Sullivan, Wilbur, and Cangir, 1975.)

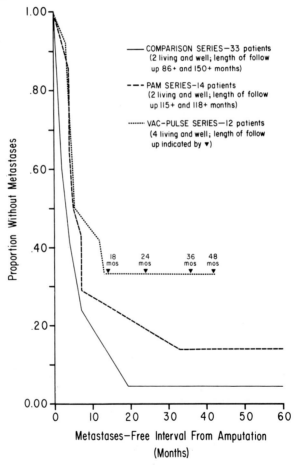

amputation in 14 children with osteosarcoma; only 2 had survived (now more than 10 years); this resulted in a control rate of 14% that was no different from published results (Sutow, Sullivan, Wilbur, and Cangir, 1975) (Fig. 1).

By 1966, the 3-drug combination of vincristine, actinomycin D, and cyclophosphamide (VAC regimen) was found to be significantly effective in children with rhabdomyosarcoma (Sutow, 1969). As a result, the combination was modified and utilized as adjuvant chemotherapy for children with osteosarcoma (Sutow, Sullivan, Wilbur, and Cangir, 1975). Following 3 pulses of cyclophosphamide, intermittent VAC pulses were continued over a 54-week period. Of 12 patients treated, 4 (33%) survive with no evidence of disease (Fig. 1).

When the effectiveness of Adriamycin in patients with osteosarcoma was established (Gottlieb *et al.*, 1972; Cortes, Holland, Wang, and Glidewell, 1972), Adriamycin was added to the VAC combination. Actinomycin D was omitted and PAM was substituted. This resulted in the regimen acronymically designated as CONPADRI-I (Sutow, 1975a) (Fig. 2). The drugs were given intermittently in several combinations, with the entire course extending over a 72-week period. The total cumulative dose of Adriamycin was 390 mg/M².

Of the 43 patients treated with CONPADRI-I thus far, 22 (51%) remain disease-free (Sutow *et al.*, 1976). These patients have been observed from 22 to 72 months, with a median of 45 months. Of the first 18 patients treated, 10 are surviving with no evidence of tumor now, 4 to 6 years from time of diagnosis (Fig. 3).

Djerassi and colleagues first developed, in 1967, the technique of

Fig. 2.—Schematic representation of CONPADRI-I regimen for adjuvant chemotherapy in osteosarcoma. CYT = cyclophosphamide, 10 mg/kg daily × 7 per course. VCR = vincristine, 0.05 mg/kg. ADR = Adriamycin, 1.5 mg/kg/dose *(heavy arrow)* and 1.0 mg/kg/dose *(thin arrow)*. PAM = phenylalanine mustard, 0.3 mg/kg/dose.

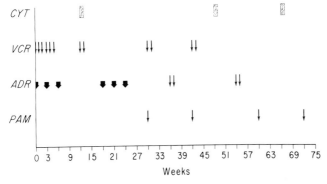

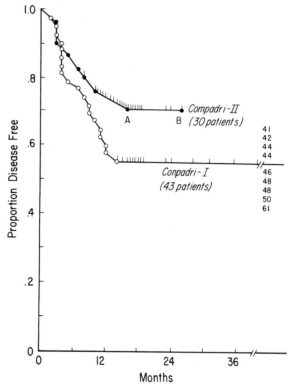

Fig. 3.—Disease-free survival curves from CONPADRI-I and COMPADRI-II adjuvant chemotherapy regimens in osteosarcoma. Each vertical bar represents a living patient. The bank of numbers at right of graphs indicates duration of follow-up studies (in months) for the 9 patients beyond 40 months. A and B indicate 2 patients who developed late metastases after 16 months from time of diagnosis. (Courtesy of Sutow, *et al.*, 1976.)

administering methotrexate in massive doses in conjunction with "leukovorin rescue" (Djerassi, Farber, Abir, and Neikirk, 1967; Djerassi, 1975). Later, this regimen was utilized in patients with metastatic osteosarcoma, and significant responses were reported (Jaffe *et al.*, 1973). The administration of massive doses of methotrexate requires considerable expertise and experience (Djerassi, 1975) as well as adequate facilities for monitoring and treating drug-related problems (Proceedings of the High Dose Methotrexate Meeting, 1975).

The CONPADRI-I regimen has been modified to include administration of methotrexate courses (COMPADRI-II and COMPADRI-III) (Fig. 4). The first 30 patients treated with the COMPADRI-II regimen

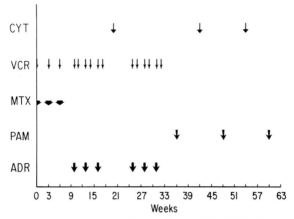

Fig. 4.—Schematic representation of multidrug COMPADRI-III regimen. CYT = cyclophosphamide, 10 mg/kg/day × 5. VCR = vincristine, 0.05 mg/kg/dose. MTX = methotrexate, 75 mg/M² (first pulse), 100 mg/M² (second pulse), and 150 mg/M² (third pulse). PAM = phenylalanine mustard, 0.3 mg/kg/dose. ADR = Adriamycin 60 mg/M² per pulse.

showed control rates during the first 18 months that were comparable or superior to those achieved by CONPADRI-I (Fig. 3). However, it was noted that among 19 patients who had been observed for more than 18 months, 4 had developed late metastases (Sutow, 1976). COMPADRI-III represents intensification of methotrexate and Adriamycin doses (Fig. 4).

All over the country, 3 general types of adjuvant chemotherapy regimens are being investigated in different medical centers (Handelsman and Carter, 1975). The regimens include: (1) the administration of Adriamycin as a single agent (Cortes *et al.*, 1974; Cortes *et al.*, 1975); (2) the use of high-dose methotrexate with leukovorin (Jaffe, Frei, III, Traggis, and Bishop, 1974; Jaffe, 1975); and (3) the use of multidrug chemotherapy regimens (Sutow *et al.*, 1976; Rosen, 1975; Wilbur *et al.*, 1975; Pratt, Hustu, and Shanks, 1974; Rosen *et al.*, 1974).

The clinical experience up to this time does not justify the selection of any 1 program as being the best. Table 1 indicates the number of patients being treated by various regimens and the projected disease-free rate at 18 months. In many studies, the follow-up observation periods are relatively short, and the question of late metastases remains (Burchenal, 1974). The optimum dosages, combinations, and schedules of drug administration continue under investigation.

TABLE 1.—PROJECTED DISEASE-FREE RATES AT
18 MONTHS FOR SEVERAL CURRENT PROGRAMS OF
ADJUVANT CHEMOTHERAPY IN OSTEOSARCOMA.*

PROGRAM	NUMBER OF PATIENTS	NED AT 18 MONTHS (%)
CONPADRI-I	43	55%
COMPADRI-II	58	65%
Memorial Hospital (New York)†	60	63%
Group B	45	65%
Stanford‡	24	50%
St. Jude§	31	55%
Farber Institute (I)	12	58%
Farber Institute (II)	22	60%

*Current data were obtained by telephone contact with the principal investigator of each study.
†Rosen, 1976.
‡Wilbur, 1976.
§Pratt, 1976.
NED—No evidence of disease.

Summary

Chemotherapy of several types has developed into an effective component of the primary treatment program for patients with osteosarcoma. Adjuvant chemotherapy has significantly improved the disease-free survival rate for these patients. Furthermore, the strategic administration of drugs has permitted innovative surgical approaches such as the en bloc resection of the tumor with prosthetic replacement of bone and preservation of limb (Rosen *et al.*, 1976). Finally, the results of therapy in patients with metastatic disease have engendered cautious optimism about increasingly successful outcomes in the presence of extensive disease (Jaffe *et al.*, 1976; Rosen *et al.*, 1975; Beattie, Martini, and Rosen, 1975; Sutow *et al.*, 1975).

REFERENCES

Beattie, E. J., Jr., Martini, N., and Rosen, G.: The management of pulmonary metastases in children with osteogenic sarcoma with surgical resection combined with chemotherapy. Cancer, 35:618-621, March 1975.
Burchenal, J. H.: A giant step forward—if. . . . (Editorial) New England Journal of Medicine, 291:1029–1031, November 7, 1974.
Cortes, E. P., Holland, J. F., Wang, J. J., and Glidewell, O.: Adriamycin (NSC-123127) in 87 patients with osteosarcoma. Cancer Chemotherapy Reports, (Part 3) 6:305–313, October 1975.
Cortes, E. P., Holland, J. F., Wang, J. J., and Sinks, L. F.: Doxorubicin in disseminated osteosarcoma. Journal of the American Medical Association, 221: 1132–1138, September 4, 1972.

Cortes, E. P., Holland, J. F., Wang, J. J., Sinks, L. F., Bloom, J., Senn, H., Bank, A., and Glidewell, O.: Amputation and Adriamycin in primary osteosarcoma. New England Journal of Medicine, 291:998–1000, November 7, 1974.

Djerassi, I.: High-dose methotrexate (NSC-740) and citrovorum factor (NSC-3590) rescue: background and rationale. Cancer Chemotherapy Reports, (Part 3) 6:3–6, July 1975.

Djerassi, I., Farber, S., Abir, E., and Neikirk, W.: Continuous infusion of methotrexate in children with acute leukemia. Cancer, 20:233–242, February 1967.

Friedman, M. A., and Carter, S. K.: The therapy of osteogenic sarcoma: current status and thoughts for the future. Journal of Surgical Oncology, 4: 482–510, October 1972.

Gottlieb, J. A., Baker, L. H., Quagliana, J. M., Luce, J. K., Whitecar, J. P., Jr., Sinkovics, J. G., Rivkin, S. E., Brownlee, R., and Frei, E., III: Chemotherapy of sarcomas with a combination of Adriamycin and dimethyl triazeno imidazole carboxamide. Cancer, 30:1632–1638, December 1972.

Handelsman, H., and Carter, S. K.: Current therapies in osteosarcoma. Cancer Treatment Reviews, 2:77–83, 1975.

Jaffe, N.: The potential of combined modality approaches for the treatment of malignant bone tumors in children. Cancer Treatment Reviews, 2:33–53, 1975.

Jaffe, N., Farber, S., Traggis, D., Geiser, C., Kim, B. S., Das, L., Frauenberger, G., Djerassi, I., and Cassady, J. R.: Favorable response of metastatic osteogenic sarcoma to pulse high-dose methotrexate with citrovorum rescue and radiation therapy. Cancer, 31:1367–1373, June 1973.

Jaffe, N., Traggis, D., Cassady, J. R., Filler, R. M., Watts, H., and Frei, E.: Multidisciplinary treatment for macrometastatic osteogenic sarcoma. British Medical Journal, 2:1039–1041, Ocotober 30, 1976.

Jaffe, N., Frei, E., III, Traggis, D., and Bishop, Y.: Adjuvant methotrexate and citrovorum-factor treatment of osteogenic sarcoma. New England Journal of Medicine, 291:994–997, November 7, 1974.

Livingston, R. B., and Carter, S. K.: Single agents in cancer chemotherapy. New York, New York–Washington, D.C.–London, England, IFI/Plenum, 1970, 405 pp.

Pratt, C. B., Hustu, H. O., and Shanks, E.: Cyclic multiple drug adjuvant chemotherapy for osteosarcoma. (Abstract) Proceedings of the American Association for Cancer Research, 15:19, March 1974.

Pratt, C. B.: Personal communication. September 1976.

Proceedings of the High Dose Methotrexate Meeting, December 19, 1974. Cancer Chemotherapy Reports, (Part 3) 6:1–82, July 1975.

Rosen, G.: The development of an adjuvant chemotherapy program for the treatment of osteogenic sarcoma. Frontiers of Radiation Therapy and Oncology, 10:115–133, 1975.

Rosen, G.: Personal communication. September 1976.

Rosen, G., Murphy, M. L., Huvos, A. G., Gutierrez, M., and Marcove, R. C.: Chemotherapy, en bloc resection, and prosthetic bone replacement in the treatment of osteogenic sarcoma. Cancer, 37:1–11, January 1976.

Rosen, G., Suwansirikul, S., Kwon, C., Tan, C., Wu, S. J., Beattie, E. J., Jr., and Murphy, M. L.: High-dose methotrexate with citrovorum factor rescue and

Adriamycin in childhood osteogenic sarcoma. Cancer, 33:1151–1163, April 1974.

Rosen, G., Tefft, M., Martinez, A., Cham, W., and Murphy, M. L.: Combination chemotherapy and radiation therapy in the treatment of metastatic osteogenic sarcoma. Cancer, 35:622–630, March 1975.

Sullivan, M. P., Sutow, W. W., and Taylor, G.: L-phenylalanine mustard as a treatment for metastatic osteogenic sarcoma in children. Journal of Pediatrics, 63:227–237, August 1963.

Sutow, W. W.: Chemotherapeutic management of childhood rhabdomyosarcoma. In Neoplasia in Childhood (The University of Texas M. D. Anderson Hospital and Tumor Institute at Houston, 12th Annual Clinical Conference on Cancer). Chicago, Illinois, Year Book Medical Publishers, Inc., 1969, pp. 201–208.

Sutow, W. W.: Combination chemotherapy with adriamycin (NSC-123127) in primary treatment of osteogenic sarcoma. Cancer Chemotherapy Reports, (Part 3) 6:315–317, October 1975a.

Sutow, W. W.: Inferences and projections regarding current clinical capabilities for the control of osteogenic sarcoma. Progress in Clinical and Biological Research, 4:297–307, 1975b.

Sutow, W. W.: Late metastases in osteosarcoma. (Letter) Lancet, 1:856, April 17,1976.

Sutow, W. W., Fernandez, C. H., Mountain, C. F., King, O. Y., Rivera, R. L., and Mumford, D. M.: Multimodal treatment of pulmonary metastases in osteogenic sarcoma. (Abstract) Proceedings of the American Association for Cancer Research, 16:39, 1975.

Sutow, W. W., Gehan, E. A., Vietti, T. J., Frias, A. E., and Dyment, P. G.: Multidrug chemotherapy in primary treatment of osteosarcoma. Journal of Bone and Joint Surgery, 58A:629–633, July 1976.

Sutow, W. W., Sullivan, M. P., Wilbur, J. R., and Cangir, A.: Study of adjuvant chemotherapy in osteogenic sarcoma. Journal of Clinical Pharmacology, 15: 530–533, July 1975.

Sutow, W. W., Vietti, T. J., Fernbach, D. J., Lane, D. M., Donaldson, M. H., and Lonsdale, D.: Evaluation of chemotherapy in children with metastatic Ewing's sarcoma and osteogenic sarcoma. Cancer Chemotherapy Reports, 55:67–78, February 1971.

Uribe-Botero, G., Russell, W. O., Sutow, W. W., and Martin, R. G.: Primary osteosarcoma of bone: A clinicopathologic investigation of 243 cases with necropsy studies in 54. American Journal of Clinical Pathology. (In press.)

Wilbur, J. R., Etcubanas, E., Long, T., Glatstein, E., and Leavitt, T.: Four drug therapy and irradiation in primary and metastatic osteogenic sarcoma. (Abstract) Proceedings of the American Association of Cancer Research and American Society of Clinical Oncology, 15:188, 1975.

Wilbur, J. R.: Personal communication. November 1976.

Intramarrow Spread of Osteosarcoma

WILLIAM F. ENNEKING, M.D., and ABBOTT KAGAN, II, M.D.

W. Thaxton Springfield Center for Orthopaedic Study and Research, Department of Orthopaedic Surgery, University of Florida, Gainesville, Florida

IN 1975, WE REPORTED 10 CASES of "skip" metastases occurring in a prospective study of 40 patients with osteosarcomas of the extremities. A "skip" metastasis was defined as a solitary separate focus of osteosarcoma occurring synchronously with a primary osteosarcoma in the absence of anatomic extension, pulmonary metastasis, exposure to toxic substances, or Paget's disease (Enneking and Kagan, 1975 a,b) (Fig. 1). The purpose of this report is to update that series and to comment on significance of "skip" metastasis.

From May 1972 to August 1976, an additional 24 cases of primary osteosarcoma meeting the above criteria were studied, bringing the series total to 64. The method of study included preoperative roentgenograms, lung and lesion tomograms, bone scans, angiography, dissection, and microscopic review of histologic macrosections. This method has been previously detailed (Enneking and Kagan, 1975 a, b). The present series of "skip" metastases consists of 12 lesions in 64 patients, an incidence of 19%.

Discussion

The age of incidence and the site of primary osteosarcomas associated with "skip" lesions are similar to those published for the series of osteosarcomas. The age range was from 7 to 66, with an average age of

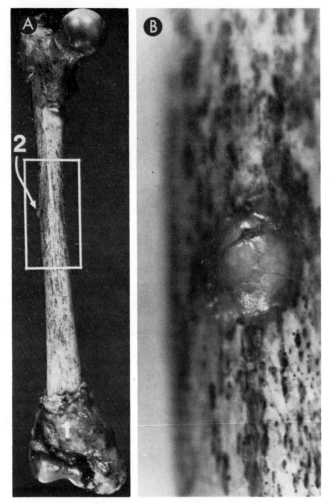

Fig. 1.—Example of an intracortical skip metastasis: **A**, the femur following dissection. (1) the primary tumor, (2) the skip metastasis. **B**, close-up of the skip metastasis. (Courtesy of Enneking and Kagan, 1975b.)

20; there was a peak incidence in the second decade of life. The site of incidence was the distal femur in 6 of 12 patients and the proximal tibia in 2 of 12. There was 1 lesion each in the proximal femur, distal tibia, proximal humerus, and distal radius. The relevant details of the 12 cases are shown in Table 1.

The preoperative diagnosis of skip metastasis is difficult. Only 3 of 12 lesions were evident on initial X-ray examinations or polytomograms; 2 of these were bone-producing lesions and 1 was a destructive lesion. Bone scanning with ^{99m}Tc polyphosphate was of no benefit in the preoperative diagnosis or localization of radiologically occult skip metastasis. At the time of definitive surgery, most lesions were evident on gross examination of the cut specimen (9 of 12) or with tetracycline labeling and examination of the tissue with ultraviolet light. However, in 3 of 12 cases, the skip lesions were only seen on histologic examination of macrosections. Clearly, preoperative studies in an attempt to define skip metastases are beneficial only when they are positive. The rate of false-negatives is high (9 of 12) (Fig. 2).

Fig. 2.—Example of a skip metastasis which was not evident on plain X-ray film, ^{99m}Tc polyphosphate bone scan, or tomograms. **A,** shows the lateral X-ray film. (1) the proximal extent of the primary lesion. (2) the region of the skip. The X-ray film is normal. On the macrosection, **B,** the proximal extent of the tumor (1) is seen with no evidence of extension to the region of the 1 cm diameter skip lesion (2). (Hematoxalin and eosin, × 3.) (Courtesy of Enneking and Kagan, 1975b.)

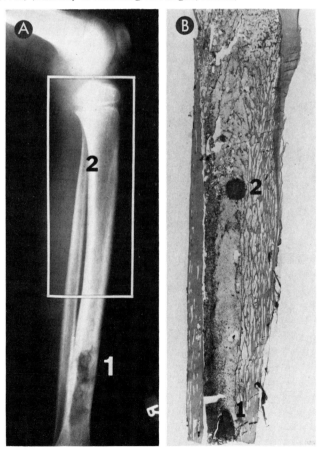

The clinical behavior of skip metastasis is variable. The route of metastasis may be either intraosseous, involving the same bone (6 of 12), or transarticular, involving an adjacent bone (6 of 12). Further, the "skip" may occur proximal (8 of 12) or distal (4 of 12) to the primary osteosarcoma.

Study of the course of patients with skip metastases reveals 6 patients with local recurrence following ablation proximal to the site of the skip lesion. Three of these had had adoptive immunotherapy, 1 had radiation therapy, 1 had chemotherapy, and 1 had no adjunctive therapy. This rate is considerably higher than the 15% recurrence rate which would be expected according to a large published series of osteosarcomas (McKenna, Schwinn, Soong, Higinbotham, 1966). All but 1 patient in the series are known to have developed pulmonary metastases; the mean interval to metastasis was 6 months.

TABLE 1.—CLINICAL DETAILS OF PATIENTS

CASE	PATIENT	AGE	SEX	SITE OF PRIMARY	"SKIP" CHARACTERISTICS	ROUTE
1	RB	18	M	proximal femur	5 cm. extraosseus intrapelvic	transarticular
2	SG	8	M	distal tibia	1 cm. central proximal tibial metaphasis	intraosseus
3	JC	7	M	distal femur	2 cm. proximal tibial epiphysis	transarticular
4	RR	15	M	proximal tibia	2.5 cm. cortical distal femoral metaphysis	transarticular
5	AT	35	F	distal femur	1 cm. cortical proximal femoral diaphysis	intraosseus
6	BH	24	M	proximal humerus	1 cm. central distal humeral metaphysis	intraosseus
7	RK	13	F	distal radius	0.6 cm. central proximal radial metaphysis	intraosseus
8	MB	66	F	proximal tibia	1 cm. central distal femoral metaphysis	transarticular
9	CH	20	M	distal femur	4 cm. central proximal tibial metaphysis	transarticular
10	GP	10	F	distal femur	0.5 cm. central proximal femoral metaphysis	intraosseus
11	AD	19	F	distal femur	1 cm. proximal tibial epiphysis	transarticular
12	MR	14	M	distal femur	1–2 cm. multiple nodules prox. femur, ilium	transarticular & intraosseus

(Adapted from Enneking and Kagan, 1975b.)

Additionally, the mean survival of this group of patients was 13 months, with 2 patients alive at 52 and 84 months postsurgery. Since different modes of therapy were employed (e.g., radiation therapy, chemotherapy, immunotherapy), statistical comparison of these figures with other published series is not possible. A more accurate representation of the clinical course of the patients with skip metastases is the disease-free interval (Fig. 3). The mean disease-free interval for these patients was 6 months, whereas for classical osteosarcoma it was 15 months. Moreover, no patient was free of disease at 2 years.

The obvious surgical implication of skip metastasis is that residual tumor is the source of stump recurrence. Clinically, this is supported by the 15% overall recurrence rate of osteosarcoma following ablation, both through the involved bone and via disarticulation above the proximal joint, a figure similar to the incidence of skip lesions (McKenna, Schwinn, Soong, Higinbotham, 1969). On the empirical

WITH SKIP METASTASES

TREATMENT	RECURRENCE	DISTANT METASTASES	SURVIVAL
hemipelvectomy	ilium — 12 mo.	lungs — 4 mo.	died — 12 mo.
above knee amputation	none — 21 mo.	lungs — 20 mo.	died — 34 mo.
irradiation 4300 R. 12 mo. later hip disarticulation	pelvis — 12 mo.	none — 12 mo.	alive — 84 mo.
above knee amputation	pelvis — 17 mo.	lungs — 17 mo.	died — 24 mo.
hip disarticulation	none — 4 mo.	lungs — 1 mo.	died — 4 mo.
regional excision followed by fore-quarter amputation	resection — 5 mo. site	widespread — 3 mo. skeletal lungs	died — 16 mo.
above elbow amputation	proximal — 4 mo. humerus	widespread — 2 mo. skeletal lungs	died — 4 mo.
hip disarticulation	none — 4 mo.	lungs — 1 mo.	died — 4 mo.
above knee amputation	none — 1 mo.	none — 1 mo.	alive — 52 mo.
hip disarticulation	none — 1 mo.	none — 1 mo.	died — 18 mo.
hip disarticulation	none — 13 mo.	lung — 4 mo.	died — 13 mo.
hemi-pelvectomy	sacrum — residual	lung — 2 mo.	died — 2 mo.

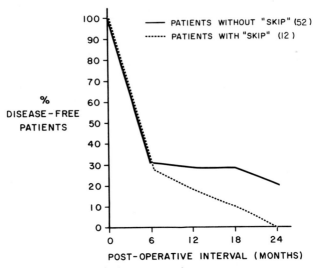

Fig. 3.—Disease-free interval of patients with osteosarcoma. No patient with a skip metastasis was free of disease at 2 years.

basis that there were no recurrences following disarticulation proximal to the tumor, compared to a 30% recurrence rate for through-bone amputation, Sweetnam (1973) recommended hip disarticulation for distal femoral osteosarcomas. The converse of this approach is to risk skip metastasis (20%) and perform the most distal ablation possible to preserve better function. Whether this risk is justifiable is speculative; at present, the role of adjunctive chemotherapy in suppressing residual micrometastasis is unknown, and offers an area for further investigation.

Summary

This report updates our experience with "skip" metastases to August, 1976. Sixty-four cases of osteosarcomas of the extremities have been prospectively studied, and a 19% incidence of skip metastasis noted. Preoperative diagnosis of skip metastasis is difficult, with a high percentage of false-negative studies. Intramarrow spread of osteosarcoma appears to be consistent with the behavior of a certain number of "classical" osteosarcomas, and is associated with a high recurrence rate, short interval to pulmonary metastasis, and early death of the patient. Patients with known "skip" metastasis constitute a significant variable and should not be included in prospective clinical therapeutic trials.

REFERENCES

Enneking, W. F., and Kagan, A.: The implication of "skip" metastasis in osteosarcoma. Clinical Orthopaedics and Related Research, 111:33–41, September 1975a.

Enneking, W. F., and Kagan, A.: "Skip" metastasis in osteosarcoma. Cancer, 36:2192–2205, December 1975b.

McKenna, R. J., Schwinn, C. P., Soong, K. Y., and Higinbotham, N. L.: Sarcomata of the osteogenic series (osteosarcoma, fibrosarcoma, chondrosarcoma, parosteal osteogenic sarcoma, and sarcomata arising in abnormal bone)—An analysis of 552 cases. Journal of Bone and Joint Surgery, 48A: 1–26, January 1966.

Sweetnam, R.: Amputation in osteosarcoma. Disarticulation of the hip or high thigh amputation for lower femoral growth. Journal of Bone and Joint Surgery, 55B:189–192, February 1973.

Ewing's Sarcoma: An Ultrastructural Study

ALBERTO G. AYALA, M.D., and BRUCE MACKAY,
M.D., Ph.D.

Department of Pathology,
The University of Texas System Cancer Center
M. D. Anderson Hospital and Tumor Institute,
Houston, Texas

SINCE THE ORIGINAL REPORT by James Ewing in 1921, Ewing's sarcoma has been accepted as a distinct clinicopathological entity. It is generally defined as a primary malignant neoplasm of bone composed of round or oval cells, compactly grouped with little intercellular connective tissue. Diagnosis of the primary bone lesion is usually not difficult, particularly when the histology is correlated with the clinical presentation and radiologic picture; however, confusion may occur with primary lymphoma of bone and, on occasion, with metastatic small cell tumors. Recognition of Ewing's sarcoma can be considerably more difficult when the tumor presents in a metastatic location, and other round cell tumors such as rhabdomyosarcoma or neuroblastoma are of significance in the differential diagnosis (Friedman and Hanaoka, 1971). The diagnostic problem is compounded by the possibility that an extraskeletal neoplasm simulating Ewing's sarcoma (Angervall and Enzinger, 1975) may arise de novo in the soft tissues.

Previous reports on the ultrastructure of Ewing's sarcoma (Friedman and Gold, 1968; Takayama and Sugawa, 1970; Hou-Jensen, Priori, and Dmochowski, 1972; Rice, Cabot, and Johnston, 1973) have not included many cases, although there is basic agreement on the fine structural features of the tumor cells. In order to consolidate these

179

previous observations and better define the ultrastructural features, we studied the fine structure of 40 well-documented cases of Ewing's sarcoma seen at M. D. Anderson Hospital since 1969.

Observations

By light microscopy, the tumors in this series conformed to the generally accepted histologic criteria for Ewing's sarcoma. The tumor cells were small, uniform, and round or oval, but rarely elongated. They were compactly grouped, and connective tissue stroma was minimal. Areas of necrosis were frequent. Occasionally, a semblance of rosette formation was encountered, but for the most part the tumors were devoid of architectural organization.

One micron section of the Epon-embedded tissue for electron microscopy was examined with the light microscope after staining with methylene blue to confirm that the tissue was representative and that preservation was acceptable. Thin sections from the selected tissue blocks were stained with lead hydroxide and uranyl acetate, and a Zeiss EM 9-S electron microscope was used for the study.

The compact arrangement of the tumor cells noted by light microscopy was evident at the ultrastructural level. Cell membranes typically possessed smooth contours, and those of adjacent cells were closely apposed (Fig. 1). Irregularities of the cell surfaces, such as indentation, infoldings, or microvillous projections, were uncommon. In most tumors, focal thickenings of apposed cell membranes could be found in occasional areas (Fig. 2), but true desmosomes with intermediate lines or tonofilaments were never seen. The cells were round or oval, and variations in size were not striking.

A single nucleus was usual, although occasional cells contained 2 nuclei. The nuclear profiles were characteristically smooth and regular; small indentations were often seen, but deep clefting was not common. A distinctive feature was the finely dispersed character of the nuclear chromatin (Figs. 1 and 3). Clumping was only seen in cells where there was a considerable admixture of degenerating cells. The nucleoli were small, but they appeared conspicuous within the background of dispersed chromatin.

The quantity of cytoplasm varied among the tumors in the series, but it was never abundant. Paucity of organelles was the rule, although groups of mitochondria were sometimes seen. Endoplasmic reticulum was invariably sparse, and most of the ribosomes were unattached. A golgi complex was never conspicuous. Cytoplasmic lipid droplets were infrequent, but most tumor cells contained glycogen.

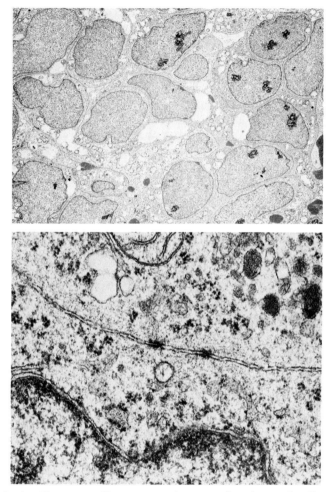

Fig. 1 (top).—The tumor cells are compactly arranged, with smooth cell and nuclear membrane contours. One or 2 nucleoli are present, and the chromatin is finely dispersed. Cytoplasmic glycogen is noted as electron lucent areas. (×4,300)

Fig. 2 (bottom).—This close-up view demonstrates a portion of 2 adjacent cells. The cell membranes display small focal thickenings. (×24,000)

The amount varied, and in many tumors all the cells were occupied by extensive lakes of cytoplasmic glycogen (Fig. 4), compressing the other constituents into small areas. It was equally common, however, to find tumors in which glycogen was only visible in some of the cells of a particular section (Fig. 1). In these situations, the glycogen was typically aggregated into discrete pools. Glycogen was absent only in

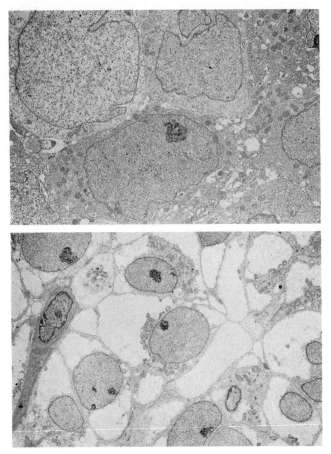

Fig. 3 (top).—Note the evenly distributed fine chromatin. The nuclear contour appears smooth and round with an occasional cleft. (×6,200)

Fig. 4 (bottom).—The cytoplasm contains large amounts of glycogen which appears as extensive electron lucent pools. The organelles are compressed into small groups. (×4,300).

the tumors of 2 patients who had received therapy prior to tissue becoming available for electron microscopy.

Discussion

Precision in the diagnosis of Ewing's sarcoma of bone is important in evaluating prognosis and selecting therapy. The outlook for a patient with a primary reticuloendothelial neoplasm of bone is considerably better (Boston, Dahlin, Ivins, and Cupps, 1974) than it is for the patient with Ewing's sarcoma. It is probable that most cases of Ewing's sarcoma of bone can be accurately diagnosed when adequate tissue is available from the primary lesion. It may be difficult or impossible to diagnose when the only available material is an artefactually distorted or extensively necrotic biopsy specimen. Provision of adequate material is essential for a valid assessment of the ultrastructural features of the tumor cells. One of the virtues of electron microscopy is the small quantity of tissue that is required for ultrastructural evaluation, permitting diagnosis from needle biopsies or aspiration procedures.

The findings from the present study support a number of conclusions reached by previous investigators, notably the presence of cytoplasmic glycogen (Friedman and Gold, 1968) emphasized by Schajowicz (1959). Cells in all the tumors we studied, with the exception of 2 previously treated cases, contained cytoplasmic glycogen, and it was frequently present in copious quantities within the cytoplasm. The ultrastructural features of the nucleus of a Ewing's sarcoma cell are also distinctive. The chromatin is typically fine and evenly distributed, and the 1 or more small nucleoli are, therefore, clearly visible. Where we encountered clumping of chromatin, the nuclei were often irregular in shape, and other degenerative phenomena were also present. The significance of the focal thickenings of apposed cell membranes is difficult to evaluate. Poorly defined desmosomes in undifferentiated neoplasms can present a similar appearance, although we have not seen true desmosomes in an established case of Ewing's sarcoma. These small membrane densities can be helpful in differentiating Ewing's sarcoma from a reticuloendothelial lesion, but failure to demonstrate their presence does not contraindicate the diagnosis. Confusion between Ewing's sarcoma and a primary lymphoma of bone is rarely a problem where adequately preserved tissue is available for electron microscopy. Cytoplasmic glycogen and finely dispersed chromatin are not characteristics of lymphoma cells (Friedman and Hanaoka, 1971).

The range of diagnostic possibilities is broader when Ewing's sarcoma presents as a metastatic focus in soft tissue, but other round cell neoplasms can usually be ruled out by electron microscopy. Neuroblastoma cells possess dendritic processes containing small membrane-bound granules, and desmosomes are frequently found between the cells and their processes (Mackay, Masse, and Butler, 1975). Probably the most difficult problem in differentiation is between Ewing's sarcoma and a round cell rhabdomyosarcoma. Both tumors contain glycogen, and while the glycogen apparently tends to be more abundant and more circumscribed in Ewing's sarcoma cells, a similar appearance and distribution may be seen in some rhabdomyosarcomas. Demonstration of skeletal muscle myofilaments can be invaluable, but they are often absent. The nuclear profile of rhabdomyosarcoma cells may be of help since it is commonly irregular and the chromatin is often clumped (Morales, Fine, and Horn, 1972 and personal communication). At the present time, it appears that there are occasional cases where it is not possible to determine whether a neoplasm is Ewing's sarcoma or a round cell rhabdomyosarcoma. It is hoped that more precise criteria will evolve as data from studied cases accrue.

Various hypotheses have been advanced to explain the histogenesis of Ewing's sarcoma, including origin from endothelial (Ewing, 1921), myelogenous (Kadin and Bensch, 1971), reticulum cells (Takayama, 1970; Friedman, 1968), or a transitional cell related to pericytes and vascular smooth muscle cells (Kojima, 1976). Our observations would not support any of these suggestions, but we are unable to offer a feasible alternative, and the histogenesis of Ewing's sarcoma remains an enigma.

Acknowledgments

The Zeiss EM 9-S electron microscope which was used for study was purchased with the aid of a generous grant from the Kelsey and Leary Foundation.

REFERENCES

Angervall, L., and Enzinger, F. M.: Extraskeletal neoplasm resembling Ewing's sarcoma. Cancer, 36:240–251, July 1975.

Boston, H. C., Jr., Dahlin, D. C., Ivins, J. C., and Cupps, R. E.: Malignant lymphoma (so called reticulum cell sarcoma) of bone. Cancer, 34:1131–1137, October 1974.

Ewing, J.: Diffuse endothelioma of bone. Proceedings of the New York Pathology Society, 21:17–24, 1921.

Friedman, B., and Gold, H.: Ultrastructure of Ewing's sarcoma of bone. Cancer, 22:307–322, August 1968.

Friedman, B., and Hanaoka, H.: Round-cell sarcomas of bone. A light and electron microscopic study. The Journal of Bone and Joint Surgery, 53(A):1118–1136, September 1971.

Hou-Jensen, K., Priori, E., and Dmochowski, L.: Studies on ultrastructure of Ewing's sarcoma of bone. Cancer, 29:280–286, February 1972.

Kadin, M. E., and Bensch, K. G.: On the origin of Ewing's tumor. Cancer, 27:257–273, February 1971.

Kojima: Cytological characterization and histogenesis of Ewing's sarcoma. Acta Pathologica Japonica, 26:167–190, 1976.

Mackay, B., Masse, S. R., King, O. Y., and Butler, J. J.: Diagnosis of neuroblastoma by electron microscopy of bone marrow aspirates. Pediatrics, 56: 1045–1049, 1975.

Morales, A. R., Fine, G., and Horn, R. C., Jr.: Rhabdomyosarcoma: An ultrastructural appraisal. Pathology Annual, 7:81–106, 1972.

————: Personal communication.

Rice, R. W., Cabot, A., and Johnston, A. D.: The application of electron microscopy to the diagnostic differentiation of Ewing's sarcoma and reticulum cell sarcoma of bone. Clinical Orthopedics, 91:174–185, 1973.

Schajowicz, F.: Ewing's sarcoma and reticulum cell sarcoma of bone. With special reference to the histochemical demonstration of glycogen as an aid to the differential diagnosis. Journal of Bone and Joint Surgery, 41A: 349–356, March 1959.

Takayama, S., and Sugawa, I.: Electron microscopy observations of Ewing's sarcoma. A case report. Acta Pathologica Japonica, 20:87–101, 1970.

Past Experiences and Future Considerations with T-2 Chemotherapy in the Treatment of Ewing's Sarcoma

GERALD ROSEN, M.D.

Associate Attending Pediatrician,
Department of Pediatrics,
Memorial Sloan-Kettering Cancer Center,
New York, New York

IN 1974, we reported on the favorable results obtained in the treatment of children with Ewing's sarcoma using 4-drug adjuvant chemotherapy in conjunction with radiation therapy delivered to the primary local tumor site (Rosen *et al.*, 1974). This study was prompted by the uniformly poor results of treating Ewing's sarcoma with therapy directed at the primary tumor only (Bhansali and Desai, 1963; Dahlin, Coventry, and Scanlon, 1961; Falk and Alpert, 1967; Phillips and Higinbotham, 1967; Wang and Schultz, 1953) which showed an approximate 10% 5-year survival following radiation therapy or surgical therapy for the primary tumor with no adjuvant chemotherapy. The rationale for selecting the 4 drugs, dactinomycin, Adriamycin, cyclophosphamide, and vincristine, was based on earlier investigations showing that these agents are of value in treating metastatic Ewing's sarcoma (Senyszyn, Johnson, and Curran, 1970; Oldham and Pomeroy; 1972; Tan *et al.*, 1972; Samuels and Howe, 1967; Haggard, 1967; Sutow and Sullivan, 1962; Sutow, 1968). At that time, other investigators were also beginning to use adjuvant chemotherapy to treat metastatic microfoci of disease presumed to be present at the time of diagnosis to eradicate, it was hoped, microscopic foci of disease in the hope of increasing the 5-year survival rate (Johnson and Humphreys, 1969; Freeman et al., 1972; Hustu, Pinkel, and Pratt, 1972; Johnson and Pomeroy, 1972). We had decided to use 4 drugs, including Adriamycin, based on the Phase I studies conducted at Memorial Sloan-Kettering Cancer Center, which had demonstrated the efficacy of Adriamycin (Tan et al., 1972) in treating advanced Ewing's sarcoma. This report concerns a 2 to 6 + year follow-up of children with Ewing's sarcoma treated with this 4-drug chemotherapy (T-2), namely, dactinomycin, Adriamycin, cyclophosphamide, and vincristine, combined with radiation therapy or surgical therapy for the treatment of the primary tumor. It will document the efficacy of this 4-drug chemotherapy in dramatically increasing the disease-free survival rate in children with Ewing's sarcoma, with attention focused on the minority of patients who failed to respond to treatment, so that guidelines for future improved therapy can be developed. In addition, the late problems of combined treatment with radiation therapy and 4-drug chemotherapy on the function and rehabilitation of children who are surviving will be discussed so that future treatment considerations will take into account the possible late side effects of this form of treatment.

Treatment Plan

The initial treatment plan called for either surgical ablation of the primary tumor or radiation therapy to a dose of 6,000–7,000 rads to the entire involved bone. This was based on the improved survival noted by Phillips and Higinbotham (1967) utilizing megavoltage radiation therapy to the entire involved bone for patients with Ewing's sarcoma. Concomitant with the start of radiation therapy, or approximately 2 weeks following surgical treatment, the patient was begun on the 4-drug protocol, starting with dactinomycin (Fig. 1). Initially, the protocol incorporated 2 courses of Adriamycin following dactinomycin (Rosen et al., 1974), and was given for a total of 8 cycles, or approximately 20 months. However, the finding that large cumulative doses of Adriamycin were capable of producing cardiomyopathy (Gilladoga et al., 1975) led us to delete 1 of the courses of Adriamycin after the first 2 cycles of T-2 chemotherapy (Fig. 1). This limited the total cumulative dose of Adriamycin to 600 mg/m². Further reductions to limit the cumulative dose of Adriamycin to 500 mg/m² were made by deleting Adriamycin in the last 2 cycles if the patients were to receive concomitant pulmonary irradiation for established metastatic disease in the chest. Further experience with the combined treatment protocol indi-

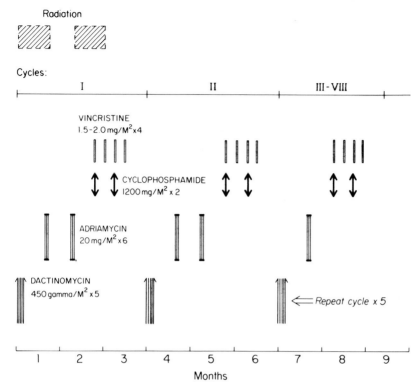

Fig. 1.—Multidiscipline protocol used for the treatment of Ewing's sarcoma (T-2). After the first 2 cycles of treatment, 1 of the two 3-day courses of Adriamycin is deleted. The total cumulative dose of Adriamycin received by patients treated with T-2 chemotherapy was further limited to 480 mg/m². However, patients treated earlier received higher doses of Adriamycin. The interval between the first day of treatment with one drug to the first day of treatment with the next drug was 2 weeks, with the exception of vincristine, which was given weekly. Treatment was continued for 8 cycles, or approximately 20 months.

cated that children receiving radiation therapy concomitantly with chemotherapy required a rest period in the radiation therapy due to severe skin erythema and soft tissue reaction at about the dose level of 3,000–4,000 rads (Tefft *et al.*, 1976). Prior to beginning treatment, all patients were discussed at a multidisciplinary conference including surgeon, radiation therapist, and pediatric oncologist. If metastatic disease was present at the time of diagnosis in solitary areas, these areas were usually irradiated as well. Radiation therapy to the lungs for metastatic pulmonary disease was given to 4 patients (whole lung irradiation to 1,400 rads in 2 patients, mediastinal irradiation to 2,100 rads for hilar disease in 1 patient, and coned-down irradiation for local disease in an additional patient). Two patients received irradiation to existing bone metastases. Radiation therapy to metastatic sites was also started concomitantly with T-2 chemotherapy.

Methods

Twenty-eight previously untreated patients with Ewing's sarcoma were treated with T-2 chemotherapy; 20 presented with primary tumor only, and 8 presented with primary tumor plus metastatic disease. Prior to the beginning of treatment, histologic sections of the biopsy material were reviewed for all patients. The clinical, roentgenographic, and histologic sections of the biopsy material were reviewed and the diagnosis confirmed by the multidisciplinary treatment team (Rosen, 1976). All patients were fully evaluated with a chest roentgenogram, skeletal survey, and ^{18}F or technetium diphosphonate bone scan, cytologic evaluation of the cerebrospinal fluid, urinary catecholamine and VMA determinations, and bone marrow examination for extrinsic cells. Treatment consisted of either surgical ablation of the involved bone or radiation therapy to the entire involved primary tumor-bearing bone to a planned dose of 6,000–7,000 rads (megavoltage). The technique of radiation therapy used has been previously described (Tefft, Chabora, and Rosen, in press). In addition, patients presenting with metastatic disease received additional radiation therapy to clinically or roentgenographically confirmed metastatic tumor-bearing areas. Concomitantly with the start of radiation therapy, or 2 weeks following surgical ablation of the tumor, the patient was begun on adjuvant chemotherapy (T-2) (Fig. 1).

Dactinomycin was given intravenously at the dosage of 450 micrograms/m²/day for 5 days. Adriamycin was given intravenously at the dosage of 20 mg/m²/day for 3 days. Cyclophosphamide was given by intravenous drip over one-half hour at a dosage of 1,200 mg/m² during a 3-hour period of intravenous hydration with electrolyte solution, in an effort to prevent hemorrhagic cystitis. Vincristine was given at the dose of 1.5 mg/m² and escalated to 2.25 mg/m² with a maximum dose of 2.5 mg. Each drug was given following a minimum of 2 weeks from the first day of administration of the previous drug, which was usually the time required for hematologic recovery between each course of chemotherapy. Two weeks following the fourth dose of vincristine, the patient was recycled on the same protocol. Patients were treated with this chemotherapy protocol for a total of 8 cycles, which usually took between 18 and 20 months to complete.

Patients were followed up with routine blood counts and serum biochemical profiles, as well as with monthly chest roentgenograms and roentgenograms of other involved or clinically indicated areas. A bone scan was repeated every 3–6 months, and electrocardiograms were done prior to each course of Adriamycin. Echocardiograms were done prior to treatment, and at appropriate times during treatment, to try to detect early signs of Adriamycin-related cardiomyopathy.

Toxicity

The toxicity of T-2 chemotherapy has been well described previously (Rosen *et al.*, 1974; Rosen, 1976), and includes the immediate effects of chemotherapy: nausea and vomiting, stomatitis, alopecia, leukopenia and thrombocytopenia, transient electrocardiographic changes, and erythema in the irradiated fields. Side effects also include the delayed complications occurring in the primary tumor site receiving radiation therapy, which consist of tendon contractures, edema of the extremity, cessation of growth of the extremity, fractures which delayed healing (requiring amputation in 3 patients), and infection of the biopsy site. Transient electrocardiographic changes consisting of mild S-T and T wave abnormalities were noted immediately following administration of Adriamycin in approximately 20% of the Adriamycin courses given. This abnormality usually returned to normal within 1 month following Adriamycin administration (Tan *et al.*, 1975). Lowering the maximum cumulative dose of Adriamycin to 600 mg/m², and 500 mg/m² in patients receiving incidental cardiac irradiation, resulted in no subsequent patient developing evidence of cardiomyopathy. However, 2 patients previously reported (Rosen *et al.*, 1974) developed severe Adriamycin-related cardiomyopathy. Both patients were treated with digitalis preparations, diuretics, and restricted activity. One of these patients was the first patient treated on the protocol and received a cumulative Adriamycin dose in excess of 900 mg/m². This patient developed Adriamycin cardiomyopathy and was treated for cardiac failure for more than 53 months. He died, with severe intractable heart failure, with no evidence of recurrent Ewing's sarcoma at 74 months from the time of starting treatment. The second patient had received 720 mg/m² of Adriamycin and had radiation therapy (2,100 rads to the mediastinum) at the onset of therapy because of pulmonary hilar metastases noted at the time of diagnosis. This patient's disease is well-controlled on digitalis and diuretics at 58 months from the time of starting treatment.

Results

Since June 1970, 20 patients with primary Ewing's sarcoma were treated with adjuvant T-2 chemotherapy. Sixteen of these patients had radiation therapy to the entire involved bone, and 4 had surgical ablation of their primary tumors. The results of adjuvant chemotherapy in this group are shown in Table 1. Of a total of 20 patients placed on adjuvant chemotherapy, 15 have been continually free of disease for from 24 + to 75 + months (median 40 + months) from the time of diagnosis and the start of treatment. The first patient to be treated in this group recently died, with no evidence of disease, of severe cardiomyopathy related to Adriamycin 74 months from the time of diagnosis and start of treatment. The actuarial disease-free survival of this group of 20 patients receiving adjuvant T-2 chemotherapy is depicted in Figure 2. At 5 years, the actuarial disease-free survival is calculated at 76%.

Less encouraging is the disease-free survival in patients with Ewing's sarcoma presenting with widespread metastatic disease. In this group of 8 patients, all of whom were treated with "curative" therapy to the primary tumor (radiation therapy in 7 patients and surgery in 1 patient), all went into complete remission while on T-2 chemotherapy (Table 2). The period of complete remission was from 4 to 58+ months. All but 1 of these patients relapsed and subsequently died of their disease. The 1 patient remaining free of disease received radiation therapy to the mediastinum for pulmonary hilar metastases (2,100 rads). This patient was one of the early patients treated on the T-2 protocol; he also received 720 mg/m^2 of Adriamycin and subsequently developed congestive heart failure. However, this patient is doing well, being managed on digitalis and diuretics. He remains free of disease at 58+ months from the start of treatment.

Of the 5 patients with primary disease only who relapsed, 2 relapsed with local recurrence in the primary site, 2 with pulmonary metastases, and 1 with pulmonary and bone metastases. Of the patients with metastatic disease who relapsed, 2 relapsed with local recurrence in the primary tumor site (both had received radiation therapy to the lungs for pulmonary metastases), 4 suffered relapse in the site of original bone metastases, and 1 relapsed in the site of original pulmonary metastases that were not irradiated, because they briefly disappeared after the initial course of chemotherapy (dactinomycin). One of the 2 patients with pulmonary metastases noted to relapse in the primary bone tumor site following radiation therapy to the primary tumor and pulmonary irradiation (1,400 rads – 200 rads × 7) had recurrence in the primary site (ilium), discovered incidentally at autopsy

TABLE 1.–ADJUVANT CHEMOTHERAPY (T-2) FOR PRIMARY EWING'S SARCOMA

TREATMENT OF PRIMARY TUMOR	NO. OF PTS.	NO. RELAPSED	% RELAPSED	TIME OF RELAPSE°	NO. NED	% NED†	TIME NED (MEDIAN)
Radiation therapy	16	4	15	7–38	12	75	25+–75+ (48+)
Surgery	4	1‡	25	26	3	75	24+–30+ (25+)
Total	20	5	25	7–38	15	75	24+–75+ (40+)

NED – No evidence of disease.
°Time in months from the start of treatment.
†1 patient died of cardiomyopathy related to Adriamycin at 74 months.
‡This patient is now with NED 10 mos. following thoracotomy, radiotherapy, and continued chemotherapy.

TABLE 2.–CHEMOTHERAPY (T-2) FOR METASTATIC EWING'S SARCOMA

TREATMENT OF PRIMARY TUMOR	NO. PTS.	NO. RESPONDING TO CHEMOTHERAPY	DURATION OF RESPONSE	NO. NED (DURATION)	NO. AWD (MOS. FROM DIAGNOSIS)	NO. DOD (MOS. FROM DIAGNOSIS)
Surgery	1	1	26 mos.	–	–	1 (29 mos.)
Radiation therapy	7	7	4–58+ mos.	1° (58+ mos.)	1 (22+ mos.)	5 (17–32 mos.)
Total	8	8	4–58+ mos.	1	1	6 (Med. survival 21 mos.)

°Patient received concomitant radiation therapy to lungs.
NED – No evidence of disease; AWD – Alive with disease; DOD – Died of disease.

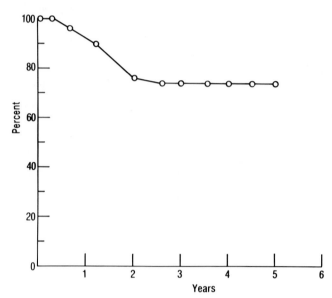

Fig. 2. — T-2 adjuvant chemotherapy: actuarial disease-free survival in 20 children with primary Ewing's sarcoma. In this series, no patient has relapsed after being off chemotherapy for more than 6 months. However, 1 patient recently expired at 74 months with no evidence of disease, due to severe heart failure secondary to Adriamycin. (He was the first patient treated on the protocol and was given Adriamycin at a higher dose. His cumulative dose was in excess of 900 mg/m².)

(she had died of disease secondary to pulmonary fibrosis), the onset of which occurred 3 months after the completion of her radiation therapy to the lungs.

Table 3 lists the 12 patients who relapsed following T-2 chemotherapy (5 presented with primary tumor only, and 7 presented with primary tumor and metastatic disease). The majority of patients suffering relapse did so after the cessation of T-2 chemotherapy, indicating that in these patients, chemotherapy may merely have delayed the reoccurrence of disease both in metastatic sites and in the primary tumor-bearing site as well.

Of the group of relapsing patients, 6 went on to develop spinal cord compression due to the epidural extension of systemic metastases. However, examination of the cerebrospinal fluid in all these patients failed to show the presence of extrinsic cells or positive cytologic findings on examination of the cell block.

In an attempt to analyze the results of combined therapy for the primary tumor, both permanent tumor control and limb function in patients receiving radiation therapy for their primary tumor were as-

TABLE 3.—PATIENTS WITH RECURRENT EWING'S SARCOMA
AFTER CHEMOTHERAPY (T-2)

PT.	SITE ORIGINAL METASTASES	SITE OF RELAPSE	TIME OF RELAPSE[†]	COMMENT
B.B.	—	Bone, lung	38 mos.	Metastases after chemotherapy completed
C.C.	—	Lung	20 mos.	Metastases at completion of chemotherapy
F.A.	—	Primary tumor (ischium)	13 mos.	Chemotherapy stopped at 8 mos. because of severe soft tissue reaction in irradiated field
D.W.	—	Primary tumor (tibia)	24 mos.	Biopsied for positive bone scan after chemotherapy stopped
L.P.	—	Lung	20 mos.	Relapsed (2 mos.) after chemotherapy stopped
C.M.	Bone	Bone	21 mos.	Chemotherapy stopped at 15 mos. because of severe soft tissue reaction in irradiated field
E.M.	Lung	Lung	17 mos.	Delays and dose reduction in chemotherapy
T.S.	Lung[°]	Primary tumor (femur)	27 mos.	Relapsed after chemotherapy completed. Posterior portion of primary tumor received less than planned 6,000 rads
F.F.	Lung Bone	Primary tumor (pelvis)	19 mos.	Had 1,400 rads pulmonary irradiation. Died of pulmonary fibrosis, local recurrence found at autopsy
S.S.	Bone	Bone	26 mos.	Metastases recurred after chemotherapy stopped (20 mos.)
S.W.	Bone	Primary tumor (foot)	18 mos.	Foot amputated for painful gait and positive bone scan. Distant metastases at 20 mos.
C.G.	Bone[°]	Lung	7 mos.	Interruption and delay in chemotherapy

[°]Received radiation therapy to metastatic site.
[†]Time from start of chemotherapy.

sessed (Table 4). We defined a functional failure as that in which a surviving patient would have had better limb function had he received a primary amputation rather than combination radiation therapy and chemotherapy. It had been noted previously that patients surviving for more than 2 years following radiation therapy, alone or

TABLE 4.—EWING'S SARCOMA
RADIATION THERAPY AND T-2 CHEMOTHERAPY FOR CONTROL OF
THE PRIMARY TUMOR IN 23 PATIENTS* (7 PATIENTS WITH
METASTATIC DISEASE)

	NO. PTS.	PERCENT	SITE—NO.	PRESENT STATUS
Successfully Treated	12/23	52%	Sacrum—2 Femur—2 Tibia—1 Foot—1 Humerus—2 Ulna—2 Radius—1 Jaw—1	10/12‡ NED (25+−75+ mos.) 2/12 Died of metastatic disease (17 mos. and 35 mos.)
Functional Failure†	6/23	26%	Pelvis—1 Femur—2 Tibia—2 Foot—1	3/6 Required amputation and are with NED (46+−58+ mos.) 3/6 Died of metastatic disease (29−55 mos.)
Local Recurrence	5/23	22%	Pelvis—2 (11, 18 mos.) Femur—1 (20 mos.) Fibula—1 (24 mos.) Foot—1 (18 mos.)	3/5 Died of disease (18, 19, 21 mos.) 2/5 Alive with disease after amputation (18 and 27 mos.)

*All patients received 5,000–7,000 rads to the primary tumor site.
†A functional failure indicates that the patient would have had better function with a primary amputation than with the result obtained by combined radiotherapy and chemotherapy.
‡One patient expired at 74 months due to cardiomyopathy (related to Adriamycin).

combined with chemotherapy, had poor limb function with a high percentage of "functional failure," particularly in the weight-bearing lower extremity (Lewis, Marcove, and Rosen, in press).

Table 4 lists the 23 patients (16 with primary tumor only and 7 with primary tumor and metastatic disease) in whom "curative" radiation therapy to the primary tumor had been attempted. Only 12 of the 23 patients (52%) were defined as successfully treated from the point of view of valuable function of the limb and lack of local recurrence. Six of the 23 patients (26%) were defined as functional failures. Their lesions were all in the lower extremity. One functional failure was in a patient whose foot required amputation because of a painful gait and nonhealing fracture. This patient has done well following amputation of her foot. Two functional failures were in the tibia, both in patients who now have excessive leg-length discrepancies and will need amputations to be able to walk properly. Two functional failures were in the femur, and 1 in the pelvis where extreme hip flexion contractures have made it impossible for the patient to walk. Of this group of functional failures, 3 of 6 subsequently required amputations and are free of disease at 46 to 58 + months. An additional 3 of these patients have died of metastatic disease at 29 to 55 months following the start of treatment. Two of these patients relapsed after having their chemotherapy prematurely stopped because of severe soft tissue reaction in the irradiated site (C.M. and E.M. – Table 3). Five of 23 patients (22%) had local recurrences. Two patients had a local recurrence in pelvic lesions (noted at 11 and 18 months following the start of treatment), 1 patient in the femur (20 months), 1 patient in the fibula (24 months), and 1 patient in the foot (18 months). Of these patients, 3 of 5 died of disease at 18, 19, and 21 months, and 2 are alive with disease following amputation at 18 and 27 months (Table 4).

Discussion

The 76% actuarial 5-year disease-free survival rate reported here in patients with primary Ewing's sarcoma treated with adjuvant T-2 chemotherapy, including dactinomycin, Adriamycin, cyclophosphamide, and vincristine, continues to represent one of the most encouraging treatment regimens for Ewing's sarcoma of those reported in the recent literature (Rosen *et al.*, 1974; Johnson and Pomeroy, 1975). Our continued surveillance of the cerebrospinal fluid both in patients with metastatic disease involving the spine, and patients continuously free of disease on systemic therapy, demonstrates that "sanctuary" disease and meningeal sarcomatosis does not occur in our experience in Ewing's sarcoma, and we have not incorporated "prophylactic" CNS treatment, with its uncertain future risk, into the treatment of this disease, as have other investigators (Johnson and Pomeroy, 1975).

Of the 8 patients with metastatic disease initially treated with dactinomycin (the first drug utilized in T-2 chemotherapy), 4 had evaluable disease prior to the addition of radiation therapy. These patients demonstrated an objective initial response to dactinomycin, confirming the usefulness of this drug in the treatment of Ewing's sarcoma.

Experience with the use of T-2 adjuvant chemotherapy and radiation therapy has drawn our attention to various problem areas to be considered in future treatment plans for children with Ewing's sarcoma. The majority of patients relapsing did so following the completion of chemotherapy, and, therefore, one may conclude that more aggressive chemotherapy is needed to completely eradicate all microfoci of metastatic disease. In addition, 4 of the 7 patients who relapsed with metastatic disease did so in the original metastatic sites, and it is our belief that more aggressive local therapy (radiation therapy) should be given to solitary or well-circumscribed metastatic sites when present at diagnosis. Thus, patients with metastatic disease in the lungs should receive radiation therapy to the lungs. However, in patients with metastatic disease in the bone marrow, we might have to rely on more aggressive chemotherapy to fully control this situation. If patients do not have metastatic disease in the lungs, it may not be necessary to give prophylactic radiation therapy to the lungs, since there is a risk of morbidity in this technique (although admittedly it is small if radiation therapy is limited to 1,400 rads in fourteen 100-rad fractions (Chabora *et al.*, in press) and not given concomitantly with radiosensitizing drugs). The argument against prophylactic radiation therapy to the lungs is that Ewing's sarcoma is a systemic disease that can just as readily occur in bones and other sites as in the lungs. However, once there is evidence of pulmonary disease, coned-down high-dose radiation therapy to the disease and prophylactic radiation therapy to the remainder of the lung fields, which would then be defined as being at a high risk, should be contemplated.

The finding that 11 of 23 patients who received "curative" radiation therapy to their primary tumors were treatment failures (6 functional failures and 5 local recurrences) makes it imperative that we re-examine the role of curative radiation therapy in patients with lower-extremity lesions (Lewis, Marcove, and Rosen, in press), since there was a total failure rate of 48% in this group (26% functional failures and 22% local recurrences). There has been a great deal of concern about the combined effect of radiation therapy and chemotherapy producing enhanced morbidity in normal tissues (Tefft, Chabora, and Rosen, in press), and therefore lower doses of radiation therapy have been advocated for patients receiving combination chemotherapy, including radiosensitizing agents such as dactinomycin and Adriamycin. This was a tenable suggestion for the treatment of Ewing's sarcoma when it had appeared that the local recurrence rate with radiation therapy and T-2 chemotherapy was lower than that observed with radiation therapy alone (Tefft, Chabora, and Rosen, in press; Fernandez, Lindberg, Sutow, and Samuels, 1974). However, the prolonged follow-up of patients receiving radiation therapy and T-2 chemotherapy (who have also witnessed severe soft tissue reactions) indicates that the local recurrence rate is increasing, and is now 22% as reported in this series, with all of the local recurrences being discovered from 18 to 27 months following the start of therapy. Therefore, we can conclude that aggressive chemotherapy is merely delaying the local recurrence rate, and if more patients are surviving longer, we might expect the local recurrence rate to reach that which has been reported with radiation therapy alone. Therefore, the need is to be more aggressive with the treatment of the primary tumor rather than less aggressive, even with the combination of chemotherapy with radiation therapy.

The avoidance of late recurrence of disease might be possible by the use of more aggressive combination chemotherapy regimens with agents that are synergistic, rather than by the use of sequential single-agent chemotherapy. Chemotherapy will have to be aggressive, with more intensive support programs for patients experiencing severe hematologic depression due to the more intensive nature of the chemotherapy. The problem of radiation treatment failures of primary tumor might be circumvented by the more judicious sparing of normal soft tissue outside the margin of the affected area, with an attempt to deliver the maximum dose of radiation therapy to the entire tumor-bearing bone and soft tissue mass. In addition, patients with large bulky tumors should perhaps undergo subsequent biopsies following the completion of radiation therapy to determine whether the tumor has been completely microscopically destroyed in an attempt to identify potential early local recurrence; it has been our experience that once local recurrence has become clinically manifest, the widespread dissemination of disease is imminent. The experience with this group of patients indicates that the period of high risk for recurrence of disease is within the first year after completion of chemotherapy. During this period, it is important to judiciously follow the chest roentgenogram, and it has been our practice to repeat a technetium diphosphonate bone scan at 3-month intervals, since the roentgenogram of the treated bone tumor is of very little value in detecting local bone recurrence if the bone has received 6,000–7,000 rads. The finding of a minimally positive bone scan in the area of the primary tumor, where the bone scan has previously been negative following aggressive treatment is an ominous indication of local recurrence, and one or even multiple biopsies should be performed at that time to try to rule out local recurrence.

The finding of functional failure in the majority of patients with lower extremity lesions in the weight-bearing bones, when patients survive and are followed long enough, makes it imperative that we develop more effective means of dealing with the primary tumor from the standpoint of future function and to decrease the increasing number of late local recurrences. To this end, we have embarked on a program of noncurative radiation therapy and surgical excision of the primary tumor in this group of patients. Surgical excision may be performed on the tumor-bearing portion of the bone, followed by non-curative radiation therapy of 4,000 rads to the remainder of the bone. Amputation should be considered if the future needs of the individual patient make it evident that, should the patient survive, function would be better than had the patient received "curative" radiation therapy. For instance, a young child with an extremity lesion involving most of the femur (Fig. 3) would probably do best with an amputation since, should the patient survive without local recurrence, the amount of radiation therapy required to produce her survival would make future rehabilitation impossible; the extent of the irradiated field would preclude future amputation should such a young patient survive to adulthood and require amputation for a small atrophic limb. This assumes that local recurrence or the occurrence of a secondary sarcoma does not occur during this period. Again, all patients must be individualized and treated by a knowledgeable, multidisciplinary team consisting of orthopedic surgeon, radiation therapist, and pediat-

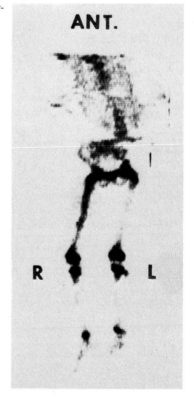

Fig. 3.—Technetium[99] bone scan of a 4-year-old child with Ewing's sarcoma. The entire right femur, including the hip joint, was involved with a very large bulky primary tumor. It was our feeling at the time of presentation that should this patient survive her disease, her rehabilitation would eventually be easier if she underwent primary surgery rather than "curative" radiation therapy to the entire femur and hip joint. She subsequently had a hemipelvectomy, completed adjuvant chemotherapy, and is free of all evidence of disease at over 30 months from the start of treatment.

ric oncologist. In general, we have developed the following guidelines (Lewis, Marcove, and Rosen, in press):

(1) Noncurative radiation therapy combined with surgery for the primary tumor is indicated in patients with pelvic lesions where curative pelvic irradiation would cause excessive morbidity in terms of bowel and bladder function, and where the local recurrence rate is very high. (No patient with a primary tumor in the ilium or ischium in this series has survived, although 2 patients with small sacral primary tumors have been successfully treated with radiation therapy.)

(2) Patients with proximal femur lesions where curative radiation therapy might lead to unacceptable hip flexion contractures would do better with noncurative radiation therapy to the total bone followed by resection of the tumor-bearing proximal femur and the insertion of a metallic prosthesis.

(3) Young patients with lesions about the knee or the tibia, where projected leg-length discrepancy (should they survive) will be excessive and eventually require an amputation, should not be put through the risk of local recurrence and the small, although real, risk of secondary bone sarcoma; these patients probably should have an amputation as their primary therapy.

(4) Patients with lesions in the foot, where curative radiation therapy might be expected to produce poor function with a painful gait, would function much better with surgical treatment of their tumors.

Many of these proposed studies are now underway at Memorial Sloan-Kettering Cancer Center in the hope of obtaining better therapeutic and functional results. The 76% five-year disease-free survival rate for children with primary Ewing's sarcoma with the therapy reported here is indeed encouraging, but the delayed effects and careful scrutiny of our failures, as well as the poor survival rate of patients with metastatic disease, make it imperative that we not only increase the aggressiveness of our treatment for this disease but also direct our attention to the delayed effects of treatment in those patients who are surviving, so that they will be better rehabilitated to lead more functional lives. Future studies should also be directed at the possible delayed effects of chemotherapy upon endocrine and intellectual function as well as at the social and emotional growth and development in the long-term survivors of childhood cancer.

Addendum

At the time of printing, no additional patients treated with adjuvant chemotherapy have relapsed, and the minimum follow-up on these patients is now 32+ months. In this series of patients, no patient has relapsed after being off chemotherapy for over 6 months. However, all 5 of the patients developing local recurrence in their primary tumor site following radiation therapy have subsequently died of disease. This fact serves to strengthen our feeling that local recurrence, no matter how early it is detected, is an ominous occurrence, and if the long-term rehabilitative considerations for a patient include surgery, if he is to survive, primary surgery should not be put off to a later date with the substitution of interim radiation therapy with the feeling that "surgery can always be done at a later date."

REFERENCES

Bhansali, S. K., and Desai, P. B.: Ewing's sarcoma. Observation on 107 cases. Journal of Bone and Joint Surgery, 45A:541–553, April 1963.

Chabora, B. M., Lattin, P. B., Rosen, G., Chu, F. C. H., and Herskovic, A.: Whole lung irradiation in the pediatric age group: Low-dose vs. conventional fractionation with multidrug chemotherapy. (In press.)

Dahlin, D. C., Coventry, M. B., and Scanlon, P. W.: Ewing's sarcoma. A critical analysis of 165 cases. Journal of Bone and Joint Surgery, 43A:185–192, March 1961.

Falk, S., and Alpert, M.: Five-year survival of patients with Ewing's sarcoma. Surgery, Gynecology and Obstetrics, 124:319–324, February 1967.

Fernandez, C. H., Lindberg, R. D., Sutow, W. W., and Samuels, M. L.: Localized Ewing's sarcoma—Treatment and results. Cancer, 34:143–148, July 1974.

Freeman, A. I., Sachatello, C., Gaeta, J., Shah, N. K., Wang, J. J., and Sinks, L. F.: An analysis of Ewing's tumor in children at Roswell Park Memorial Institute. Cancer, 29:1563–1569, June 1972.

Gilladoga, A. C., Manuel, C., Tan, C., Wollner, N., and Murphy, M. L.: Cardiotoxicity of Adriamycin (NSC-123127) in children. Cancer Chemotherapy Reports, 6:75–80, 1975.

Haggard, M. E.: Cyclophosphamide (NSC-26271) in the treatment of children with malignant neoplasms. Cancer Chemotherapy Reports, 51:403–405, 1967.

Hustu, H. O., Pinkel, D., and Pratt, C. B.: Treatment of clinically localized Ewing's sarcoma with radiotherapy and combination chemotherapy. Cancer, 30:1522–1527, December 1972.

Johnson, R. E., and Pomeroy, T. C.: Evaluation of therapeutic results in Ewing's sarcoma. American Journal of Roentgenology, Radium Therapy and Nuclear Medicine, 123:583–587, March 1975.

———: Integrated therapy for Ewing's sarcoma. American Journal of Roentgenology, Radium Therapy and Nuclear Medicine, 114:532–535, March 1972.

Johnson, R., and Humphreys, S. R.: Past failures and future possibilities in Ewing's sarcoma—Experimental and preliminary clinical results. Cancer, 23:161–166, 1969.

Lewis, R. J., Marcove, R. C., and Rosen, G.: Ewing's sarcoma: Functional effects of radiation therapy. (In press.)

Oldham, R. K., and Pomeroy, T. C.: Treatment of Ewing's sarcoma with actinomycin (NSC-123127). Cancer Chemotherapy Reports, 56:635–639, 1972.

Phillips, R. F., and Higinbotham, N. L.: The curability of Ewing's endothelioma of bone in children. Journal of Pediatrics, 70:391–397, March 1967.

Rosen, G.: Management of malignant bone tumors in children and adolescents. Pediatric Clinics of North America, 23:183–213, 1976.

———: Multidisciplinary management of Ewing's sarcoma. In Donaldson, M., and Sydel, G., Eds.: *Trends in Childhood Cancer.* New York, New York, J. Wiley and Sons, 1976, pp. 89–105.

Rosen, G., Woolner, N., Tan, C., Wu, S. J., Hajdu, S. I., Cham, W., D'Angio, G. J., and Murphy, M. L.: Disease-free survival in children with Ewing's sarcoma treated with radiation therapy and adjuvant 4-drug sequential chemotherapy. Cancer, 33:384–393, February 1974.

Samuels, M. L., and Howe, C. D.: Cyclophosphamide in the management of Ewing's sarcoma. Cancer, 20:961–966, June 1967.

Senyszyn, J. J., Johnson, R. E., and Curran, R. E.: Treatment of metastatic Ewing's sarcoma with actinomycin D (NSC-3053). Cancer Chemotherapy Reports, 54:103–107, 1970.

Sutow, W. W.: Vincristine (NSC-67574) therapy for malignant solid tumors in children (except Wilms' tumor). Cancer Chemotherapy Reports, 52: 485–487, 1968.

Sutow, W. W., and Sullivan, M. P.: Cyclophosphamide therapy in children with Ewing's sarcoma. Cancer Chemotherapy Reports, 23:55–60, October 1962.

Tan, C., Etcubanas, E., Wollner, N., Rosen, G., Murphy, M. L., and Krakoff, I. H.: Adriamycin in children with acute leukemia and other neoplastic diseases. In Carter, S. K., DiMarco, A., Ghione, M., Krakoff, I. H., and Mathe, G., Eds.: *International Symposium on Adriamycin.* Berlin and Heidelberg, West Germany, and New York, New York, Springer-Verlag, 1972, pp. 204–212.

Tan, C., Gilladoga, A. C., Ghavimi, F., Rosen, G., Haghbin, M., Wollner, N., Helson, L., and Murphy, M. L.: Adriamycin alone and in combination in the treatment of childhood neoplastic diseases. In Ghione, M., Fetzer, J., and Maier, H., Eds.: *Ergebnisse Der Adriamycin Therapie.* Berlin and Heidelberg, West Germany, and New York, New York, Springer-Verlag, 1975, pp. 71–82.

Tefft, M., Chabora, B., and Rosen, G.: Radiation in bone sarcomas—A reevaluation in the era of intensive systemic chemotherapy. (In press.)

Tefft, M., Lattin, P. B., Jereb, B., Cham, W., Ghavimi, F., Rosen, G., Exelby, P. R., Marcove, R. C., Murphy, M. L., and D'Angio, G. J.: Treatment of rhabdomyosarcoma and Ewing's sarcoma of childhood: Acute and late effects on normal tissue following combination therapy with emphasis on the role of irradiation combined with chemotherapy. Cancer, 37:1201–1213, 1976.

Wang, C. C., and Schultz, M. D.: Ewing's sarcoma—A study of fifty cases treated at the Massachusetts General Hospital, 1930–1952 inclusive. New England Journal of Medicine, 248:571–576, 1953.

Metabolic and Endocrine Alterations in Osteosarcoma Patients

MARK A. GOODMAN, M.D.,† JAMES H. McMASTER,
M.D.,* ALLAN L. DRASH, M.D.,‡ PETER E. DIAMOND,
M.D.,† GEORGE S. KAPPAKAS, M.D.,† and
PIERCE E. SCRANTON, Jr., M.D.†

*Associate Professor, Orthopaedic Surgery, University
of Pittsburgh School of Medicine and Director,
Department of Orthopaedic Surgery, Allegheny General
Hospital, Pittsburgh, Pennsylvania;† Research Fellows,
Orthopaedic Surgery, University of Pittsburgh School of
Medicine, Pittsburgh, Pennsylvania;‡ Associate
Professor, Pediatrics, Children's Hospital of
Pittsburgh, Pittsburgh, Pennsylvania

Introduction

THE ASSOCIATION OF ENDOCRINE ABNORMALITIES with neoplasia
has been recognized for nearly a century, with Freund (1885) first
reporting hypoglycemia in cancer patients in 1885. Brown (1928) observed hyperadrenocorticism secondary to a functioning oat cell carcinoma in 1928. Subsequently, numerous metabolic abnormalities have
been linked to tumors of varying histologic types. The clinical manifestations, resulting from the production of metabolically active substances by neoplasms, have been labeled "paraneoplastic syndromes."
Such syndromes have been noted in association with the ectopic production of insulin (Cahill, 1974), nonsuppressible insulin-like activity
factors (NSILA) (Megyesi and Kahn, 1974), adrenocorticotropic hor-

205

mones (ACTH) (Amatruda and Upton, 1974), parathyroid hormone (PTH) (Nathanson and Hall, 1974), gonadotropins (Jones, 1974), and numerous other metabolic factors.

The literature contains relatively little information regarding such "syndromes" in association with tumors of mesodermal origin. The first association was made by Glicksman and Rawson (1956) who noted a 25% incidence of "diabetes" in patients with sarcomas of bone. Marcove and Francis (1963) found hyperglycemia in 85% of their chondrosarcoma patients, and Turner and Horne (1970) reported similar abnormalities associated with fibrosarcoma. This study of adolescent patients with primary osteosarcoma was undertaken to further define abnormalities in carbohydrate metabolism seen with this tumor and to assess pituitary, adrenal, and gonadal functions.

Materials and Methods

PATIENT POPULATION. — This study was composed of 18 patients with histologically proven osteosarcoma who presented to the Health Center Hospitals of the University of Pittsburgh between January 1973 and January 1976. Admission to the study was limited to patients in the first 3 decades of life, which corresponds to the peak incidence of this tumor (Cade, 1955; Coventry and Dahlin, 1957).

The patients ranged in age from 6 to 25 years with an equal sex distribution. No patient had clinical evidence of a primary endocrinologic abnormality during this study. Eighty percent of the primary lesions were in the femur, with the remainder in the tibia, clavicle, and skull. Two patients presented with multiple lesions (Table 1).

Seventeen of 18 patients underwent surgical ablation of their primary tumors, and an equal number were placed on adjunctive chemotherapy. Seven patients had their tumors irradiated.

METHODS. — After an overnight fast, a 21-gauge butterfly needle was inserted into a peripheral vein and attached to a syringe filled with heparinized saline via a 3-way stopcock. All samples were drawn after the heparin solution was aspirated from the tubing and needle.

Fasting bloods were drawn from baseline glucose, insulin, and growth hormone (GH) determinations. Additional samples were obtained for serum cortisol, estradiol (E2), follicle stimulating hormone (FSH), luteinizing hormone (LH), testosterone, somatomedin, cholesterol, and triglyceride levels, and for lipoprotein electrophoresis. Glucose was measured by a glucose oxidase technique (Fales, 1974), while radioimmunoassay was used to measure insulin and GH (Herbert, 1965), cortisol (Foster and Dunn, 1974), FSH (Raiti and

TABLE 1.—PROFILE OF PATIENTS
WITH OSTEOSARCOMA

PATIENT	SEX	AGE	TANNER STAGE	LOCATION OF LESION
K.J.	F	6	1	Femur
W.J.	M	7	1	Femur
L.P.	F	7	1	Femur, shoulder
J.L.	M	11	2	Femur
K.Jo.	F	12	4	Femur, shoulder
M.R.	M	12	2	Tibia
N.Z.	F	13	4	Femur
J.B.	F	15	5	Femur
D.P.	F	15	5	Femur
M.W.	F	15	5	Femur
H.H.	M	16	5	Femur
L.M.	M	16	5	Femur
R.S.	F	16	5	Skull
J.T.	F	16	5	Femur
D.Po.	M	18	5	Femur
F.K.	M	20	5	Femur
R.St.	M	20	5	Femur
R.K.	M	25	5	Clavicle

Blizzard, 1968), LH (Bagshawe, Wilde, and Orr, 1966), testosterone (Endocrine Sciences, 1972), and E2 (Hotchkiss, Atkinson, and Knobil, 1971). Somatomedin was assayed by Van Wyk's (1971) technique utilizing rat cartilage. Lipid screening was carried out in accordance with the methods of Bragdon (1953), Sperry and Webb (1950), and Lees and Hatch (1963).

Following the withdrawal of fasting blood samples, the patient ingested Glucola (carbonated preparation for postprandial and glucose tolerance test, Ames Company, Elkhart, Indiana) (1.75 gm of glucose per kilogram body weight, up to a total of 100 gm). Samples for glucose insulin and growth hormone were taken at $1/2$, 1, 2, 3, 4, and 5 hours. A concomitant 24-hour urine sample was assayed for 17 hydroxy (17-OH) and 17 keto (17-K) steroids by the methods of Sanghvi and Wight (1973) and Sunderman and Sunderman (1967), respectively.

Eight patients were studied prior to biopsy. The remaining 10 were sampled during the course of their disease, with at least 2 weeks elapsing between surgical or chemotherapeutic procedures and endocrine evaluation. Whenever possible, all studies were repeated at 3-month intervals throughout the course of the disease; however, this schedule could not be rigidly followed. Variations in laboratory capabilities prevented the routine performance of all tests. Data were analyzed utilizing standard statistical tests.

Results

GLUCOSE, INSULIN, AND GROWTH HORMONE. — Six of 18 patients had only 1 glucose tolerance test, and 12 patients had 2 or more tests for a total of 53 sets of data. Within any 1 parameter, a significant abnormality was defined as 2 or more values greater than 2 standard deviations from the mean of control observations. Mean values were based on 31 normal adolescents. Single variations of more than 2 standard deviations from the mean were considered chance phenomena, and therefore of no significance.

Two patients had completely normal response curves, and 2 additional patients had only single variations from the norm. Glucose response curves were abnormal in 7 patients (39%). Abnormalities were present in the insulin and growth hormone responses in 5 (28%) and 10 (56%) patients, respectively. Six patients demonstrated changes in 2 parameters and 1 patient was abnormal in all 3 areas investigated. The overall incidence of abnormal responses to glucose loading was 78%.

The mean group response to glucose loading and the wide range of values obtained are shown in Figures 1, 2, and 3. Variations were statistically significant at the 0.02 level for the 3- and 5-hour glucose values, at the 0.05 level for the 0- to 3-hour insulin values, and at the 0.01 level for all but the 4-hour growth hormone response.

A regression analysis of the ratio of insulin to glucose over 3 hours $(\Delta I/\Delta G_{0-3})$ was used to assess the relative imbalance of these 2 factors.

Fig. 1.—Mean glucose response to oral glucose loading in 18 patients with osteosarcoma and 31 normal adolescents. Variations are significant at 3 and 5 hours (P < 0.02).

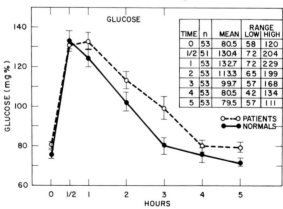

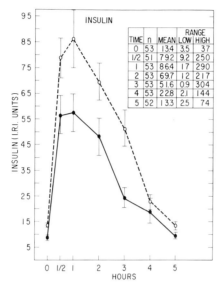

TIME	n	MEAN	RANGE	
			LOW	HIGH
0	53	13.4	3.5	37
1/2	51	79.2	9.2	250
1	53	86.4	17	290
2	53	69.7	12	217
3	53	51.6	0.9	304
4	53	22.8	2.1	144
5	52	13.3	2.5	74

Fig. 2.—Mean insulin response to oral glucose loading in 18 osteosarcoma patients and 31 normal adolescents. Significant deviations are seen at 0 to 3 hours (P < 0.05).

Danowski has defined the range of normal values to be between 1.0 and 4.0 (Danowski, personal communication). Thirty-nine percent of the calculated values fell within the normal range, while 10% were greater than 4.0, and 51% were less than 1.0.

The values for $\Delta I/\Delta G_{0-3}$ were compared with the absolute values for

Fig. 3.—Mean growth hormone response to oral glucose loading in 18 patients with osteosarcoma and 31 normal adolescents. Deviations from the norm are significant at 0 to 3 and 5 hours (P < 0.01).

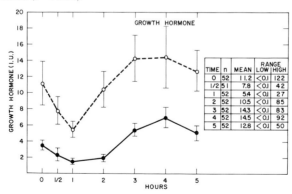

TIME	n	MEAN	RANGE	
			LOW	HIGH
0	52	11.2	<0.1	12.2
1/2	51	7.8	<0.1	42
1	52	5.4	<0.1	27
2	52	10.5	<0.1	85
3	52	14.3	<0.1	83
4	52	14.5	<0.1	92
5	52	12.8	<0.1	50

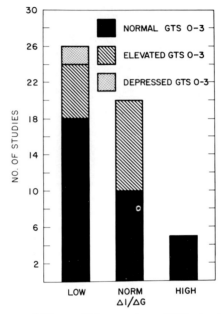

Fig. 4. — A comparison of Glucose Tolerance Sums (GTS$_{0-3}$) to high, normal, and low insulin: glucose ratios ($\Delta I/\Delta G_{0-3}$).

glucose (GTS$_{0-3}$) over the same 3-hour period. The upper limit of normal was taken as 450 mg/dl. At this level Khurana reported a 2% overall incidence of diabetes in children (Khurana and Drash, 1973). No consistent relationship was noted between these 2 parameters (Fig. 4).

CORTISOL. — The 8 a.m. fasting serum cortisol levels were studied in 10 patients, 4 of whom were tested twice. The normal values reported by Williams (1974) were applied to the results obtained since these values have never been reported to be age- or sex-dependent (Tanner, 1969, and Nelson, 1975). Cortisol levels in the patient population ranged from 4.6 μg/dl to 32.8 μg/dl with a mean of 17.3 ± 7.1 μg/dl. This did not vary significantly from the mean value for the normal population of 18.0 ± 5.5 μg/dl. Both patients with abnormal results were normal when retested (Table 2).

17 HYDROXYSTEROIDS AND 17 KETOSTEROIDS. — The urinary excretion of 17-OH and 17-K steroids was investigated in 5 patients. Normal levels of 17-K steroids were noted in all. A subnormal amount of 17-OH steroid was excreted by patient M. R., but this was not a statistically significant finding (P < 0.1) (Table 2).

ESTRADIOL. — Eight patients were studied for serum estradiol lev-

TABLE 2.—STUDY OF STEROID
HORMONES IN PATIENTS WITH
OSTEOSARCOMA

PATIENT	SERUM CORTISOL°	17 HYDROXY-STEROID†	17 KETO-STEROID†
W.J.	4.5 ↓	1.5 N	4.8 N
L.P.	8.0 N	2.5 N	1.8 N
L.P.	15.7 N	—	—
J.L.	18.4 N	1.7 N	4.0 N
K.J.	—	3.2 N	4.5 N
M.R.	21.3 N	0.5	2.5 N
M.W.	12.6 N	—	—
L.M.	22.9 N	—	—
R.S.	32.8 ↑	—	—
R.S.	21.3 N	—	—
D.Po.	18.8 N	—	—
R.St.	12.6 N	—	—
R.St.	21.7 N	—	—
R.K.	18.3 N	—	—

°Serum cortisol in μg/dl.
†Urinary steroids in mg/24 hrs.
N—Normal; ↑—Elevated; ↓—Depressed.

els, and all 8 were within 2 standard deviations of the norm for their age and sex (Table 3).

TESTOSTERONE.—Twelve samples, obtained from 9 patients, were assayed for testosterone. Patient L. P. demonstrated an elevated level on 1 occasion, which was considered to be insignificant (Table 3).

FOLLICLE-STIMULATING HORMONE AND LUTEINIZING HORMONE. —The patient group assayed for testosterone was also studied for FSH

TABLE 3.—STUDY OF GONADAL AND
GONADOTROPIC HORMONES IN
OSTEOSARCOMA PATIENTS

PATIENT	ESTRADIOL°	FSH°	LH°	TESTOSTERONE†
W.J.	5.0 N	5.3 N	19.0 N	33 N
L.P.	10.1 N	1.6 ↓	2.7 ↑	43 ↑
J.L.	5.0 N	—	—	—
K.J.	10.0 N	3.0 N	1.1 N	61 N
M.R.	4.7 N	2.1 N	4.4 N	414 N
M.W.	—	—	7.9 N	79 N
L.M.	—	3.8 N	4.9 N	645 N
R.S.	19.6 N	3.2 N	5.2 N	81 N
D.Po.	15.8 N	1.5 N	1.5 N	371 N
R.St.	19.2 N	2.4 N	5.4 N	1220 N

°Reported in ng/ml.
†Reported in ng/dl.
N—Normal; ↑—Elevated; ↓—Depressed.

TABLE 4.—LIPID SCREENING IN PATIENTS
WITH OSTEOSARCOMA

PATIENT	CHOLESTEROL[°]	TRIGLYC-ERIDES[°]	ALPHA LIPOPROTEIN	PRE-BETA LIPOPROTEIN	BETA LIPOPROTEIN
W.J.	150	15	N	N	N
L.P.	128	155	N	↑	N
J.L.	120	45	N	N	N
K.Jo.	120	50	↓	N	N
M.R.	100	35	N	N	N
L.M.	190	73	N	N	N
R.S.	180	60	N	N	N
D.Po.	144	35	N	N	N
R.St.	236	90	N	N	↑
Mean	151.6	62.0			
± SEM	±13.9	±13.8			

[°]Lipids in mg/dl.
N—Normal; ↑—Elevated; ↓—Depressed.

and LH. A single variation was noted in the FSH values obtained, and 1 value for LH was outside the normal range. Neither of these variations was significant (Table 3).

LIPIDS.—Lipid screening was done in 9 patients. The mean cholesterol value, 151.6 ± 13.9 mg/dl varied significantly from the adolescent norm of 170.0 ± 3.5 mg/dl reported by Drash ($P < 0.01$) (Drash and Hengstenberg, 1972). The mean triglyceride value, 62.0 ± 13.8 mg/dl, did not vary significantly from the normal, 69.0 ± 7.0 mg/dl, and no significant variations were present in alpha, pre-beta, or beta lipoproteins (Table 4).

SOMATOMEDIN.—Serum somatomedin was assayed in 7 patients and reported in plasma equivalent units (pl. eq.). One unit corresponds to the quantity of ^{3}H-methyl thymidine (New England Nuclear

TABLE 5.—SERUM SOMATOMEDIN LEVELS
IN OSTEOSARCOMA PATIENTS

PATIENT	^{3}H-THYMIDINE[°]	^{35}SULFATE[°]
J.B.	1.17	1.30
K.J.	1.40	1.47
F.K.	0.65	1.49
L.M.	3.28	2.89
D.P.	0.35	1.66
J.T.	1.51	1.42
N.Z.	1.32	0.56

[°]Reported in plasma equivalent units.
Normal—0.5–1.5 pl. eq.

Corporation, Boston, Massachusetts) or [35]sulfate (Cambridge Nuclear Inc., Billeria, Massachusetts) incorporated by hypophysectomized rat cartilage in the presence of 1 cc of pooled normal serum (Van Wyk and Hall, 1971). Two patients had elevated somatomedin levels, and 3 additional patients demonstrated values at the upper border of normal (Table 5).

Discussion

"Paraneoplastic syndromes" are abnormalities in metabolic function associated with nonendocrine system neoplasms. These disorders run the gamut of endocrinopathies and are unrelated to the histology of the primary tumor. The abnormalities noted, associated with primary osteosarcoma, may constitute a new "paraneoplastic syndrome."

The most pronounced abnormalities are in response to glucose loading, with 78% of the study population showing deviant responses in glucose, insulin, or growth hormone levels. Serial tests showed these abnormalities to be inconsistent over time in any patient. No clinical correlation was noted between the activity of the primary or metastatic tumors and the patient's response to glucose loading. Likewise, no mode of therapy produced consistent changes.

A two-by-two paradigm was used to test the association of each factor with the others. The statistical "Z" tests were not significant, implying that only a chance association exists between any of these 3 factors. Thus no one factor is indentifiable as the primary defect and the cause of the other variations seen. An additional, as yet unidentified, factor may be postulated linking together all the abnormalities seen in response to glucose loading.

An analysis of the relation of I/G_{0-3} to GTS_{0-3} demonstrates 3 distinct groups. The first group shows normal variations with consistent changes in both values. The second group demonstrates an augmentation of insulin action with a I/G_{0-3} below 1.0, indicative of an insulin deficiency, yet a concomitant normal or low GTS_{0-3}. Some other substance, not measured by radioimmunoassay technique, appears to be aiding in glucose transport. This insulin-like activity (ILA) has been noted in tissue cultures of osteosarcoma cells and in the serum of patients with this disease (Poffenbarger and Scranton, unpublished data).

The third group demonstrates elevated GTS_{0-3} values in the presence of normal insulin ratios, or normal GTS_{0-3} values associated with elevated I/G_{0-3}. Both can be attributed either to a relative lack of insulin, or to insulin resistance. Insulin antibodies were not specifically studied, but the radioimmunoassay technique used did not indicate their presence. Thus, it is unlikely that antibodies are responsible for the insulin resistance noted.

Another possible explanation for these observations is the induction of insulin resistance at the cellular level. Although many glucose tolerance curves resemble those seen in obese diabetics, mechanical changes in insulin receptor sites are not likely to be the cause. One can postulate that some chemical change has been brought about in the receptor itself, or perhaps a nonfunctional insulin analogue has been produced which has bound to the receptor site. No data are available on these theories, and much work remains to be done to explain these observations.

It is difficult to hypothesize a unified model which would explain these conflicting relationships. However, this type of model may be unnecessary. Farber (1973) has proposed an evolutionary concept of cancer which would allow for a number of discrete cell populations to coexist within a single, clinically apparent tumor. Each population could have unique metabolic requirements and would produce its own products. The relative size of each clone would define the metabolic changes seen in a patient at a given point in time. This cellular evolution is believed to continue until the death of either the tumor or the host.

The theory of continued evolution can explain the inconsistent picture seen clinically. At one moment ILA-producing cells may predominate, and at another moment cells producing resistance factors may be dominant. Neither may be significant, or their effects may be mutually exclusive at another time, thereby producing no clinical derangement in carbohydrate metabolism.

Somatomedin is a polypeptide hormone produced in the liver and kidneys in response to circulating growth hormone. Several different somatomedins are known to exist, each with tissue specific growth-stimulating potential.

Elevated somatomedin is known to be associated with accelerated growth and increased levels of circulating growth hormone. Five of 7 patients studied had high somatomedin levels. All of these patients were above the fiftieth percentile in height for their age, as were all other patients in this study. This corresponds to the tall stature of osteosarcoma patients noted by Dahlin (1967), Fraumeni (1967), and Scranton (1975). Of 6 patients who were concomitantly tested for growth hormone, 5 had significantly elevated responses, and 1 had a single abnormal value. Thus, growth hormone was uniformly elevated in this subgroup. The numbers are too small to allow for meaningful statistical analysis, but it seems likely that the elevated somatomedin levels seen correlate with the accentuated growth hormone responses observed in these patients.

Steroid hormones are important factors in the cellular utilization of glucose and in the release of insulin and growth hormone. This lead to the investigation of 8 a.m. fasting serum cortisol levels and 24-hour 17-OH and 17-K steroid excretion. With the exception of 3 isolated abnormalities, the results were within normal limits. Therefore, no link seems to exist between the deviations noted in carbohydrate metabolism and the secretion of steroid hormones in this population.

The high incidence of osteosarcoma at the time of the pubertal growth spurt produced questions regarding sexual development among patients with this lesion as compared to their peers. Tanner staging of clinical development and laboratory investigations of gonadal and gonadotropic hormones were carried out. All patients fell within their expected Tanner stage, thus failing to demonstrate either precocious or retarded sexual development. Laboratory studies were essentially normal as well. It should be noted that the laboratory methods used are inaccurate at the low ends of their scales, so little can be said regarding the underproduction of these factors; hyperfunctioning, however, has been ruled out.

Lipid disorders are often associated with variations in sugar metabolism. Changes in free fatty acids are known to accompany changes in insulin levels as well. In these patients, no significant abnormalities were uncovered in serum triglyceride or lipoprotein values. Cholesterol values, while within the range of normal for each individual, were, as a group, significantly lower than for normal adolescents. This finding cannot be explained at the present time, and additional investigation into its cause and significance is needed.

Conclusion

Adolescent patients with primary osteosarcoma demonstrate abnormal glucose, insulin, and growth hormone responses to oral glucose loading in 78% of the study population. No statistical association exists between any 2 of the 3 factors and therefore no primary abnormality can be identified.

High somatomedin levels were noted in 72% of the group studied, accompanied by simultaneous elevations of growth hormones.

Studies of adrenal, gonadal, and gonadotropic hormones were essentially normal, thereby ruling these out as associated endocrine abnormalities.

The evolutionary concept of tumor growth may explain the inconsistent nature of these abnormalities and their variability. Some additional factor or factors may be present and the cause of the derangements seen. These may be produced by the tumor or by the body in response to the tumor. Additional work is underway to define and characterize these substances.

The consistency of these findings in association with primary osteosarcoma characterizes an abnormality in carbohydrate metabolism which fulfills the definition of a "paraneoplastic syndrome."

Acknowledgments

All somatomedin samples were assayed by Dr. Thomas Foley, Jr., Department of Pediatrics, University of Pittsburgh School of Medicine, Pittsburgh, Pennsylvania.

The authors wish to acknowledge the assistance given by Mrs. Diane Anthony, Miss Cathy Richards, Mrs. Fay Hengstenberg, and Mrs. Mamie Moore of the CORE Laboratory of Children's Hospital of Pittsburgh. Sincere appreciation is also expressed to the staff of the Clinical Research Unit of Children's Hospital.

This work was supported in part by the John M. Olin Foundation, the Orthopaedic Research and Education Foundation, the American Cancer Society, The Arthritis Foundation, Western Pennsylvania Chapter, and the National Institutes of Health.

References

Amatruda, T., and Upton, G.: Hyperadrenocorticism and ACTH-releasing factors. Annals of the New York Academy of Sciences, 230:168–180, 1974.

Bagshawe, K. D., Wilde, C. E., and Orr, A. H.: Radioimmunoassay for human chorionic gonadotropin and luteinizing hormone. Lancet, 1:1118–1121, May 21, 1966.

Bragdon, J.: Colorimetric determination of blood lipids. Journal of Biological Chemistry, 190:513–517, 1953.

Brown, W.: A case of pluriglandular syndrome: "Diabetes in a bearded woman." Lancet, 2:1022–1023, 1928.

Cade, S.: Osteogenic sarcoma. Journal of the Royal College of Surgeons, 1:79–111, 1955.

Cahill, G., Jr.: Hyperglycemia. Annals of the New York Academy of Sciences, 230:161–167, 1974.

Coventry, M. B., and Dahlin, D. C.: Osteogenic sarcoma. A critical analysis of 430 cases. Journal of Bone and Joint Surgery, 39A:741–758, July 1957.

Dahlin, D. C., and Coventry, M. B.: Osteogenic sarcoma. A study of six hundred cases. Journal of Bone and Joint Surgery, 49A: 101–110, January 1967.

Danowski, T.: Personal communication, 1976.

Drash, A., and Hengstenberg, F.: The identification of risk factors in normal children in the development of atherosclerosis. Annals of Clinical and Laboratory Science, 2:348–359, Sept.–Oct., 1972.

Endocrine Sciences: Plasma testosterone radioimmunoassay procedure. Tarzana California, Endocrine Sciences Co., 1972.

Fales, F.: Glucose oxidase technique for the measurement of serum glucose. Methods of Clinical Chemistry, 4:1974.

Farber, E.: Carcinogenesis—cellular evolution as a unifying thread: Presidential address. Cancer Research, 33:2537–2550, November 1973.

Foster, L. B., and Dunn, R. T.: Single-antibody technique for radioimmunoassay for cortisol in unextracted serum or plasma. Clinical Chemistry, 20: 365–368, 1974.

Fraumeni, J.: Stature and malignant tumors of bone in childhood and adolescence. Cancer, 20:967–973, 1967.

Freund, E.: Zur Diagnose des Carcinoms. Wien Medizinische Blatter, 8: 268–269, 1885.

Glicksman, A. S., and Rawson, R. W.: Diabetes and altered carbohydrate metabolism in patients with cancer. Cancer, 9:1127–1134, Nov.–Dec., 1956.

Hebert, V., Lau, K.-S, Gottlieb, C. W., and Bleicher, S. J.: Coated charcoal immunoassay of insulin. Journal of Clinical Endocrinology, 25:1375–1384, October 1965.

Hotchkiss, J., Atkinson, L. E., and Knobil, E.: Time course of serum estrogen and luteinizing hormone (LH) concentrations during the menstrual cycle of the rhesus monkey. Endocrinology, 89:177–183, 1971.

Jones, K.: Feminization, virilization and precocious sexual development that result from neoplastic processes. Annals of the New York Academy of Sciences, 230:195–203, 1974.

Khurana, R. C., Drash, A., Howland, J., and Danowski, T. S.: Glucose tolerance sums and glucose: Insulin ratios in children. Metabolism, 22:295–305, February 1973.

Lees, R. S., and Hatch, F. T.: Sharper separation of lipoprotein species by paper electrophoresis in albumin-containing buffer. Journal of Laboratory and Clinical Medicine, 61:518–528, March 1963.

Marcove, R. C., and Francis, K. C.: Chondrosarcoma and altered carbohydrate metabolism. New England Journal of Medicine, 268:1399–1400, June 20, 1963.

Megyesi, K., Kahn, C. R., Roth, J., and Gorden, P.: Hypoglycemia in association with extrapancreatic tumors: Demonstration of elevated plasma NSILA-s by a new radioreceptor assay. Journal of Clinical Endocrinology and Metabolism, 38:931–934, May 1974.

Nathanson, L., and Hall, T.: Lung tumors: How they produce their syndromes. Annals of the New York Academy of Sciences, 230:367–378, 1974.

Nelson, W. E.: *Textbook of Pediatrics*. 10th edition, Philadelphia, Pennsylvania, W. B. Saunders Co., 1975, p. 1327.

Poffenbarger, P., and Scranton, P. E., Jr.: Unpublished data.

Raiti, S., and Blizzard, R. M.: Measurement of immunologically reactive follicle stimulating hormone in human urine by radio-immunoassay. Journal of Clinical Endocrinology, 28:1719–1723, December 1968.

Sanghvi, A., Wight, C., Parikh, B., and Desai, H.: Urinary 17-hydroxycorticosteroid determination with p-hydrazinobenzene sulfonic acid-phosphoric acid. American Journal of Clinical Pathology, 60:684–690, November 1973.

Scranton, P. E., Jr., and McMaster, J. H.: Investigation of carbohydrate metabolism and somatomedin in osteosarcoma patients. Journal of Surgical Oncology, 7:403–409, 1975.

Sperry, W., and Webb, M.: A revision of the Schoenheimer-Sperry method for cholesterol determination. Journal of Biological Chemistry, 187:97–106, 1950.

Sunderman, F., and Sunderman, F., Jr.: *Lipid and Steroid Hormones in Clinical Medicine.* Philadelphia, Pennsylvania, J. B. Lippincott Co., 1967.

Tanner, J. M.: Growth and endocrinology of the adolescent. In L. I. Gardner, Ed.: *Endocrine and Genetic Diseases of Childhood.* Philadelphia, Pennsylvania, W. B. Saunders Co., 1969, pp. 19–60.

Turner, M. A., and Horne, C. H. W.: Primary fibrosarcoma of lung and diabetes mellitus. British Journal of Surgery, 57:713–715, September 1970.

Van Wyk, J. J., Hall, K., Van den Brande, J. L., and Weaver, R. P.: Further purification and characterization of sulfation factor and thymidine factor from acromegalic plasma. Journal of Clinical Endocrinology and Metabolism, 32:389–405, March 1971.

Williams, R. H., Ed.: *Textbook of Endocrinology.* 5th edition. Philadelphia, Pennsylvania, W. B. Saunders Co., 1974, 1138 pp.

Recent Developments in the Classification of Soft Tissue Sarcomas

FRANZ M. ENZINGER, M.D.

Chief, Department Soft Tissue Pathology, Armed Forces Institute of Pathology, Washington, D.C.[°]

DESPITE SIGNIFICANT ADVANCES in the identification and diagnosis of soft tissue sarcomas over the past 20 years, development of a useful and comprehensive classification has been a relatively slow process. Clear understanding of this complex group of tumors has been hampered by 2 major difficulties: first, the comparative rarity of these neoplasms, which makes it difficult to gain much experience in this field; and second, and more importantly, the great variety and wide morphological range of soft tissue sarcomas which reflect the complexity of mesenchymal tissues.

Like any modern classification, the soft tissue classification is based on the identification of the tissue type produced by the tumor. By definition, soft tissues include all nonepithelial tissues of extraskeletal origin, with the exception of tissues of the reticuloendothelial system and the glia, and the supporting tissue of specific organs and viscera. Earlier and purely descriptive classifications, employing such terms as round cell- or spindle cell sarcoma, must be considered obsolete, since they provide no useful information as to the nature and biologic behavior of a given neoplasm.

Two major classifications of soft tissue sarcomas have been pro-

---

[°]The opinions or assertions contained herein are the private views of the author and are not to be construed as official or as reflecting the views of the Department of the Army or the Department of Defense.

posed over the past years: one is the classification presented by A. P. Stout in the Soft Tissue Fascicle of the *Atlas of Tumor Pathology,* first published in 1957 and reissued in 1967 with R. Lattes as coauthor (Stout and Lattes, 1967); the second is the classification issued by the World Health Organization (WHO) in 1969 on the basis of a review of more than 500 soft tissue tumors by an international panel of pathologists (Enzinger, Lattes, and Torloni, 1969). The main objective of this work was to provide and illustrate a widely accepted classification that would foster a more uniform language in soft tissue pathology and, thus, would promote a closer understanding and collaboration on an international basis.

The current classification of soft tissue sarcomas used at the Armed Forces Institute of Pathology is essentially an updated version of the WHO classification. As Table 1 illustrates, this classification can be divided into 3 basic groups: (1) tumors that are histologically well defined and in which the tissue type can be identified. Most of the better-known soft tissue sarcomas, such as liposarcoma, rhabdomyosarcoma, and synovial sarcoma, belong in this category. Subtypes are distinguished in some of these entities for diagnostic purposes, as in rhabdomyosarcoma, or for more accurate prediction of clinical behavior; (2) a relatively small group of sarcomas in which the exact tissue type is still unknown but which can be reliably identified by their characteristic cellular features and arrangement of the tumor cells. Alveolar soft part sarcoma is perhaps the best-known example of this group; (3) a large and diverse group of unclassified sarcomas that are

TABLE 1.—CLASSIFICATION OF PRIMARY SOFT
TISSUE SARCOMAS

TUMORS OF KNOWN HISTOGENESIS

Fibrosarcoma	Synovial sarcoma
Malignant fibrous histiocytoma	Malignant mesothelioma
Liposarcoma	Malignant schwannoma
Leiomyosarcoma	Malignant neuroepithelioma
Rhabdomyosarcoma	Extraskeletal myxoid chondrosarcoma
Hemangiosarcoma	Extraskeletal mesenchymal chondrosarcoma
Lymphangiosarcoma	Extraskeletal osteosarcoma
Malignant hemangiopericytoma	Malignant mesenchymoma

TUMORS OF SPECIFIC TYPE BUT UNCERTAIN HISTOGENESIS

Alveolar soft part sarcoma	Epithelioid sarcoma
Malignant granular cell tumor	Extraskeletal neoplasm resembling
Clear cell sarcoma	Ewing's sarcoma

TUMORS, TYPE UNDETERMINED
Sarcoma, type undetermined

too poorly differentiated for a reliable diagnosis. This group amounts to about 15 or 25% of all soft tissue sarcomas, depending upon the experience of the examining pathologists. Further investigation of these poorly differentiated neoplasms is highly desirable because the degree of cellular differentiation alone, without recognition of the tumor type, is an unreliable yardstick for the prediction of clinical behavior.

Since the preparation of the WHO soft tissue classification in 1969 several changes have become necessary. Malignant fibrous histiocytoma, carried in the classification as malignant fibroxanthoma, was placed between liposarcoma and fibrosarcoma to emphasize its close kinship to these 2 entities. Mesenchymal chondrosarcoma was added because it was realized that it not only occurs as a bone tumor but also may arise in soft tissues. Epithelioid sarcoma and an extraskeletal neoplasm resembling Ewing's sarcoma were included as newly described entities.

Since it is impossible here to review all malignant categories of the soft tissue classification, this presentation will be limited to the above entities, with the emphasis upon the most common and perhaps the most controversial of them, malignant fibrous histiocytoma.

Epithelioid Sarcoma

Although not particularly rare, this neoplasm has been slow to be recognized as a specific type of sarcoma and has been confused with a variety of benign and malignant lesions. Superficial forms of this tumor often have been mistaken for a necrotizing granulomatous process or an ulcerating squamous cell carcinoma. Deeply located ones were usually recognized as a sarcoma, but in many instances were erroneously identified as fibrosarcoma or synovial sarcoma.

Clinically, epithelioid sarcoma manifests itself as a firm, slowly growing, scar-like mass which arises from the fascia or the deep subcutis or, and less commonly, from tendon or tendon sheath. It may develop at any age, but primarily afflicts patients between 20 and 40 years of age. Following our initial report of 62 cases of this tumor (Enzinger, 1970), we have seen on consultation an additional 95 cases which essentially confirm our initial findings. Of the total 157 cases, more than half (57%) were located in the regions of the hand and forearm. More than two-thirds (70%) developed in males. A similar incidence with regard to location and age has been reported by other reviewers (Gabbiani *et al.*, 1972, Bryan *et al.*, 1974).

In most cases, the tumor can be recognized readily under the microscope. Characteristically, it consists of large mononuclear polygonal, epithelium-like cells that have vesicular nuclei and a deeply eosinophilic cytoplasm and that are arranged in an irregular multinodular pattern (Fig. 1). Unlike carcinomas, they are often separated by dense, frequently hyalinized, collagen. The cells tend to undergo degeneration or necrosis, especially in the poorly vascularized centers of the tumor nodules. Transitions between polygonal cells and plump, fibroblast-like spindle cells are common, but there is never a distinctly biphasic cellular pattern as in synovial sarcoma. Distinction from synovial sarcoma is further facilitated by the complete absence of glandular formation and intracellular mucin that stains positively with the PAS and alcian blue preparations. Collagen not only is seen between the tumor cells but also is abundant in the surrounding tissue, a feature that is responsible for the scar-like gross appearance of this tumor.

Epithelioid sarcoma has a tendency to recur before metastasis. Follow-up information of our initial series (Enzinger, 1970) revealed an 85% recurrence rate with metastasis in 30% of the cases. The lung, lymph nodes, and scalp were the most common sites of metastasis. Additional follow-up information obtained since the publication of these data suggests that the incidence of metastasis is still higher if the patients are followed for a longer period of time, preferably 10 or more

Fig. 1.—Epithelioid sarcoma showing nodular arrangement of epithelium-like tumor cells and central necrosis of the tumor nodules. (H&E, ×210, AFIP Neg. No. 72-315.)

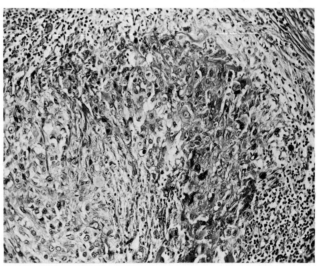

years. Early and rigorous surgical therapy is necessary to prevent recurrence and metastasis.

Extraskeletal Neoplasm Resembling Ewing's Sarcoma

During the past years, we have been impressed by the occurrence of a peculiar and hitherto unrecognized sarcoma that we tentatively classified as an "extraskeletal neoplasm resembling Ewing's sarcoma" (Angervall and Enzinger, 1975). Judging from our cases, this tumor is a fully malignant neoplasm that principally affects the soft tissues of the paravertebral region and the lower extremities and, like Ewing's sarcoma of bone, prevails in older children and young adults.

Since 1971, when we reported 39 examples of this tumor (Angervall and Enzinger, 1975), we have seen in consultation numerous additional cases that confirmed our initial impression of this neoplasm. Judging from the reviewed material, the tumor may develop at any age, but is encountered most frequently in the second and third decades of life. Its incidence in males and females is about equal. The most common locations are the paravertebral region, including the chest wall, posterior mediastinum, and retroperitoneum. Second in frequency are the lower extremities. The majority of tumors range in size from 5 to 10 cm in greatest diameter.

The microscopic picture is characterized by a coarsely lobular pattern consisting of solidly packed round and oval tumor cells exhibiting an almost monotonous degree of uniformity. The nuclei of these cells are distinctly outlined and contain finely dispersed chromatin. Their cytoplasm is scant, pale-staining, and usually poorly defined (Fig. 2). Mitotic figures occur but are much less common than one would expect to find in such a poorly differentiated neoplasm. Large and small areas of necrosis are commonly seen. The richly vascular pattern of this tumor can be discerned only with difficulty in well-differentiated areas. It becomes apparent, however, in areas of degeneration where convolutes of thick-walled vessels simulate a hemangiopericytoma or malignant hemangioendothelioma.

Special stains are helpful in reaching a diagnosis; collagen and reticulin fibers are usually confined to the fibrous trabeculae that separate the individual tumor lobules. They are rarely seen between the individual tumor cells and then only when the tumor undergoes focal fibrosis secondary to degeneration and necrosis. Intracellular glycogen, as in Ewing's sarcoma of bone (Schajowicz, 1959), is present in nearly all of the cases. Exceptional cases with little or no glycogen do occur, however, and the absence of glycogen does not necessarily rule

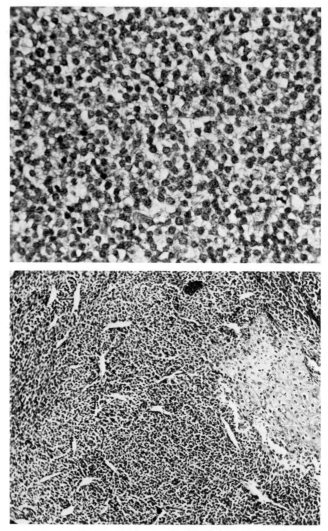

Fig. 2 (top).—Extraskeletal neoplasm resembling Ewing's sarcoma. Solidly packed rounded tumor cells of uniform appearance having an ill-defined cytoplasm and distinctly outlined nuclei. The vacuolated appearance of the cytoplasm is the result of intracellular deposition of glycogen. (H&E, ×350, AFIP Neg. No. 74-507.)

Fig. 3 (bottom).—Mesenchymal chondrosarcoma showing the characteristic biphasic pattern consisting of islands of well-differentiated cartilage and undifferentiated tumor cells. The pericytoma-like pattern is characteristic of this neoplasm. (H&E, ×150, AFIP Neg. No. 71-2443.)

out this diagnosis. In most instances, however, the glycogen is more regularly distributed than is that of rhabdomyosarcoma, a tumor that has the same age incidence and must be considered foremost in differential diagnosis.

Follow-up information in 35 of the cases revealed a fully malignant neoplasm that metastasized, chiefly to the lungs and bones, at an early stage of the disease. There was no apparent morphologic correlation between the tumors that were cured and those that metastasized despite extensive therapy. As in Ewing's sarcoma of bone, a combination of surgical excision, chemotherapy, and radiotherapy appears to be the treatment of choice.

The exact histogenesis of this tumor is still unknown. The ultrastructural findings (Szakacs, Carta, and Szakacs, 1974) suggest a neoplasm of primitive mesenchymal or reticular cells similar to those observed in Ewing's sarcoma of bone (Friedman and Gold, 1968, Takayama and Sugawa, 1970). The cells contained few organelles but, as evident under the light microscope, considerable amounts of glycogen.

Differential diagnosis includes chiefly neuroblastoma, neuroepithelioma, synovial sarcoma, and rhabdomyosarcoma. All of these entities, with the exception of rhabdomyosarcoma, usually lack a positive glycogen stain. Rhabdomyosarcoma can be recognized by its more irregular cellular pattern and, in the majority of cases, the presence of rhabdomyoblasts.

Extraskeletal Mesenchymal Chondrosarcoma

Although mesenchymal chondrosarcoma is primarily a bone tumor (Lichtenstein and Bernstein, 1959, Dahlin, Coventry, and Scanlon, 1961), its occurrence as a primary tumor in soft tissues is well-documented in the literature (Dahlin and Henderson, 1962, Salvador, Beabout, and Dahlin, 1971, Guccion, Font, Enzinger, and Zimmerman, 1973). When in bone, it affects chiefly the flat bones and the jaw; when in soft tissue, it is most commonly encountered in the regions of the head and neck. Young patients in the third and fourth decades of life are mainly involved. Males and females are about equally affected.

Grossly, the tumors are large, multilobulated, and well-circumscribed, and on cross sections are white and fleshy with blue-gray nodules of cartilage and occasional hard, yellow-tan areas of osteoid or bone.

Microscopically, mesenchymal chondrosarcoma is easily recognized by its characteristic biphasic pattern: primitive, undifferentiated mesenchymal cells that are intimately associated with rather well-circumscribed islands of malignant but well-differentiated cartilage. Commonly, the undifferentiated portions of the tumor are supplied by thin-walled, slit-like vascular channels vaguely resembling the picture of a malignant hemangiopericytoma (Fig. 3). Ossification of the cartilaginous tissue is sometimes prominent.

Mesenchymal chondrosarcoma, regardless of its location, is a fully malignant neoplasm which pursues an indolent and relentless course in most of the patients. Metastases, especially to the lung, are common. Late metastasis, 10 or more years after the initial removal of the tumor, has been observed. Judging from our material and the reports in the literature, the tumor is radioresistant and the principal mode of therapy is radical surgical excision.

Malignant Fibrous Histiocytoma

Since 1964, when O'Brien and Stout described this tumor, malignant fibrous histiocytoma (MFH) has been increasingly recognized by pathologists as a specific entity and has emerged as perhaps the most common soft tissue sarcoma to occur in older patients. In fact, many sarcomas formerly interpreted as pleomorphic fibrosarcoma, liposarcoma, or rhabdomyosarcoma are now considered to be of this type.

Malignant fibrous histiocytoma occurs principally in older patients, with the highest incidence in the age groups between 50 and 70 years. Children and young adults are afflicted occasionally, but when occurring in young patients, the disease differs in its histologic picture and is marked by a lesser degree of cellular pleomorphism (Kauffman and Stout, 1961). The prevailing anatomic site of the tumor in the AFIP material is the thigh, followed by the chest wall, shoulder region, and retroperitoneum. In most cases the tumors are deep-seated, coarsely nodular, and measure between 5 and 10 cm in greatest diameter. Their multinodular appearance often masks their invasive growth. Small, superficially located tumors, situated entirely in the dermis or subcutis, occur and, according to recent data obtained on a series of 200 cases of MFH (Weiss and Enzinger, unpublished data), have a much more favorable prognosis. It is conceivable that this provides an explanation for the benign course of atypical fibroxanthoma, a tumor that microscopically is virtually indistinguishable from MFH.

It is of some interest that a history of a previously excised epithelial or mesenchymal neoplasm, either at the same or some other site, was given in several cases. This is of dubious significance and most likely is a coincidence related to the prevalence of MFH in older patients. These cases are in addition to several instances in which a MFH developed several years after intensive radiotherapy for some other type of neoplasm such as mammary carcinoma or retinoblastoma, or in which a MFH preceded the onset of malignant lymphoma.

More than most other types of sarcomas, MFH is typified by an extremely wide range in its cellular composition and pattern, not only

Fig. 4 (top). — Malignant fibrous histiocytoma exhibiting the typical arrangement of the plump spindle cells in a storiform or cartwheel pattern. (H&E, ×165, AFIP Neg. No. 72-7184.)

Fig. 5 (bottom). — Malignant fibrous histiocytoma displaying a pattern similar to Figure 4, but showing a much greater degree of cellular pleomorphism, including occasional multinucleated giant cells. (H&E, ×180, AFIP Neg. No. 71-11513.)

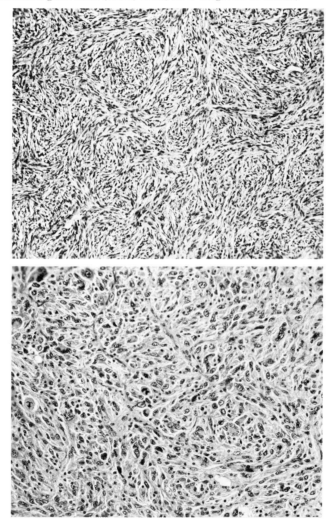

from tumor to tumor, but also often in different portions of the same tumor. If we arrange the various histologic appearances of the tumor in order of increasing cellular pleomorphism, then the least pleomorphic portion of the spectrum is occupied by a neoplasm that shows a distinct storiform or whorled pattern. This pattern resembles that of dermatofibrosarcoma protuberans (storiform fibrous histiocytoma) but differs in the larger size of the cells and their more irregular arrangement (Fig. 4). Dermatofibrosarcoma protuberans, however, is also part of the spectrum and should be considered a link between benign and malignant forms of fibrous histiocytoma.

With increasing cellular pleomorphism, the storiform or whorled pattern becomes less pronounced or occupies only a small portion of the neoplasn (Fig. 5). In these cases, giant cells with eosinophilic cytoplasm and one or more hyperchromatic nuclei, often of bizarre appearance, and with or without intranuclear vacuoles become one of the most striking features of the tumor and account for the frequent confusion of MFH with pleomorphic or adult type of rhabdomyosarcoma or pleomorphic carcinoma (Fig. 6).

Most examples of MFH are composed of several types of cells: plump fibroblast-like spindle cells, round or oval mononuclear cells resembling histiocytes, and giant cells with 1 or more nuclei. Frequently intermingled with these cells are foamy histiocytes (lipid

Fig. 6.—Malignant fibrous histiocytoma. Typical pleomorphic pattern with scattered multinucleated giant cells of variable appearance. (H&E, ×225, AFIP Neg. No. 72-1234.)

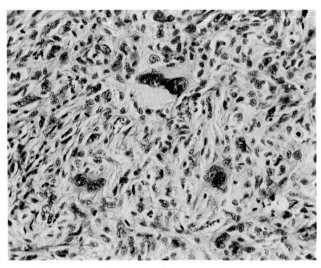

carrying macrophages) and cells storing hemosiderin (siderophages). Intermediate forms between these cells are common, implying that all or most of these cells are modifications of the same basic mesenchymal cell in different stages of functional activity. Inflammatory cells, especially lymphocytes, eosinophils, and plasma cells, unrelated to areas of necrosis, are present in most instances of MFH. Indeed, in some cases, the focal prominence of the inflammatory infiltrate makes it difficult to distinguish the tumor from Hodgkin's disease, especially since some of the giant cells have eosinophilic nucleoli and bear a close resemblance to Reed-Sternberg cells.

This mixture of cells is usually associated with a prominent vascular pattern and with varying amounts of reticulum and collagen. Highly collagenized and hyalinized portions in MFH are common, perhaps more so than in any other soft tissue sarcoma. At the other extreme, myxoid changes may be severe and may simulate a variety of soft tissue neoplasms, foremost of which is myxoma and myxoid liposarcoma.

While most examples of MFH show a mixture of the described cellular and stromal features, there are some instances in which one or the other of these features predominates. Depending upon the predominant characteristic of these tumors, we consider them as subdivisions of MFH and have tentatively classified them as giant cell, xanthomatous, and myxoid variants of MFH.

The giant cell type of MFH is used here synonymously with giant

Fig. 7.—Malignant fibrous histiocytoma, giant cell type. (H&E, ×210, AFIP Neg. No. 71-5582.)

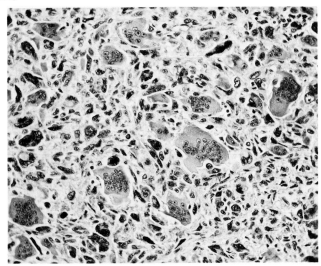

cell fascial sarcoma and malignant giant cell tumor of soft parts (Guccion and Enzinger, 1973). It is characterized by a large number of multinucleated, osteoclast-like giant cells combined with the typical picture of MFH (Fig. 7). The number of giant cells varies considerably, and in some cases the giant cells are limited to a small portion of the neoplasm. Asteroids may be present in some of the giant cells, giving support to their histiocytic origin. Association with newly formed osteoid or osseous tissue is encountered more commonly in this tumor than in the ordinary MFH. According to an AFIP review of 35 cases, superficial and deep forms do occur. Like other types of MFH, the superficially located tumors have a more favorable prognosis than do those that are deep-seated and large.

The xanthomatous type of MFH has also been described as malignant xanthogranuloma (Stout and Lattes, 1967), xanthosarcoma (Kahn, 1972), and inflammatory fibrous histiocytoma (Kyriakos and Kempson, 1976). It is composed of a striking number of xanthoma cells intimately associated with acute and chronic inflammatory elements (Fig. 8). There is some cellular pleomorphism in most of the cases, but sometimes pleomorphism is minimal, making it difficult to recognize this tumor as an aggressively growing and fully malignant neoplasm. It is likely, however, as Kahn (1972) has suggested, that most tumors described as retroperitoneal xanthogranuloma are xanthomatous variants of MFH.

The third and most common subtype is the myxoid variant of MFH. Initially we classified examples of this tumor as myxofibrosarcoma, but over the years we have become increasingly aware that this is still another type of MFH, having the same clinical setting as the ordinary MFH (Weiss and Enzinger, 1976). It is characterized by an extremely variegated pattern, ranging from that of a richly myxoid tumor resembling myxoma or nodular fasciitis to that of a pleomorphic MFH. The extremes of these patterns, the myxoid and pleomorphic changes, are often encountered in different portions of the same specimen or in different specimens obtained during the course of the disease (Fig. 9). Judging from a recent review of 80 cases at the AFIP, the myxoid type has a more favorable prognosis than ordinary MFH, especially when the tumor is confined to the subcutis without invasion of fascia or muscle. In this series, the metastatic rate was 23%, the rate of local recurrence 61%.

There is still another remarkable aspect of this tumor: areas indistinguishable from those of MFH may occur in other types of sarcomas. Liposarcomas, in particular, may contain MFH-like areas, suggesting a close relationship between these 2 neoplasms. On rare occasions we have also encountered MFH-like portions in leiomyosarcoma, osteo-

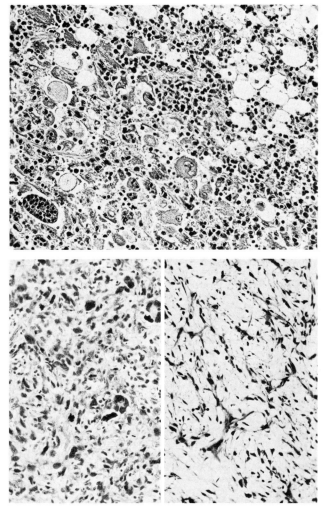

Fig. 8 (top).—Malignant fibrous histiocytoma, xanthomatous type, consisting of a mixture of xanthoma cells, histiocyte-like cells with atypical nuclei, and a large number of scattered inflammatory elements. (×210, AFIP Neg. No. 74-4821.)

Fig. 9 (bottom).—Malignant fibrous histiocytoma, predominantly of the myxoid type. (Left), pleomorphic pattern (×180, AFIP Neg. No. 76-739). (Right), myxoid pattern (×180, AFIP Neg. No. 76-740).

sarcoma, and even in carcinosarcoma. As in malignant mesenchymoma, the coexistence of several tumor types in the same neoplasm is probably explained by the great potential and versatility of mesenchyme, particularly in the uncontrolled conditions of a malignant process. In fact, electron microscopic examination of soft tissue sarcomas in general implies that cells may be transformed under changing local conditions and that the cellular composition of many sarcomas is much more complex than has been realized from studying them under the light microscope.

The histogenesis of MFH is still a matter of controversy. Kauffman and Stout (1961), when describing MFH in children, suggested that this tumor is basically a histiocytic neoplasm with some of the histiocytes acting as facultative fibroblasts. Tissue culture studies (Ozzello, Stout, and Murray, 1963) supported this concept. Ultrastructural studies later confirmed the presence of histiocytic and fibroblastic elements in MFH (Merkow *et al.*, 1971) but also revealed them to be intermixed with undifferentiated mesenchymal cells (Fu, Gabbiani, Kaye, and Lattes, 1975). This gives credence to the concept that MFH is a tumor of primitive or uncommitted mesenchymal cells differentiating mainly in a bimodal manner along histiocytic and fibroblastic lines. This concept is an attractive one because it satisfactorily explains the variegated appearance of this tumor and allows for occasional intermediate forms between MFH and other types of sarcomas.

Accurate prediction of the behavior of MFH in the individual case is difficult and depends upon a variety of histologic and clinical parameters. In general, tumors with a distinctive storiform or myxoid pattern pursue a more favorable clinical course than do the more pleomorphic variants of MFH. Absence of mitotic figures also suggests a favorable course, but increased mitotic rate, a reliable prognostic criterion in many sarcomas, appears to be of little prognostic significance. Large, deep-seated neoplasms are more likely to recur and metastasize than are small ones located entirely in the subcutis.

Data gained from a recent follow-up study of 200 cases of MFH (Weiss and Enzinger, unpublished data) indicate an overall metastatic rate of 42%. In 18% of the cases the tumor recurred prior to metastasis. The principal sites of metastatic spread were the lung (82%), lymph nodes (28%), liver (18%), and bone (15%).

Summary

Although considerable progress has been made over the past years, much of our knowledge in the field of soft tissue tumors is still incomplete, and new and more reliable methods of diagnosis will have to be employed for a more accurate evaluation and understanding of this complex group of neoplasms. For the present, however, continued efforts must be made to define the histologic picture and biologic behavior of these tumors as clearly and precisely as possible and to arrange them into an orderly and comprehensive classification. Such a classification will necessarily remain a tentative one, but will serve as a baseline for better understanding of these neoplasms and, especially, for comparison of data and sound appraisal of conventional and newly developed modes of therapy.

REFERENCES

Angervall, L., and Enzinger, F. M.: Extraskeletal neoplasm resembling Ewing's sarcoma. Cancer, 36:240–251, July 1975.

Bryan, R., Soule, E., Dobyns, J., Pritchard, E., and Lincheid, R.: Primary epithelioid sarcoma of the hand and forearm. A review of thirteen cases. Journal of Joint and Bone Surgery, 56A:458–465, April 1974.

Dahlin, D. C., Coventry, M. B., and Scanlon, P. W.: Ewing's sarcoma. A critical analysis of 165 cases. Journal of Bone and Joint Surgery 43A:185–192, March 1961.

Dahlin, D. C., and Henderson, E. D.: Mesenchymal chondrosarcoma. Further observations on a new entity. Cancer, 15:410–417, March–April 1962.

Enzinger, F. M.: Epithelioid sarcoma. A sarcoma simulating a granuloma or a carcinoma. Cancer, 26:1029–1041, November 1970.

———: *Histological Typing of Soft Tissue Tumors.* World Health Organization, Geneva, Switzerland, 1969.

Friedman, B., and Gold, H.: Ultrastructure of Ewing's sarcoma of bone. Cancer, 22:307–322, August 1968.

Fu, Y.-S., Gabbiani, G., Kaye, G. I., and Lattes, R.: Malignant soft tissue tumors of probable histiocytic origin. (Malignant fibrous histiocytomas): General considerations and electron microscopic and tissue culture studies. Cancer, 35:176–198, January 1975.

Gabbiani, G., Fu, Y.-S., Kaye, G. I., Lattes, R., and Majno, G.: Epithelioid sarcoma. A light and electron microscopic study suggesting a synovial origin. Cancer, 30:486–499, August 1972.

Goldman, R. L.: "Mesenchymal" chondrosarcoma, a rare malignant chondroid tumor usually primary in bone. Report of a case arising in extraskeletal soft tissue. Cancer, 20:1494–1498, September 1967.

Guccion, J. G., and Enzinger, F. M.: Malignant giant cell tumor of soft parts: An analysis of 32 cases. Cancer, 29:1518–1529, June 1972.

Guccion, J. G., Font, R. L., Enzinger, F. M., and Zimmerman, L. E.: Extraskeletal mesenchymal chondrosarcoma. Archives of Pathology, 95:336–340, May 1973.

Hedinger, C.: Mesenchymales Chondrosarcom der Weichteile. Schweizerische Medizinische Wochenschrift, 99:1142–1147, August 1969.

Kahn, L. B.: Retroperitoneal xanthogranuloma and xanthosarcoma (malignant fibrous xanthoma). Cancer, 31:411–421, February 1973.

Kauffman, S. L., and Stout, A. P.: Histiocytic tumors (fibrous xanthoma and histiocytoma) in children. Cancer, 14:469–482, May–June 1961.

Kempson, R. L., and Kyriakos, M.: Fibroxanthosarcoma of the soft tissues. A type of malignant fibrous histiocytoma. Cancer, 29:961–976, April 1972.

Kyriakos, M., and Kempson, R. L.: Inflammatory fibrous histiocytoma. An aggressive and lethal lesion. Cancer, 37:1584–1606, March 1976.

Lichtenstein, L., and Bernstein, D.: Unusual benign and malignant chondroid tumors of bone—A survey of some mesenchymal cartilage tumors and malignant chondroblastic tumors, including a few multicentric ones, as well as many atypical chondroblastomas and chondromyxoid fibromas. Cancer, 12: 1142–1157, November–December 1959.

Mackenzie, D. H.: *The Differential Diagnosis of Fibroblastic Disorders.* Blackwell Scientific Publications, Oxford and Edinburgh, 1970, 167 pp.

Merkow, L. P., Frich, J. C., Jr., Slifkin, M., Kzreages, C. G., and Pardo, M.: Ultrastructure of a fibroxanthosarcoma (malignant fibroxanthoma). Cancer, 28:372–383, August 1971.

O'Brien, J. E., and Stout, A. P.: Malignant fibrous xanthomas. Cancer, 17: 1445–1455, November 1964.

Ozzello, L., and Hamels, J.: The histiocytic nature of dermatofibrosarcoma protuberans: Tissue culture and electron microscopic study. American Journal of Clinical Pathology, 65:136–148, February 1976.

Ozzello, L., Stout, A. P., and Murray, M. R.: Cultural characteristics of malignant histiocytomas and fibrous xanthomas. Cancer, 16:331–344, March 1963.

Salvador, A. H., Beabout, J. W., and Dahlin, D. C.: Mesenchymal chondrosarcoma—Observations on 30 new cases. Cancer, 28:605–615, September 1971.

Santiago, H., Feinerman, L. K., and Lattes, R.: Epithelioid sarcoma. A clinical and pathologic study of nine cases. Human Pathology, 3:133–147, March 1972.

Schajowicz, F.: Ewing's sarcoma and reticulum-cell sarcoma of bone. With special reference to the histochemical demonstration of glycogen as an aid to differential diagnosis. Journal of Bone and Joint Surgery, 41A:349–356, March 1959.

Soule, E. H., and Enriquez, P.: Atypical fibrous histiocytoma, malignant fibrous histiocytoma, malignant histiocytoma and epithelioid sarcoma. A comparative study of 65 tumors. Cancer, 30:128–143, July 1972.

Stout, A. P., and Lattes, R.: Tumors of the Soft Tissues. In *Atlas of Tumor Pathology.* Second Series, Fascicle 1, Armed Forces Institute of Pathology, Washington, D. C., 1967. 196 pp.

Szakacs, J. E., Carta, M., and Szakacs, M. R.: Ewing's sarcoma, extraskeletal and of bone. Case report with ultrastructural analysis. Annals of Clinical Laboratory Science, 4:306–322, July–August 1974.

Takayama, S., and Sugawa, I.: Electron microscopic observations of Ewing's sarcoma—A case report. Acta Pathology, Japan, 20:87–101, February 1970.

Weiss, S. W., and Enzinger, F. M.: Myxoid variant of malignant fibrous histiocytoma. Cancer, 39:1672–1685, April 1977.

Weiss, S. W., and Enzinger, F. M.: Malignant fibrous histiocytoma. An analysis of 200 cases. (In press.)

Angiography and Lymphangiography in Peripheral Soft Tissue Sarcomas

LUIS A. de SANTOS, M.D., SIDNEY WALLACE, M.D., and J. BARNETT FINKELSTEIN, M.D.

Department of Diagnostic Radiology, The University of Texas System Cancer Center M. D. Anderson Hospital and Tumor Institute, Houston, Texas

WITH THE DEVELOPMENT OF MORE SOPHISTICATED forms of therapy aimed at complete eradication of the neoplasm with maximum preservation of mechanical function, more detailed radiographic information is essential for individualization of treatment of patients with soft tissue tumors (Simon and Enneking, 1976; Suit, Russell, and Martin, 1973). The radiographic evaluation is necessary to determine the nature and extent of disease, to delineate the anatomic relationship to adjacent osseous and vascular structures, to define residual or recurrent neoplasm, and, at times, to locate the optimal site for biopsy.

At M. D. Anderson Hospital, the initial radiographic work-up consists of chest radiograph and tomography examinations, examination of the specific area with bone and soft tissue techniques, including xeroradiography, and, in selected cases, radionuclide bone scanning. In specific circumstances, angiography enhanced by magnification and subtraction techniques and lymphangiography confirmed by percutaneous needle aspiration biopsy can be of considerable assistance in staging the neoplastic process. As an extension of angiography, transcatheter intravascular occlusive therapy has been employed in preoperative and palliative management of disease. Utilizing illustrative cases, the indications and contributions of angiography and lymphangiography to patients with soft tissue tumors will be presented.

Angiography

TECHNIQUE. — Arteriography is usually performed by percutaneous catheterization of the femoral artery by the Seldinger technique. Selective catheterization of the vessel of interest as close to the lesion as possible is preferable. For the lower extremity, this is accomplished in patients without significant tortuosity by contralateral retrograde catheterization around the bifurcation (Fig. 1). The selective catheterization of the axillary and brachial arteries is readily accomplished by way of the femoral artery.

At least 2 projections are necessary, especially when the underlying vascular anatomy is complex, as in the pelvis. Magnification angiography and subtraction technique enhances the presentation of the vascular structures. Pharmacoangiography, i.e., the use of vasoactive agents (dilators such as priscoline, papaverine, glucagon, and prostaglandin E_1 or constrictors including epinephrine, angiotensin, and vasopressin), is effective in the preferential visualization of tumor vascu-

Fig. 1.—Catheterization technique. Catheter curves around aortic bifurcation and descends on the opposite side. Catheter tip lies *(arrow)* in the common femoral artery. Selective catheterization of branches is easily performed by manipulation of catheter aided by guide wire.

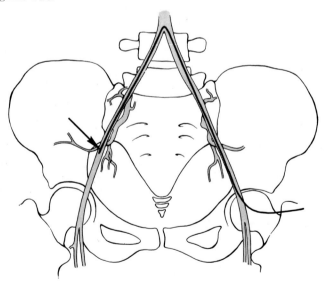

larity (Ekelund and Lunderquist, 1974; Hawkins and Hudson, 1974; Jacobs and Hanafee, 1967; Rockoff, Doppman, Block, and Ketchan, 1966). However, the value of pharmacoangiography in the differentiation of benign from malignant neoplasms is in itself not entirely reliable.

The complications of angiography are few. The most common, thromboembolism, which occurs in 0.4 to 2.3% of the patients, is minimized by systemic hyparinization by the intraarterial injection of 45 units per killigram of aqueous heparin at the onset of the procedure (Wallace, Medellin, De Jongh, and Gianturco, 1972).

Criteria

There are no absolute angiographic criteria for the diagnosis of malignancy in soft tissue tumors (Viamonte, Roen, and LaPage, 1973; Denny, 1956; Ney, Feist, Altemus, and Ordinario, 1972). The angiographic findings include:

(1) Distortion and displacement of vessels; this may be due to the presence of any mass.

(2) Hypervascularity; this is an increase in the number of opacified vessels, and is nonspecific.

(3) Tumor stain or blush; this is an increased capillary blush which is a manifestation of hypervascularity.

(4) AV shunting; this may be seen in inflammatory lesions, vascular occlusion, trauma, congenital malformations, benign and malignant neoplasms.

(5) Encasement; this is the abrupt and irregular change in caliber of vessels seen in neoplasms, but it can be present with inflammation.

(6) Pooling of contrast material outside of normal tapered vessels; this is usually a manifestation of neovascularity.

(7) Irregular, poorly defined margin of a mass; this suggests malignancy, whereas the presence of smooth, well-circumscribed border, a capsule, or a pseudocapsule is more frequently seen in the case of benign processes.

Of these findings, encasement and neovascularity are the most consistent angiographic criteria for malignant neoplasms.

Clinical Applications

NATURE OF THE DISEASE. — A specific diagnosis should not be attempted by angiography (Viamonte, Roen, and LaPage, 1973). Arteriography is most useful when applied to the resolution of a specific problem aided by the plain radiographic findings in a defined clinical setting.

Confusion is created by the hypervascularity seen in masses secondary to trauma with muscle necrosis (e.g., myositis ossificans), to infection, and to postoperative changes (Hutcheson, Klatte, and Kremp, 1972; Gronner, 1972). The gamut of vascular patterns seen in angiomatous lesions is at times difficult to differentiate from malignant neoplasm (Levin, Gordon, and McSweeney, 1976). Hemangiomas are usually composed of benign-appearing, normally tapering arteries with persistence of opacification of the vessels or lakes late into the venous phase; they are seldom associated with early venous drainage (Fig. 2). At the other end of the spectrum are the bizarre vessels found in an angiomatous hamartoma (Fig. 3). Attempts to correlate the histological diagnosis with the angiographic presentation have proven unsuccessful.

EXTENT OF DISEASE. — The intelligent treatment of the patient with a soft tissue tumor is based largely upon the determination of the extent of disease, as illustrated by the low recurrence rate (2%) when

Fig. 2 (left). — Angiomyolipoma of upper thigh. Tortuous dilated vessels are seen extending from upper thigh to obturator and pubic area. Pelvic extension of an upper thigh lesion is difficult to evaluate without angiography.

Fig. 3 (right). — Vascular hamartoma. Bizarre malignant-appearing vessels and vascular lakes are seen in this popliteal vascular lesion that proved completely benign at pathologic examination.

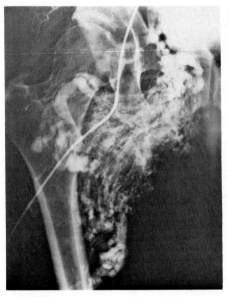 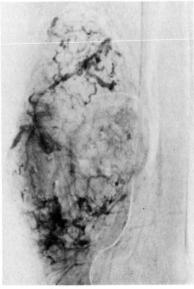

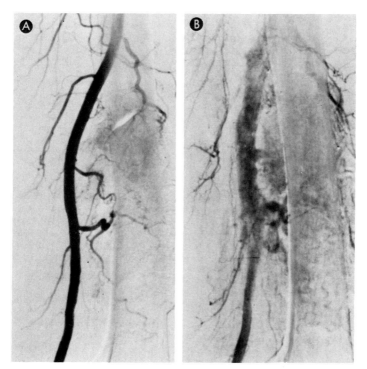

Fig. 4. – Recurrent liposarcoma. Mass effect and posterior displacement of, **A,** femoral artery and, **B,** vein are seen. At surgery, extensive tumor and encasement of femoral vein were demonstrated. The lesion could not be removed.

the neoplasm is adequately resected (Martel and Abell, 1973; Hudson, Haas, Enneking, and Hawkins, 1975). Angiography contributes greatly by demonstrating the origin of the vascular supply to the neoplasm, encroachment upon major vessels and bone, relationships to joint spaces, and integrity of adjacent fascial planes.

Displacement and distortion of the major vessels (Fig. 4) indicate that the neoplasm is beyond radical local resection. Encasement and obstruction of major vessels and involvement of nonexpendable bone usually necessitate amputation (Fig. 5).

A well-circumscribed mass is more likely the result of a slowly progressing process, and is more frequently seen in the case of a benign neoplasm which, when large enough, displaces intermuscular septi. However, pseuodoencapsulation is common with sarcomas. Benign processes, especially hemangiomas, as well as malignant processes, can violate septal planes.

Only when positive is the angiographic information significant.

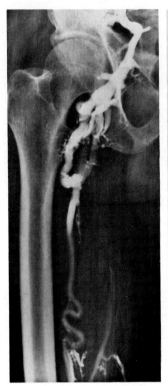 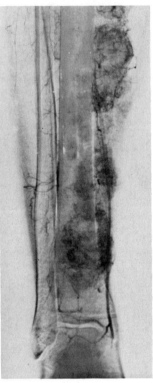

Fig. 5 (left).—Recurrent neurofibrosarcoma. A venogram performed after 2 previous operations revealed complete occlusion of the femoral vein and collateral circulation. Extensive disease, beyond resectability, was found at surgery.

Fig. 6 (right).—Recurrent fibrosarcoma. White male with recurrent fibrosarcoma after 2 consecutive operations for primary tumor in the upper leg. Present recurrent nodules in the lower leg were not palpable.

Angiography is extremely useful in demonstrating disease beyond that determined by clinical means (Fig. 6) (Hudson, Haas, Enneking, and Hawkins, 1975). At times, pelvic extension of a sarcoma of the thigh can only be defined by angiography. The delineation of microscopic disease obviously exceeds the competence of this technique.

The frequency of hepatic metastases from sarcomas (21%) (Bucalossi and Veronesi, 1973), especially in the case of large or recurrent tumors, necessitates the angiographic evaluation of the liver. The vascular pattern of metastatic disease usually mimics that of the primary tumor (Fig. 7).

SITE OF BIOPSY.— Biopsy is usually necessary to establish the histo-

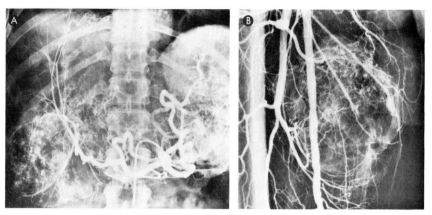

Fig. 7.—Metastatic leiomyosarcoma. **A,** vascular pattern of hepatic metastases closely resembled the primary lesion in the upper thigh (**B**).

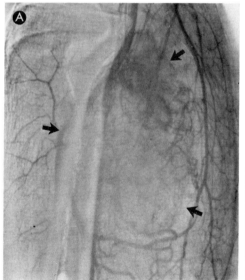

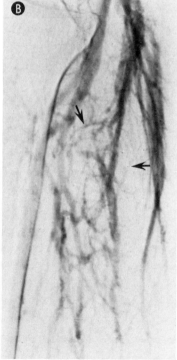

Fig. 8.—Soft tissue Ewing's sarcoma. **A,** prior to therapy, a large vascular mass is present posteriorly in the upper calf region. **B,** after chemotherapy and radiation treatment there is a marked improvement, but a small mass still remains in the area.

logic diagnosis. By defining the extent of the neoplasm, angiography can assist in demonstrating the most accessible site for biopsy. The most aggressive component of the neoplasm is usually the most vascular. Occasionally, in necrotic or hypovascular tumors, biopsy of the most vascular area is necessary to establish a diagnosis, and it may obviate repeated operations.

EFFECT OF THERAPY. — Demonstration of residual or recurrent disease is one of the primary uses of angiography in soft tissue tumors (Hudson, Haas, Enneking, and Hawkins, 1975). The angiographic criteria are the same as with primary tumors. When serial studies are

Fig. 9.—**A,** malignant fibrohistiocytoma of soft tissue before treatment. Embolization was performed in this nonsurgical candidate. The patient subsequently bled into the lesion and died. At autopsy no viable tumor was found. **B,** embolization was performed with Gelfoam and completed with metallic coil *(arrow).*

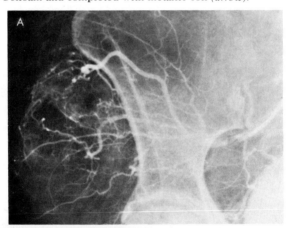

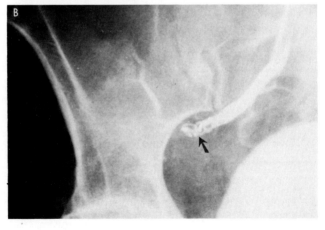

available, the angiographic pattern of the primary tumor and the residual or recurrent disease will be similar. The presence of hypervascularity and tumor stain at the site of previous surgery should be evaluated with caution. Two to 3 months should be allowed between these events to minimize confusion with the vascularity of granulation tissue. Occasionally, angiography can be of help in the evaluation of the results of either radiation therapy or chemotherapy, particularly when the primary mass is no longer palpable (Fig. 8).

TRANSCATHETER EMBOLIZATION. — Recently, the angiographic route has been employed for transcatheter intravascular occlusion of neoplasms (Bree, Goldstein, and Wallace, 1976; Wallace and Goldstein, 1976; Tadavarthy, Knight, and Ovitt, 1974; Bookstein, Chlosta, Foley, and Walter, 1974). The embolic materials used include blood clot, modified clot (with amicar, thrombin, etc.), autologous tissue, Gelfoam, oxycel, ivalon, metallic and silicone spheres, silicone rubber, cyanoacrylate, and mechanical devices (Wallace *et al.*, 1976; Gianturco, Anderson, and Wallace, 1975). This approach has been utilized for the control of hemorrhage and the relief of pain, and to decrease tumor bulk and vascularity preoperatively or for palliation. The possibility that an ischemic neoplasm may stimulate an immune response is an interesting theory. The decrease of tumor vascularity in a malignant fibrous histiocytoma by Gelfoam embolization and coil occlusion of the right internal iliac for palliative management is illustrated in Figure 9.

Lymphangiography

At M. D. Anderson Hospital, lymphangiography is routinely employed in the staging of patients with lymphomas and a variety of carcinomas. Lymphangiography, when properly used in the staging of soft tissue sarcomas, provides useful additional information as to the extent of disease.

Criteria

Rigid criteria must be used so that the diagnosis of metastases is associated with a high degree of pathologic correlation (95%) (Wallace, Jackon, Dodd, and Greening, 1965; Wallace, 1968; Wallace and Jackson, 1964; Wallace and Jing, in press). The primary criterion for the diagnosis of metastatic disease is the presence of a defect in a lymph node that is not traversed by lymphatic vessels (Fig. 10). For this, both the lymphatic and the nodal phases must be carefully studied. At times, especially with rhabdomyosarcoma, the lymphan-

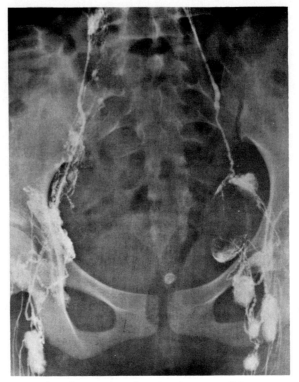

Fig. 10.—Positive lymphangiogram "carcinoma pattern." Lower-extremity liposarcoma defect within the node not transferred by lymphatics defines the carcinoma pattern of metastatic disease.

giographic pattern of metastases will be similar to that seen in lymphoma (Fig. 11). Complete replacement of lymph nodes by tumor may be associated with interruption of lymph flow, resulting in the opacification of collateral pathways, which include lymphatic to lymphatic, lymphatic to prelymphatic, and lymphatic to venous. Once the node is totally replaced, disruption of lymphatic channels is secondary evidence of nodal disease which should be confirmed by additional studies such as pyelography, venography, ultrasonography, computerized tomography, and needle biopsy.

METASTASES IN SOFT TISSUE SARCOMAS

The soft tissue sarcomas that most commonly disseminate by the lymphatic system include malignant fibrous histiocytoma, rhabdomyosarcoma, synovial sarcoma and clear cell sarcomas of the tendon

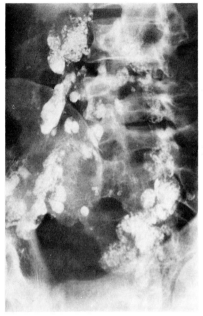

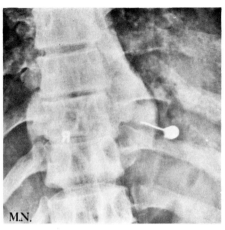

Fig. 11 (left). — Metastatic "lymphoma pattern." Rhabdomyosarcoma of fibular region multiple nodes with abnormal architecture due to metastatic disease, similar to the pattern seen in lymphoma.

Fig. 12 (above). — Metastatic osteogenic sarcoma. Paraspinal mass in a patient, under treatment, with known osteosarcoma of a lower extremity. Specimen was compatible with osteogenic sarcomatous tissue.

sheath, and aponeurosis (Dutra, 1970; Haagensen and Stout, 1943; Patton and Horn, 1962; Ariel and Pack, 1963; Soule and Enriquez, 1972).

Prior to the study of Tallroth (1976) of lymphangiography in sarcomas, no serious attempt was made to document the findings in the lymphangiography of soft tissue tumors. A number of isolated reports, however, are available (Guccion and Enfinger, 1972; Enfinger, 1965; Willis, 1973; Enterline, Culberson, Rochin, and Brady, 1960; Edland, 1968). Tallroth (1976) studied 71 patients with soft tissue sarcomas in a group of 132 skeletal malignancies. Of these 71 patients, 24 had lymph node metastases. This incidence of 33.8% is considerably higher than any previous reports. In this study, no significant metastatic spread was found in patients with fibrosarcoma and liposarcoma. Of 9 patients with rhabdomyosarcoma, particularly the pleomorphic variety, 8 demonstrated metastases to the lymph nodes. Metastases were also diagnosed in 4 of 7 patients with synovial sarcoma, and in 7 of 12 patients with neurogenic sarcoma.

At M. D. Anderson Hospital, lymphangiography was performed in 81 patients with all types of sarcomas (Thaggard, unpublished data).

In this nonrandomized group, 16 were found to have lymph node metastases. Of the 20 patients with rhabdomyosarcoma, 4 were shown to have lymph node metastases. Lymph node involvement was demonstrated in 1 of 8 patients with fibrosarcomas, 2 of 7 with unclassified sarcomas, 1 of 6 with liposarcomas, 1 of 6 with neurogenic sarcomas, and 1 each with synovial sarcomas and clear cell sarcomas. The other 5 patients with sarcomas with lymph node metastases had sarcomas that were of osseous origin.

PERCUTANEOUS TRANSPERITONEAL BIOPSY

Histologic confirmation of lymph node metastases in abdominal, retroperitoneal, and paravertebral masses has been achieved by percutaneous aspiration biopsy utilizing a 23-gauge needle with fluoroscopic guidance (Zornoza et al., in press; Dodd et al. 1976; Gothlin, 1976). The lymph node previously opacified by lymphangiography is localized fluoroscopically and the overlying skin is anesthetized. The 23-gauge needle is passed through a small skin incision into the lymph node of interest. Once in the node, side-to-side synchronous motion confirms the presence of the needle tip within the node. The stylet is removed and suction applied with a 10 cc syringe while the needle is moved up and down through an excursion of 1 cm. The suction is released and the needle withdrawn. The aspirate is placed on glass slides and fixed immediately in 95% alcohol. Experienced cytologic interpretation is imperative to the success of the procedure. The same procedure is used for percutaneous aspiration biopsy of other masses (Fig. 12).

Conclusion

A combined diagnostic effort is necessary for the adequate treatment of soft tissue tumors. Through the use of angiography and lymphangiography, radiology provides essential information in the diagnosis and follow-up of these neoplasms. Although the angiographic findings are not always specific, significant information is provided regarding the extent of disease and the presence of recurrent or residual tumor. Lymphangiography also has proven useful in staging of disease, especially rhabdomyosarcoma, synovial sarcoma, clear cell sarcoma, and malignant fibrous histiocytoma. Lymph node metastases may be confirmed by transperitoneal aspiration biopsy.

Transcatheter intravascular occlusion techniques are available preoperatively to decrease tumor vascularity, thus facilitating surgery. Palliative management of these neoplasms can also be accomplished through arterial embolization to alleviate pain by decreasing tumor bulk and to control acute or chronic hemorrhage.

REFERENCES

Ariel, I. M., and Pack, G. T.: Synovial sarcomas. Review of 25 cases. The New England Journal of Medicine, 268:1272–1275, June 6, 1963.

Bookstein, J. J., Chlosta, E. M., Foley, D., and Walter, J. F.: Transcatheter hemostasis of gastrointestinal bleeding using modified autologous clot. Radiology, 113:277–285, November 1974.

Bree, R. L., Goldstein, H. M., and Wallace, S.: Transcatheter embolization of the internal iliac artery in the management of neoplasms of the pelvis. Surgery, Gynecology and Obstetrics, 143:597–601, October 1976.

Bucalossi, P., and Veronesi, U.: Tumori dell'apparato locomotore, vascolare e di sostegno. *Oncologia Clinica*, Casa editrice Ambrosiana, Milano, 1973, p. 2561.

Denny, M. B. M.: Vascular patterns in tumors of the extremities. South African Medical Journal, 30:27–30, July 1956.

Dodd, G. D., Wallace, S., Jing, B.-S., Paulus, D. D., Jr., Goldstein, H. M., Handel, S. F. and Zornoza, J.: Diagnostic radiologic techniques in the detection, staging and treatment of neoplastic disease. In Clark, R. L., and Howe, C. D., Eds.: *Cancer Patient Care at M. D. Anderson Hospital and Tumor Institute*, Chicago, Illinois, Year Book Medical Publishers, Inc., 1976, pp. 769–823.

Dutra, F. R.: Clear cell sarcoma of the tendons and adoneurosis. Three additional cases. Cancer, 25:942–946, April 1970.

Edland, R. W.: Liposarcoma: A retrospective study of fifteen cases. A review of the literature and a discussion of radiosensitivity. The American Journal of Roentgenology, Radium Therapy and Nuclear Medicine, 103:778–791, August 1968.

Ekelund, L., and Lunderquist, A.: Pharmacoangiography with angiotensin. Radiology, 110:533–540, March 1974.

Enfinger, F. M.: Clear cell sarcoma of the tendons and adoneuroses. An analysis of 21 cases. Cancer, 18:1163–1174, September 1965.

Enterline, H. T., Culberson, J. D., Rochlin, D. B., and Brady, L. W.: Liposarcoma: A clinical and pathological study of 53 cases. Cancer, 13:932–950, September–October 1960.

Gianturco, C., Anderson, J. H., and Wallace, S.: Mechanical devices for arterial occlusion. American Journal of Roentgenology, Radium Therapy and Nuclear Medicine, 124:428–435, July 1975.

Göthlin, J. H.: Post-lymphographic percutaneous fine needle biopsy of lymph node guided by fluoroscopy. Radiology, 120:205–207, July 1976.

Gronner, A. T.: Muscle necrosis simulating a malignant tumor angiographically. Case report. Radiology, 103:309–310, May 1972.

Guccion, J. G., and Enfinger, F. M.: Malignant giant cell tumor of soft parts: An analysis of 52 cases. Cancer, 29:1518–1529, June 1972.

Haagensen, C. D., and Stout, D. P.: Synovial sarcoma. Annals of Surgery, 118:1032–1051, December 1943.

Hawkins, I. F., Jr., and Hudson, T.: Priscoline in bone and soft tissue angiography. Radiology, 110:541–546, March 1974.

Hudson, T. M., Haas, G., Enneking, W. F., and Hawkins, I. F.: Angiography in the management of musculoskeletal tumors. Surgery, Gynecology and Obstetrics, 141:11–21, July 1975.

Hutcheson, J., Klatte, E. C., and Kremp, R.: The angiographic appearance of myositis ossificans circumscripta. A case report. Radiology, 102:57–58, January 1972.

Jacobs, J. B., and Hanafee, W. N.: The use of priscoline in peripheral arteriography. Radiology, 88:957–960, May 1967.

Levin, D. C., Gordon, D. H., and McSweeney, I.: Arteriography of peripheral hemangiomas. Radiology, 121:625–630, December 1976.

Martel, W., and Abell, M. R.: Radiologic evaluation of soft tissue tumors. A retrospective study. Cancer, 32:352–366, August 1973.

Ney, F. G., Feist, J. H., Altemus, L., and Ordinario, V. R.: The characteristic angiographic criteria of malignancy. Radiology, 104:567–570, September 1972.

Patton, R. B., and Horn, R. C., Jr.: Rhabdomyosarcoma: Clinical and pathological features and comparison with human fetal and embryonal skeletal muscle. Surgery, 52:572–584, June 1962.

Rockoff, S. D., Doppman, J., Block, J. B., and Ketchan, A.: Variable response of tumor vessels to intra-arterial epinephrine: An angiographic study in man. Investigative Radiology, 1:205–213, May–June 1966.

Simon, M. A., and Enneking, W. F.: The management of soft tissue tumors of the extremities. Journal of Bone and Joint Surgery, 58A:317–327, April 1976.

Soule, E. H., and Enriquez, P.: Atypical fibrous histiocytoma, malignant fibrous histiocytoma, malignant histiocytoma and epitheloid sarcoma. A comparative study of 65 tumors. Cancer, 30:128–143, July 1972.

Suit, H. D., Russell, W. O., and Martin, R. G.: Management of patients with sarcoma of soft tissue in an extremity. Cancer, 31:1247–1255, May 1973.

Tadavarthy, S. M., Knight, L., Ovitt, T. W., Snyder, C., and Amplatz, K.: Therapeutic transcatheter arterial embolization. Radiology, 112:13–16, July 1974.

Tallroth, K.: In Paperi, J. A., and Painotuote, K., Eds. *Lymphatic Dissemination of Bone and Soft Tissue Sarcomas.* Helsinki, Finland, 1976.

Thaggard, A., Wallace, S., and Jing, B.-S.: Lymphangiography in sarcomas. Unpublished data.

Viamonte, M., Jr., Roen, S., and LaPage, J.: Nonspecificity of abnormal vascularity in the angiographic diagnosis of malignant neoplasms. Radiology, 106:59–63, January 1973.

Wallace, S.: Dynamics of normal and abnormal lymphatic systems as studied with contrast media. Cancer Chemotherapy Reports, 52:31–58, January 1968.

Wallace, S., et al.: Therapeutic vascular occlusion utilizing steel coil technique: Clinical applications. American Journal of Roentgenology, Radium Therapy and Nuclear Medicine, 127:381–387, September 1976.

Wallace, S., and Goldstein, H. M.: Intravascular occlusive therapy. Postgraduate Medicine, 59:141–146, February 1976.

Wallace, S., and Jackson, L.: Lymphangiography. Encyclopedia of Medicine, 3:307–323, 1964.

Wallace, S., Jackson, L., Dodd, G. D., and Greening, R. R.: Lymphangiographic interpretation. *Radiologic Clinics of North America,* Philadelphia, Pennsylvania, W. B. Saunders Co., December 1965.

Wallace, S., and Jing, B.-S.: Lymphangiography in carcinoma. In Clouse, M., Ed. *Golden Diagnostic Radiology.* Baltimore, Maryland, Williams and Wilkins Company. (In press.)

Wallace, S., Medellin, H., De Jongh, D. S., and Gianturco, C.: Systemic heparinization for angiography. American Journal of Roentgenology, Radium Therapy, and Nuclear Medicine, 116:204–209, September 1972.

Willis, R. A.: *The Spread of Tumors in the Human Body.* 3rd edition. London, England, Butterworth, 1973, 417 pp.

Zornoza, J., *et al.*: Transperitoneal percutaneous retroperitoneal lymph node aspiration biopsy. Radiology. (In press.)

Biopsy of Soft Tissue Tumors

MARVIN M. ROMSDAHL, M.D., Ph.D.

*Department of Surgery, The University of Texas System
Cancer Center M. D. Anderson Hospital and Tumor Institute,
Houston, Texas*

BIOPSY OF SOFT TISSUE tumors is mandatory for establishing a diagnosis and for planning a rational program of treatment. The principles relating to this important procedure, which may seem obvious, are often now acknowledged by physicians who first see the majority of patients with this problem. A standard approach to biopsy of soft tissue tumors is not practical, since their behavior and clinical presentation vary widely. Finally, a unified concept with regard to management of these tumors has not yet emerged, although there is progress toward this goal.

Fundamentally, there are 3 different procedures which are usually employed to obtain tissue from a lesion suspected of being a soft tissue sarcoma. These are: needle biopsy, incisional biopsy, and excisional biopsy.

NEEDLE BIOPSY

A needle biopsy is usually not the procedure of choice for the following reasons:

(1) The small core of tissue obtained will usually disclose only whether the tumor is malignant. One can usually determine, however, whether a lesion is a "small" cell type and, therefore, characteristic of either rhabdomyosarcoma or lymphoma. It is difficult to obtain a margin or the leading edge of the primary tumor, and specific classification is substantially compromised.

(2) Sufficient tissue is not obtained by needle biopsy to permit a

wide variety of special diagnostic stains, which are often helpful in characterizing these tumors.

(3) A needle biopsy will yield tissue from a restricted region of the tumor and it may, therefore, not be as representative of the entire tumor as tissue obtained by other types of biopsies.

Needle biopsies are helpful, however, in securing tissue to document suspected recurrence in a formerly treated wound. This may suffice to permit further definitive treatment. They are also helpful in those circumstances in which a very large lesion requires only the documentation of malignancy to institute further therapy; however, this is rare, since therapy often depends on a specific classification of the soft tissue tumor.

INCISIONAL BIOPSY

The indications for incisional biopsy are few and highly specific.

(1) The most frequent indication for incisional biopsy is in the case of large soft tissue tumors which, because of size or location, either are not resectable or are resectable only with substantial risk of deformity. It has been our practice to utilize either preoperative X-ray therapy or, occasionally, chemotherapy to reduce a large or strategically located tumor to smaller dimensions. Consequently, it is vital to obtain accurate classifications initially. While preoperative radiotherapy and chemotherapy are often effective in reducing the size of large soft tissue neoplasms, these measures can also be expected to render further attempts at classification more difficult, when complete excision is eventually performed.

(2) Incisional biopsy is the procedure of choice when a mass, whether external or within one of the major body cavities, is unresectable. Accurate histological classification will serve to determine prognosis and help to form the basis for treatment of similar tumors subsequently encountered.

EXCISIONAL BIOPSY

Excisional biopsy is the procedure of choice as the initial measure for most soft tissue sarcomas. This method is especially preferred for small lesions and those considered suitable for complete surgical extirpation (Fig. 1). In this regard, the procedure of "shelling out" a circumscribed tumor, often by blunt dissection, is strongly condemned. Excisional biopsies should include a minimum of 1 to 2 cm of normal tissue adjacent to the primary tumor mass. This will often require

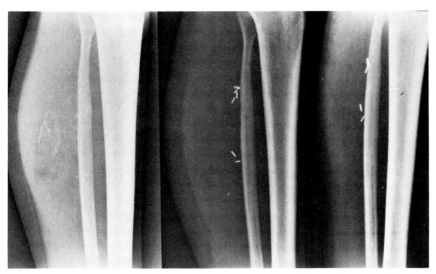

Fig. 1.—The soft tissue tumor is visualized on the left. Following excisional biopsy, with a 2 cm margin of normal tissue, the upper and lower margins of the surgical wound were referenced by the placement of small silver clips.

great care and appreciation of the 3-dimensional aspects of such tumors. While excisional biopsy, as described, may well not represent the final aspect of management, it does serve to minimize prospects for local recurrence, which commonly range from 20% to 40% (Lindberg, Martin, and Romsdahl, 1975; Cantin, McNeer, Chu, and Booker, 1968).

LENGTH AND PLACEMENT OF BIOPSY INCISIONS

LENGTH.—Biopsy incisions should ideally be only the approximate length of the presumed neoplasm. It is not good judgement to attempt excision of a soft tissue neoplasm through an incision smaller than the largest tumor diameter. Similarly, it is not necessary to make incisions considerably longer than the underlying lesion.

PLACEMENT.—Incisions are ideally placed for ease in gaining direct access to the tumor. However, when feasible, an incision may be made to one side of a lesion in order to gain a degree of remoteness from the adjacent bone or joint. In circumstances where incisional biopsies are required, it is well to anticipate possible future surgery and placement of the incision to permit its complete inclusion in subsequent resections.

CONSERVATIVE SURGERY

Radical surgery for soft tissue sarcomas has been practiced in past years at The University of Texas System Cancer Center M. D. Anderson Hospital as well as at many other cancer centers (Simon and Enneking, 1976). This approach usually will include margins of adjacent normal tissue ranging from 5 to 10 cm on all sides of the tumor, as well as entire muscles or muscle groups. Conservative surgery, on the contrary, designates excisions whereby the lesion is excised with definite, but smaller margins of normal tissue. In accomplishing this, an attempt is made to restrict the incision and field without compromising on complete extirpation of the soft tissue neoplasm. This approach serves to minimize physical deformity and also to localize the area of potential tumor recurrence by implantation of tumor cells. Conservative surgery is especially appropriate for our present program of man-

Fig. 2.— Following wide excision of a large rhabdomyosarcoma from the thigh, silver clips were used to indicate the surgical field in the anterior *(left)* and lateral views *(right)* in the postoperative period.

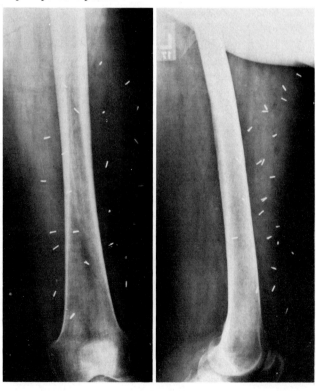

agement for soft tissue sarcomas which includes complete surgical excision followed by radiation therapy (Lindberg, Martin, Romsdahl, and McMurtrey, 1977, pages 289–298, this volume). It is feasible, therefore, to restrict the fields of radiotherapy, which should extend somewhat beyond the margins of the surgical dissection.

CONCEPT OF SUBCLINICAL OR MICROSCOPIC DISEASE

The rationale for our approach to the biopsy and subsequent management of soft tissue sarcomas is partly based on the concept of subclinical or microscopic disease (Fletcher, 1972). In this regard, the surgical field of the primary lesion is considered at high risk for contamination by either freely dispersed cancer cells or extremely small nests of tumor in adventitia, lymphatics, or vessels within the surgical area. This extension of disease is *not* apparent grossly and may even be missed by careful pathological review of excised so-called "normal tissue" boundaries. This concept is supported by the high rate of local wound recurrence for most types of sarcomas encountered in clinical practice. It is this presumed involvement for which radiotherapy is utilized as an adjunct to conservative surgery for soft tissue sarcomas at our institution.

Fig. 3.—**A,** a large soft tissue sarcoma was excised from the thigh and the wound margins identified with silver clips. The left frame in each composite was taken in the early postoperative period and the right frames were taken 9 months later. **B,** lateral views showing the lower aspects of the same operative field. Note the increased compactness of the area designated as the surgical wound on the right in both composites.

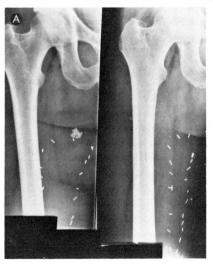
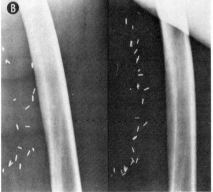

RADIOLOGICAL MARKING OF SURGICAL FIELDS

Following surgical excision of sarcoma tumors, it is feasible to outline the margins of the surgical field with small silver clips. A routine X-ray examination will then define precisely the extent of the operative procedure and assist the radiotherapist in demarcating fields for radiotherapy (Fig. 2). The position and arrangement of such clips can sometimes serve to suggest recurrence of disease, since they usually remain in a fixed position after complete wound healing (Fig. 3A and B).

Summary

A consideration of different aspects of a multidisciplinary approach to the management of soft tissue sarcomas indicates certain procedures which show promise in improving our management of this group of tumors. The physician who initially encounters the patient with a soft tissue tumor is usually the one responsible for performing the biopsy and establishing the diagnosis. The type of biopsy taken should be based on features relating to clinical presentation, but one should also consider tactical approaches to further surgical treatment and management.

Acknowledgments

This study was supported in part by funds from various donors for surgical research on sarcomas.

REFERENCES

Cantin, J., McNeer, G. P., Chu, F. C., and Booker, R. J.: The problem of local recurrence after treatment of soft tissue sarcoma. Annals of Surgery, 168:47–53, 1968.

Fletcher, G. H.: Elective irradiation of subclinical disease in cancers of the head and neck. Cancer, 29:1450–1454, 1972.

Lindberg, R. D., Martin, R. G., and Romsdahl, M. M.: Surgery and postoperative radiotherapy in the treatment of soft tissue sarcomas in adults. The American Journal of Roentgenology, Radium Therapy and Nuclear Medicine, 123:123–129, 1975.

Lindberg, R. D., Martin, R. G., Romsdahl, M. M., and McMurtrey, M. J.: Conservative surgery and radiation therapy for soft tissue sarcomas. In *Current Concepts in the Management of Primary Bone and Soft Tissue Tumors* (The University of Texas System Cancer Center M. D. Anderson

Hospital and Tumor Institute, 21st Annual Clinical Conference on Cancer). Chicago, Illinois, Year Book Medical Publishers, Inc., 1977, pp. 289–298.

Simon, M. A., and Enneking, W. F.: The management of soft tissue sarcomas of the extremities. Journal of Bone and Joint Surgery, 58A:317–327, 1976.

Electron Microscopy of Soft Tissue Tumors

BRUCE MACKAY, M.D., Ph.D.

Department of Pathology, The University of Texas
System Cancer Center M. D. Anderson Hospital and Tumor Institute,
Houston, Texas

THE BASIC PRINCIPLE of diagnostic electron microscopy in oncology is the identification of ultrastructural features of normal cells that are recapitulated in the neoplastic cells. A number of the soft tissues of the body possess unique morphologic features, and consequently, electron microscopy is helpful in identifying cell types and classifying the soft tissue neoplasms. Since at least 15% of the malignant soft tissue tumors cannot be adequately classified by light microscopy (Martin, Lindberg, Sinkovics, and Butler, 1976), the role of electron microscopy in the diagnosis of sarcomas is one of practical significance to the surgical pathologist and clinician. Despite the interesting challenge they present, sarcomas have not been extensively studied by electron microscopy; probably many pathologists with access to an ultrastructural laboratory experience difficulty in obtaining numbers of adequately preserved specimens.

The practical value of a sound subclassification of neoplasms of the soft tissues might be debated by clinicians to whom the diagnosis of benign or malignant soft tissue tumor is all that is required to determine selection of therapy, but it is to be hoped that a more enlightened attitude is developing. Assessment of biologic behavior and response to various forms of therapy must be related to the type of tumor. At the present time, this is particularly relevant as the effectiveness of chemotherapeutic agents in the treatment of the soft tissue tumors is evaluated.

In any ultrastructural study, it is mandatory that material be representative and suitably preserved and processed. Small amounts of tissue are acceptable, but while a needle biopsy may be adequate for identification of cell type, it will not reflect the range of histologic variation that may be present within a large tumor. The potential of thin needle biopsies as a source of material for diagnostic electron microscopy has not yet been adequately explored. At present, most specimens are obtained from open biopsies or surgical resections. Our routine practice is to obtain the tissue promptly and to select an area from a freshly exposed cut surface that shows no evidence of hemorrhage or necrosis. A slender wedge, not more than 1 mm in maximum thickness, is sliced from the tissue, using a clean scapel or razor blade, and is immersed in 2% buffered glutaraldehyde. The electron micrographs in this paper are of Epon-embedded thin sections, stained with lead hydroxide and uranyl acetate, and photographed using a Zeiss EM 9-S electron microscope.

The tumors that are discussed were selected somewhat arbitrarily, but it is hoped that they will illustrate the contribution that electron microscopy can provide as a supplement to light microscopy in the study of soft tissue tumors as well as demonstrate that information so obtained is not merely of academic interest, but that electron microscopy is a practical new dimension in diagnostic oncology.

Fibrosarcoma, Leiomyosarcoma, Liposarcoma

The ultrastructural features of the cells of most fibrosarcomas, leiomyosarcomas, and liposarcomas should serve to identify all but the least differentiated tumors. It is now apparent, however, that some tumors are composed of cells whose morphology is intermediate among these established entities; possibily it would be correct to view them as fitting within a spectrum of interrelated neoplasms.

Figure 1 shows part of a cell from a spindle cell tumor that was infiltrating the submandibular gland and surrounding soft tissues in a 2-month-old boy. The electron micrograph demonstrates the profusion of irregularly distended cisternae of granular endoplasmic reticulum that characterizes normal fibroblasts and the cells of most normal fibrosarcomas. The number of cisternae decreases with dedifferentiation. Evidence of collagen production can usually be seen in the presence of precollagen filaments in the peripheral cytoplasm, and the stroma often contains dense bundles of collagen fibrils.

In cells of the benign and better differentiated malignant smooth

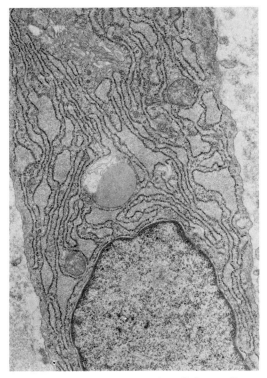

Fig. 1.—Electron micrograph showing part of a cell from a fibrosarcoma infiltrating the submaxillary gland of a 2-month-old boy. The cytoplasm contains numerous cisternae of granular endoplasmic reticulum. (×19,000.)

muscle tumors (Morales, Fine, Pardo, and Horn, 1975), the endoplasmic reticulum is confined to a small number of cisternae aggregated close to the poles of the nucleus, together with a few mitochondria and a golgi complex. The cytoplasm contains longitudinally aligned, slender (approximately 60 Å) filaments with interspersed small densities similar to those seen in normal smooth muscle cells. Dense zones are also present at the cell membrane, with varying numbers of pinocytotic vesicles.

Cells having ultrastructural features of both fibroblasts and smooth muscle cells have been described and called myofibroblasts. They have the basic fine structure of fibroblasts, but also contain bundles of smooth muscle myofilaments. The filaments are confined to the peripheral cytoplasm, and they vary in quantity. Cells of this type have been reported in hypertrophic scars (Kischer, 1974) and granulation tissue (Ryan *et al.*, 1974); an interesting aspect is the apparent attachment of the outer surface of the cell membrane to surrounding stroma by slender bundles of fine filaments (Fig. 2). It has been suggested that myofibroblasts may be responsible for scar contracture (Gabbiani and Majno, 1972). We have encountered these cells in benign and malignant tumors that were considered to be neoplasms of fibroblasts by light microscopy.

In cells of liposarcomas, it is common to find cytoplasmic lipid droplets, but they vary in number and size. Collagen fibrils in the electron-lucent stroma are usually restricted to scattered small bundles. Since lipid droplets may also be found in small numbers of fibrosarcomas and other tumors, their presence is not diagnostic. In some liposarcomas, lipid droplets are not conspicuous, but the endoplasmic reticulum is plentiful and the cisternae are distended with finely granular material that may show central condensations. More information is needed about the cytophysiology of adipose cells in order to explain the ultrastructural appearances seen in liposarcomas. Figure 3 shows

Fig. 2 (left).—Myofibroblast. In addition to the granular reticulum, the cytoplasm contains peripheral smooth muscle filaments, and a slender bundle of filaments continues from the cell surface out into the adjacent stroma. (×20,000.)

Fig. 3 (right).—Finely granular, moderately electron-dense material fills cisternae of granular endoplasmic reticulum in the cytoplasm of a liposarcoma cell. (×23,000.)

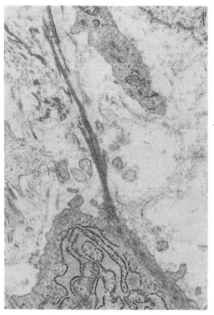 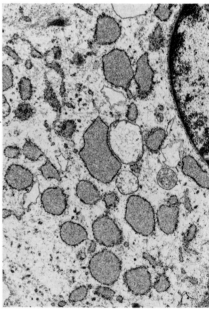

distended granular reticulum in a cell from a liposarcoma of the thigh in a 55-year-old woman.

There appears to be considerable overlap between the morphology of liposarcomas and that of malignant fibrous histiocytomas. Electron-dense material may accumulate within the endoplasmic reticulum of some malignant fibrous histiocytomas and the so-called atypical fibrous xanthomas (Fig. 4). The cells of most malignant fibrous histio-cytomas that we have studied have resembled fibroblasts, although they show more variation in size and shape; some are multinucleated, and the nuclei have irregular profiles (Fig. 5). The cytoplasm may show evidence of lipid production. Lysosomes are sometimes present, and histiocytes are commonly intermingled with the tumor cells, al-though they are not a proven neoplastic component (Soule and Enri-quez, 1972). On occasion, it is not possible to determine by either light or electron microscopy whether a particular tumor is a malignant fibrous histiocytoma or a liposarcoma.

Fig. 4 (left).—Round condensations of material are present in the cisternae of this tumor cell from a crusting lesion of the temple skin in a 78-year-old man. The differ-ential diagnosis was between atypical fibrous xanthoma and malignant fibrous histio-cytoma, and because of the degree of mitotic activity, the latter diagnosis was favored. (×8,200.)

Fig. 5 (right).—Part of a multinucleated cell from a malignant fibrous histiocytoma demonstrating the irregular nuclear profiles. (×4,500.)

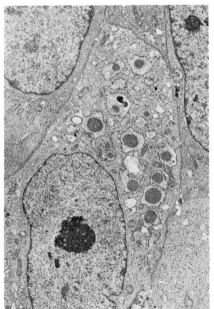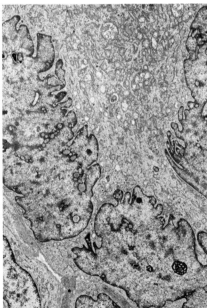

Sarcomas Ascribed to Cells of Synovium or Tendon Sheath

Synovial sarcomas do not always occur in relation to a joint, and there has been speculation whether these tumors are in fact derived from synovial lining cells (Cadman, 1965). The ultrastructural similarities between cells of the glandular and spindle components in biphasic tumors raise the possibility that the 2 may be related. Figure 6 shows an electron micrograph of part of a glandular aggregate from a pulmonary metastasis of a synovial sarcoma that occurred in the region of the knee in a 16-year-old boy. The tumor was biphasic in both locations, but the epithelial component predominated in the metastasis. The cells form a typical acinar grouping, limited by a basal lamina. Adjacent cells are united by desmosomes, and junctional complexes are present at the luminal margin. Microvilli are common, but they vary in size, shape, and number. We have observed some similarities between cells of synovial sarcoma and those of normal human synovi-

Fig. 6.—Metastatic synovial sarcoma in lung. The cells in a glandular aggregate are united by junctional complexes at the luminal margin. (×18,000.)

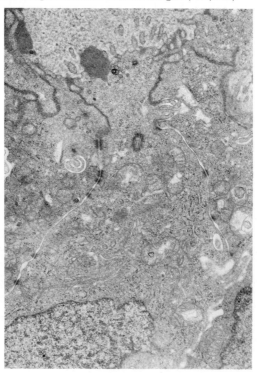

al membrane (Mackay, in press), but the histogenesis of synovial sarcoma remains controversial.

The term epithelioid sarcoma was introduced by Dr. Franz Enzinger in 1970. These neoplasms are composed of cells with acidophilic cytoplasm; they commonly occur in the extremities, are often superficial and ulcerated, have a multinodular growth pattern, and tend to extend along fascial planes (Enzinger, 1977, see pages 219–234, this volume). They may readily be confused with epithelial neoplasms, melanoma, or granulomatous inflammation, and recognition is important since they tend to recur and will metastasize if the primary lesion is not promptly and effectively treated. Figure 7 shows the light microscopic appearance of an epithelioid sarcoma from the ankle of a 50-year-old man who also had tumor in his groin and who has subsequently died with disseminated metastases. An electron micrograph of tumor cells from a chest wall metastasis in the same patient is shown in Figure 8. There are probably no specific ultrastructural features that will definitely distinguish epithelioid sarcoma from other neoplasms that it may simulate by light microscopy, but the combined light and electron microscopy, taken in conjunction with the clinical

Fig. 7 (left).—Epithelioid sarcoma of the ankle in a 50-year-old man. (×400.)
Fig. 8 (right).—Cell from chest wall metastasis of the tumor shown in the preceding figure. Organelles are sparse, and the cytoplasm contains fine filaments. (×18,000.)

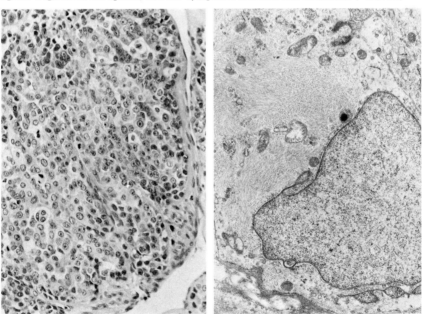

setting, should be sufficient to establish the diagnosis. The tumor cells are round or polygonal, and are usually closely apposed. Elongated cells may occur. The cytoplasm contains the usual organelles; they are not numerous, but mitochondria may be present in groups. A feature that we have observed in several cases is the presence of slender filaments in irregular bundles that may be concentrically oriented and are often more numerous in the perinuclear cytoplasm (Fig. 8). The filaments are only found in some cells of a particular tumor, and their significance is not known.

Tendon sheath has been implicated as a possible tissue of origin for the so-called clear cell sarcoma (Enzinger, 1965). Lucent cytoplasm can result from accumulation of glycogen or lipid, or from overhydration and other degenerative changes, and there is a tendency to misuse the diagnosis. The nature of clear cell sarcoma, or its existence as a specific entity, consequently, are unsettled issues. Figure 9 shows the light microscopic appearance of a tumor of the foot in a 29-year-old woman who died within 4 months of diagnosis with widely dissemi-

Fig. 9 (left).— Sarcoma of the foot in a 29-year-old woman. The tumor was called a clear cell sarcoma by light microscopy. Electron microscopy demonstrated the presence of premelanosomes in the tumor cells. (×400.)

Fig. 10 (right).— Numerous closely apposed cytoplasmic processes of cells of an intra-abdominal neurosarcoma. (×16,000.)

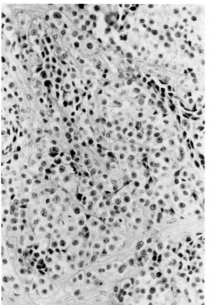 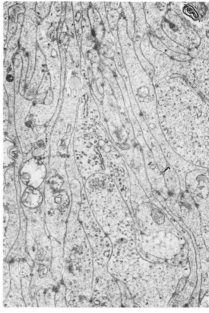

nated metastases. The tumor was called clear cell sarcoma by light microscopy, but an intriguing finding was the presence of premelanosomes in the cytoplasm of the tumor cells by electron microscopy. A tumor cell line was established by Dr. Joseph Sinkovics, and premelanosomes could still be demonstrated after 4 passages. We have seen other tumors with a similar appearance by light and electron microscopy, and the occurrence of melanin in tumors designated clear cell sarcomas has been reported (Bearman, Noe, and Kempson, 1975; Hoffman and Carter, 1973). Conceivably, melanocytes might become diverted during their embryonic migration from neural crest to epidermis, and become attached to deeper tissues where neoplastic transformation could later develop (DasGupta, 1969).

Peripheral Nerve Sheath Tumors

Benign tumors of the peripheral nerves are readily identified by light microscopy, and their ultrastructure has been documented (Waggener, 1966). In contrast, the histologic spectrum of related sarcomas is poorly defined, and the diagnosis of neurosarcoma often depends on a history of neurofibromatosis or the development of malignant change within a benign tumor. Delineation of electron microscopic criteria for the recognition of neurogenic sarcomas would thus be useful to the surgical pathologist.

Some pertinent data can be gleaned from observations of benign neoplasms. Schwannoma and neurofibroma cells possess cytoplasmic extensions that can be many times the length of the cell body, and zones of the neoplasm may be occupied by these branching processes. In an area of palisading, the rows of nuclei are separated by bands of acidophilic material in light microscopic sections, and these areas are largely occupied by parallel or interweaving processes. Elongated mitochondria, longitudinally oriented microtubules, and fine filaments may be found in the processes, and it is common to find an investing basal lamina, but Schwannian cytoplasm is often absent.

We have now seen a number of sarcomas with electron microscopic features similar to those of benign nerve sheath tumors, suggesting that they are neurosarcomas (malignant schwannomas). One case is discussed in the Ninth Annual Special Pathology Program (1977, see pages 433–464, this volume). The long cytoplasmic extensions may run parallel, or pursue a tortuous course among processes of other cells, and a basal lamina is frequently absent. Microtubules and filaments occur in some processes. The cells may be loosely arranged in a relatively structureless matrix which corresponds to the myxoid zones seen by light microscopy. More often they are compactly grouped, and the tendency is then for close apposition of the processes (Fig. 10). Apposed cell membranes are commonly joined by cell membrane specializations that simulate interneuronal synapses. The common organelles are present in the cytoplasm of the cell body, but they are sparse in the processes. Straight or curved rows of nuclei separated by intervening zones of processes and scanty stroma can create a distinctive appearance by light microscopy that resembles the typical palisading architecture of many benign nerve sheath tumors. An analogy may be seen in the rosette formation of neuroblastomas, where the interior of the rosette is occupied by a tangle of dendritic processes of the neuroblastoma cells (Mackay, Luna, and Butler, 1976). Unlike the neuroblastomas, however, the cells of neurosarcomas do not contain significant numbers of neurosecretory granules.

In this paper, it has only been possible to focus on a small number of the soft tissue tumors that we have so far examined by correlated light and electron microscopy. In order to define the range of ultrastructural appearances of the various tumor types, and to provide clues for some of the persisting histogenetic puzzles, many more cases must be studied. Collaborative ventures between pathologists and clinicians have the potential to broaden our understanding of the relationships of these tumors, and their behavior, and can lead to the development of selective therapeutic regimens so that the patients will be the ultimate beneficiaries.

Acknowledgments

The technical assistance of Mrs. Joyce Cox, Miss Diana Garza, and Mrs. Mary Seeley is gratefully acknowledged.

The Zeiss electron microscope was purchased with the aid of a generous grant from the Kelsey and Leary Foundation.

REFERENCES

Ayala, A. G., and Enzinger, F.: Soft Tissue Neoplasms: A clinicopathologic discussion. In *Management of Bone and Soft Tissue Tumors* (The University of Texas System Cancer Center M. D. Anderson Hospital and Tumor Institute, 21st Annual Clinical Conference on Cancer). Chicago, Illinois, Year Book Medical Publishers, Inc., 1977, pp. 433–464.

Bearman, R. M., Noe, J., and Kempson, R. L.: Clear cell sarcoma with melanin pigment. Cancer, 36:977–984, September 1975.

Cadman, N. L., Soule, E. H., and Kelly, P. J.: Synovial sarcoma. An analysis of 134 tumors. Cancer, 18:613–627, May 1965.

DasGupta, T. K., Brasfield, R. D., and Paglia, M. A.: Primary melanomas in unusual sites. A collective review. Surgery, Gynecology, and Obstetrics, 12: 841–848, April 1969.

Enzinger, F. M.: Clear cell sarcoma of tendons and aponeuroses. An analysis of 21 cases. Cancer, 18:1163–1174, September 1965.

———: Epithelioid sarcoma. A sarcoma simulating a granuloma or a carcinoma. Cancer, 26:1029–1041, November 1970.

———: Recent developments in the classification of soft tissue sarcomas. In *Management of Bone and Soft Tissue Tumors* (The University of Texas System Cancer Center M. D. Anderson Hospital and Tumor Institute, 21st Annual Clinical Conference on Cancer). Chicago, Illinois, Year Book Medical Publishers, Inc., 1977, pp. 219–234.

Gabbiani, G. and Majno, G.: Dupuytren's contracture: Fibroblast contraction? An ultrastructural study. American Journal of Pathology, 66:131–138, January 1972.

Hoffman, G. J., and Carter, D.: Clear cell sarcoma of tendons and aponeuroses with melanin. Archives of Pathology, 95:22–25, January 1973.

Kischer, C. W.: Fibroblasts of the hypertropic scar, mature scar and normal skin. A study by scanning and transmission electron microscopy. Texas Reports on Biology and Medicine, 32:699–709, Fall and Winter 1974.

Mackay, B.: Soft tissue tumors. In Bennington, J. L., Ed.: *Major Problems in Pathology.* (In press.)

Mackay, B., Luna, M. A., and Butler, J. J.: Adult neuroblastoma. Electron microscopic observations in 9 cases. Cancer, 37:1334–1351, March 1976.

Martin, R. G., Lindberg, R. D., Sinkovics, J. C., and Butler, J. J.: Soft-tissue sarcomas. In Clark, R. L., and Howe, C. D., Eds.: *Cancer Patient Care at M. D. Anderson Hospital and Tumor Institute.* Chicago, Illinois, Year Book Medical Publishers, Inc., 1976, pp. 473–483.

Morales, A. R., Fine, G., Pardo, V., and Horn, R. C., Jr.: The ultrastructure of smooth muscle tumors with a consideration of the possible relationship of glomangiomas, hemangiopericytomas, and cardiac myxomas. Pathology Annual, 10:65–92, 1975.

Rayn, G. B., Cliff, W. J., Gabbiani, G., Irle, C., Montandon, D., Statkov, P. R., and Majno, G.: Myofibroblasts in human granulation tissue. Human Pathology, 5:55–67, January 1974.

Soule, E. H., and Enriquez, P.: Atypical fibrous histiocytoma, malignant fibrous histiocytoma, malignant histiocytoma, and epithelioid sarcoma. A comparative study of 65 tumors. Cancer, 30:128–143, July 1972.

Waggener, J. D.: Ultrastructure of benign peripheral nerve sheath tumors. Cancer, 19:699–709, May 1966.

Staging Soft Tissue Sarcoma

Review from the American Joint Committee Task Force on
Soft Tissue Sarcoma

WILLIAM O. RUSSELL, M.D., JONATHAN COHEN,
M.D., FRANZ ENZINGER, M.D., STEVEN I. HAJDU,
M.D., HERMAN HEISE, B.S., RICHARD G. MARTIN,
M.D., WILLIAM MEISSNER, M.D., WALLACE T.
MILLER, M.D., ROBERT L. SCHMITZ, M.D., and
HERMAN D. SUIT, M.D.

M. D. Anderson Hospital, Houston, Texas
Children's Hospital Medical Center, Boston,
Massachusetts
Armed Forces Institute of Pathology, Washington, D.C.
Memorial Hospital for Cancer and Allied Disease, New
York, New York
National Cancer Institute, Bethesda, Maryland
M. D. Anderson Hospital, Houston, Texas
New England Deaconess Hospital, Boston,
Massachusetts
Hospitals of the University of Pennsylvania,
Philadelphia, Pennsylvania
University of Illinois Mercy Hospital and Medical
Center, Chicago, Illinois
Massachusetts General Hospital, Boston, Massachusetts

Introduction

AT PRESENT, NO CLASSIFICATION EXISTS for staging soft tissue sarcomas based on clinical as well as pathologic data. Such a classification is needed for the purpose of planning therapy to be administered in cooperative therapeutic centers. It also is needed to allow quality control of data for analysis and reporting end results. These needs have increased substantially in the past years as a result of the greatly increased application of radiotherapy, chemotherapy, and immunotherapy. During the past 8 years, a Soft Tissue Sarcoma Task Force appointed by the American Joint Committee for Cancer Staging and End Results Reporting (A.J.C.) has developed and tested a clinical and pathological staging system for these tumors (American Joint Committee for Cancer Staging and End Results Reporting, in press; Russell *et al.*, in press).

This presentation will review the staging system developed by the (A.J.C.) Task Force on Soft Tissue Sarcoma, delineating the 4 stages employed, with the basis for their determination and clinical use. The reader is referred to the Task Force report for further details of the staging system and its evolution (Russell *et al.*, in press).

Materials and Methods

The system was constructed and evaluated from a retrospective study of 1,215 cases of histologically confirmed soft tissue sarcomas seen over a 15-year period. Each case was followed by a 5-year interval to provide a minimum of 5 years follow-up. The material was obtained from 13 institutions. In 600 of the cases, slide review was done by the pathologists of the Task Force; malignancy grade was determined in 437 cases. The T(tumor)-N(nodes)-M(metastases) system was augmented to include the malignancy grade of the tumor as G (grade). In the staging of soft tissue sarcoma, the type of tumor, its size, and its malignancy grade are fundamental parameters. The grade levels used in the system are the results of assessment of malignancy made by the pathologist from the histologic study of representative biopsy specimens of the tumor. With the pathologists' histologic input, soft tissue sarcoma staging became the G-T-N-M system.

The 1,215 sarcomas on which the staging system was based included extraskeletal mesenchymal neoplasms, but did not include either those sarcomas arising within the confines of the dura mater, including the brain, or those sarcomas arising in parenchymatous organs and hollow viscera. Kaposi's hemorrhagic sarcoma, a tumor primarily of soft parts, also was excluded from the angiosarcoma group because of its multiple sites of origin and its bizarre pattern of progression and extension. Finally, dermatofibrosarcoma and fibrosarcoma Grade 1 (desmoid type) were also excluded because metastasis rarely if ever occurs with these lesions and the prognosis, therefore, is uniformly favorable.

The following 13 soft tissue sarcomas have been evaluated and tested for this staging system:

1. Alveolar soft parts sarcoma
2. Angiosarcoma
3. Extraskeletal chondrosarcoma
4. Extraskeletal osteosarcoma
5. Fibrosarcoma.
6. Leiomyosarcoma ,
7. Liposarcoma .
8. Malignant fibrohistiocytoma
9. Malignant mesenchymoma
10. Malignant schwannoma
11. Rhabdomyosarcoma.
12. Synovial sarcoma
13. Sarcoma, type not designated

For 10% of soft tissue lesions that we found definable only as "sarcoma" but not recognizable as an established type, we used the term "sarcoma, type not designated." This group of so-called hard core of unclassifiable lesions, therefore, becomes a working category and, in fact, a tumor type.

SOFT TISSUE SARCOMA STAGING SYSTEM OF THE AMERICAN JOINT COMMITTEE

The definitions of the G-T-N-M categories for soft tissue sarcoma are as follows:

G — Pathologic Grade Of Malignancy

G_1, low
G_2, moderate
G_3, high

The grade of malignancy given by the pathologist is a malignancy assessment of the tumor, taking into account such factors as cellularity, cellular pleomorphism, number of mitotic figures, capsule formation, vascularity, necrosis, and the production of indentifiable intra- and extracellular substances. Other factors include the age of the patient and the location of the tumor. There are some tumors, such as rhabdomyosarcoma and certain types of angiosarcoma and synovial sarcoma, that were designated as Grade 3 neoplasms because of their established high-level aggressiveness, even though they may have lacked the advanced histologic characteristics of Grade 3 neoplasms. The patient's age also was a factor because fibrosarcomas in childhood have a more favorable prognosis than do the adult forms. Superficially located tumors obviously have a more favorable outlook than deep-seated ones. For simplicity's sake, these factors were considered part of the malignancy evaluation and became integral factors used, together with histological features, in determining the G (grade), which was added to the T-N-M designations.

T — Primary Tumor

T_1, Tumor less than 5 cm

T_2, Tumor greater than 5 cm

T_3, Tumor which grossly invades a bone, a major vessel, or a major nerve

N — Regional Lymph Nodes

N_0, No histologically verified metastases to lymph nodes

N_1, Histologically verified lymph node metastases

M — Distant Metastases

M_0, No distant metastases

M_1, Distant metastases

Because of the difficulty in obtaining histologic verification of the nature of distant metastases in parenchymatous viscera, such verification was not required. Rather, roentgenographic evidence, isotopic scan, lymphangiograms, and angiograms, when positive, were accepted as evidence of disseminated disease.

Staging

With these definitions for G, T, N, and M, 4 stages were identified, based on 702 cases of the series in which complete information for staging was available, and including 423 cases histologically reviewed and graded by 4 pathologists on the Soft Tissue Task Force.

Stage I

Stage Ia

$G_1 T_1 N_0 M_0$ A Grade 1 tumor less than 5 cm in diameter, with no regional lymph node or distant metastases.

Stage Ib

$G_1 T_2 N_0 M_0$ A Grade 1 tumor 5 cm or greater in diameter, with no regional lymph node or distant metastases.

The distinction between the stage designations of Ia and Ib is based solely on the 5 cm size factor.

Stage II

Stage IIa
$G_2 T_1 N_0 M_0$ — A Grade 2 tumor less than 5 cm in diameter, with no regional lymph nodes or distant metastases.

Stage IIb
$G_2 T_2 N_0 M_0$ — A Grade 2 tumor 5 cm or greater in diameter, with no regional lymph nodes or distant metastases.

As in Stage I, the distinction between IIa and IIb is based on the 5 cm size factor of the primary tumor, the G_2 being the sole qualification.

Stage III
Stage IIIa
$G_3 T_1 N_0 M_0$ — A Grade 3 tumor less than 5 cm in diameter, with no regional lymph nodes or distant metastases.

Stage IIIb
$G_3 T_2 N_0 M_0$ — A Grade 3 tumor greater than 5 cm in diameter, with no regional lymph nodes or distant metastases.

Stage IIIc
Any G or $T_{1-2} N_1 M_0$ — A tumor of any malignancy grade or size (no invasion) with regional lymph node metastases, but no distant metastases.

It was necessary to spread the gradation into 3 subgroups for Stage III. The G_3 classification is the largest single determinant, and is the common factor for stages IIIa and IIIb; the N_1 classification functions as a sole determinant for Stage IIIc.

Stage IV
Stage IVa
Any G $T_3 N_{0-1} M_0$ — A tumor of any grade which grossly invades a bone, a major vessel, or a nerve, with or without regional lymph node metastases, but without distant metastases.

Stage IVb
Any G T $N_{0-1} M_1$ — A tumor with distant metastases. The involvement of bone, nerve, or vessel indicates an extremely poor prognosis, but not as poor as does the presence of distant metastases. This conclusion regarding

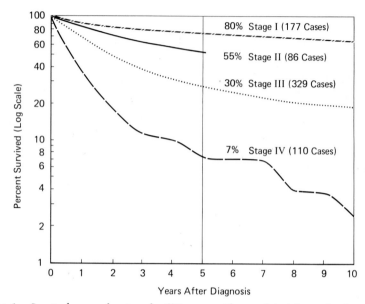

Fig. 1. — Survival curves by stage for 702 cases, with complete information for staging (423 cases with slide review, 279 cases without). The curve for Stage II was not plotted beyond 5 years, since at that point the standard error was 5% or higher.

prognosis was based on the personal experiences of the Task Force, because these data on prognosis were not collected in the retrospective study.

The determination of the stages and substages was constructed from the information obtained from the retrospective study of the 1,215 cases, with 702 cases having complete staging information. The consideration resulted in the reflection of each stage as a biological entity with a definable prognosis. Data for Stages I through IV have been plotted for the 702 cases with complete computer staging information. As shown in Figure 1, each stage shows a grouping differentiation to clearly define it as a characteristic biologic group.

CHECKLIST FOR SOFT TISSUE SARCOMAS

To assist in determining the stage, a checklist for collection of clinical and pathological information was developed by the A.J.C. Soft Tissue Sarcoma Task Force (Appendix).

Comment

In this staging system, the importance of information from the pathologist deserves special consideration. The precise identification of the histologic type and the accuracy of the malignancy grading assessment are pivotal to the staging schema. The pathologist's identification of the type of tumor, leading to the grade assessment, is no better than the reliability of sampling of the tissue submitted for examination. Soft tissue lesions are notorious for their extreme variations in growth patterns from 1 part of a tumor to another. For example, a liposarcoma may have a pure fibroblastic growth pattern in 1 sizeable area of the tumor. When this area is taken out of context with the whole tumor, it may be confused with fibrosarcoma, malignant fibrohistiocytoma, or even rhabdomyosarcoma.

Therefore, the size and representativeness of the sample taken are extremely important in obtaining the maximal reliability of designation of grade. A needle biopsy has the lowest reliability; an incisional biopsy is better. However, the excisional biopsy, whenever possible, allows the pathologist access to the total picture for diagnosis and grade assessment; the entire tumor may be sectioned to eliminate sampling error, special stains may be employed, and ultrastructural studies may be made.

By itself, the histologic grade of soft tissue sarcomas has been shown to be a reliable index of survival and prognosis for patients with some types of soft tissue tumors. This is well-documented in the literature (Broders, Hargrave, and Meyerding, 1939; Pritchard, Soule, Taylor, and Ivins, 1974; Russell *et al.*, in press; Shiu, Castro, Hajdu, and Fortner, 1975; Stout, 1948; Suit, Russell, and Martin, 1975; van der Werf-Messing and Unnik, 1965). The inclusion, therefore, of histologic grade information is essential for any successful staging system of soft tissue lesions. However, the staging system devised allows a far broader application of all relevant information as compared to that allowed by the purely histological evaluation of the tumor.

Appendix

SITE FOR SPECIFIC DATA FORM FOR SOFT SARCOMA

CLINICAL

Anatomic Site

☐ Head and Neck
☐ Trunk
☐ Extremities
   ☐ Shoulder and/or arm
   ☐ Elbow and/or below
   ☐ Buttocks and/or thigh
   ☐ Knee and/or below
☐ Retroperitoneum or Mediastinum
☐ Other _____
    (specify)

Localization

☐ Confined to anatomic site   ☐ Blood vessels
☐ Subcutaneous
☐ Muscle   ☐ Other _____ ☐ Nerves
    (specify)

Tumor Site, (largest dimension in cm.)

☐ Less than 5
☐ 5 or more
☐ Exact Dimensions _____

Regional Lymph Node Metastisis

☐ None
☐ Regional
☐ Distant

Metastases

☐ None
☐ Bone
☐ Lymph node
☐ Lung
☐ Liver
☐ Other _____
    (specify)

PATHOLOGIC

Site of Origin

☐ Subcutis   ☐ Tendon, Fascia
☐ Muscle   ☐ Major nerve
☐ Other _____
   (specify)

Histological Type

☐ Alveolar soft part sarcoma
☐ Angiosarcoma
☐ Estraskeletal osteosarcoma
☐ Extraskeletal chondrosarcoma
☐ Fibrosarcoma
☐ Leiomyosarcoma
☐ Liposarcoma
☐ Malignant fibrohistiocytoma
☐ Malignant mesenchymoma
☐ Malignant schwannoma
☐ Rhabomyosarcoma
☐ Synovial sarcoma
☐ Sarcoma, type not designated

Tumor Invades

☐ Skin   ☐ Nerve
☐ Subcutis   ☐ Bone
☐ Muscle   ☐ Viscus
☐ Blood vessel   ☐ Other _____
    (specify)

Grade of Malignancy

☐ Grade I (Low)
☐ Grade II (Moderate)
☐ Grade III (High)

Tumor Size (largest dimension in cm.)

☐ Less than 5   ☐ 5 or more
☐ Exact Dimensions _____

Regional Lymph Node Involvement

☐ None   ☐ Regional
☐ Negative results

Distant Metastisis

☐ None   ☐ Bone   ☐ Lymph node
☐ Lung   ☐ Liver
☐ Other _____
    (specify)

REFERENCES

American Joint Committee for Cancer Staging and End Results Reporting: *Classification and Staging of Cancer – by Site, a Handbook.* (In press.)

Broders, A. C., Hargrave, R., and Meyerding, H. W.: Pathologic features of soft tissue sarcoma. Surgery, Gynecology, and Obstetrics, 69:267 – 280, 1939.

Pritchard, D. J., Soule, E. H., Taylor, W. F., and Ivins, J. C.: Fibrosarcoma – A clinicopathologic and statistical study of 199 tumors of the soft tissues of the extremities and trunk. Cancer, 33:888 – 897, March 1974.

Russell, W. O., Cohen, J., Enzinger, F., Hajdu, S. I., Heise, B. S., Martin, R. G., Meissner, W., Miller, W. T., Schmitz, R. L., and, Suit, H. D.: A clinical and pathological staging system for soft tissue sarcomas. Cancer. (In press.)

Shiu, M. H., Castro, E. B., Hajdu, S. I., and Fortner, J. G.: Surgical treatment of 297 soft tissue sarcomas of the lower extremity. Annals of Surgery, 182: 597 – 602, November 1975.

Stout, A. P.: Fibrosarcoma: The malignant tumor of fibroblasts. Cancer, 1: 30 – 63, May 1948.

Suit, H. D., Russell, W. O., and Martin, R. G.: Sarcoma of soft tissue: Clinical and histopathologic parameters and response to treatment. Cancer, 35: 1478 – 1483, May 1975.

van der Werf-Messing, B., and Unnik, J. A. M.: Fibrosarcoma of the soft tissues – A clinicopathologic study. Cancer, 18:1113 – 1123, 1965.

Surgical Management of Soft Tissue Sarcomas

RICHARD G. MARTIN, M.D.
Department of Surgery, The University of Texas System
Cancer Center M. D. Anderson Hospital and Tumor Institute,
Houston, Texas

THE NATURE AND LOCATION of soft tissue sarcomas determine their surgical management. Also essential in the management of these lesions is understanding the use of combined surgery, X-ray therapy, and chemoimmunotherapy (Martin, Lindberg, Sinkovics, and Butler, 1976). This chapter will deal strictly with the surgical management of soft tissue sarcomas and will present the "pro's and con's" of given surgical procedures.

The soft tissue sarcomas discussed here are those lesions arising in the soft tissues which surround the skeletal structure (sarcomas arising in organs are not included). These soft tissue tumors usually present as innocuous nodules; they may or may not be painful, and when very small, they are often considered to be simple, benign lesions until excised and examined histologically.

Surgical Management

The role of surgical management of soft tissue tumors today is based on the treatment emphasized by George Pack, i.e., amputation or wide en bloc resection whenever possible (Pack, Miller, and Ariel, 1964; Pack and Ariel, 1964).

The majority of soft tissue tumors appear to be encapsulated; however, when examined microscopically, the capsule or "pseudocapsule" is actually found to be a layering of tumor cells compressing other cell layers into what appears to be a capsule (Clark, Martin, White, and Old, 1957; Clark, Martin, and White, 1959). Often these encapsulated tumors are "shelled out," only to rapidly recur locally. By enucleating such a lesion, microscopic cells are left behind and the tumor recurs. For this reason, an adequate amount of normal tissue must be removed along with the tumor in order to prevent recurrences.

The recurrence rate for an encapsulated tumor that has been "shelled out" is more than 75% (Clark, Martin, and White, 1959). The use of radical excisions, such as en bloc local resection, "muscle-bundle" resection, or amputation results in a lowering of the recurrence rate to 9% (Clark, Martin, and White, 1959). The 5-year survival rate for such procedures is approximately 40% (Martin, Butler, and Albores-Saavedra, 1965).

Because of the nature of these soft tissue sarcomas, the following surgical procedures are considered adequate for treating these sarcomas:

Local excision may be done for small superficial lesions (Fig. 1), which are usually in the skin or subcutaneous tissues. Excisions should be wide, leaving a margin of 3-5 cm around the tumor. The superficial fascia over the underlying muscle should be included. Such a procedure may require skin flaps or skin grafts in order to close the wound properly.

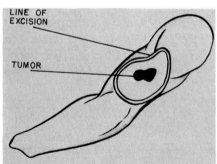

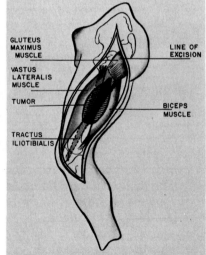

Fig. 1 (above).— Diagram of local excision for soft tissue tumor of the upper arm. (Courtesy of Clark, Martin, White, and Old, 1957.)

Fig. 2 (right).— Diagram of a "muscle-bundle" resection for soft tissue tumor in the thigh. (Courtesy of Clark, Martin, White, and Old, 1957.)

"Muscle-bundle" resection is required for lesions involving muscles or located in muscle bundles; the procedure involves excising the muscles from organ to insertion (Fig. 2). Because these lesions are deeper, much normal tissue must be removed with the lesion and there may, or may not, be some weakness in the use of the extremity involved. This type of procedure is suitable for lesions occurring in the thigh, buttocks, calf, and trapezius muscle area.

Local and/or wide en bloc resection may be accomplished on lesions occurring in the chest wall. When removal of ribs and the entire thickness of the chest wall becomes necessary, the defect may be closed with Marlex mesh and a skin flap. A portion, or all, of the scapula may be resected together with the tumor when in the area of the posterior shoulder in order to preserve a functional limb (Fig. 3).

Amputation is necessary for lesions around joints where there is not a large amount of soft tissue, making a wide en bloc resection impossible. The site of amputation should be above the level of origin or insertion of the muscle involved. A lesion below or at the knee would require a mid-thigh amputation (Fig. 4) and a lesion of the foot, a below-the-knee amputation. A large lesion of the thigh often necessitates a hip disarticulation (Fig. 5) and a lesion high in the thigh, protruding into the lower pelvis, a modified hemipelvectomy. The modi-

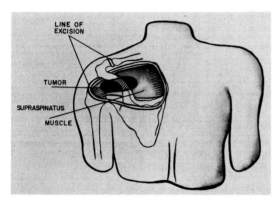

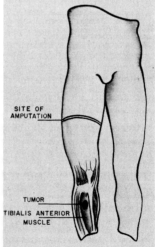

Fig. 3 (above).— Diagram of resection for soft tissue tumor together with a portion of the scapula, preserving functional limb. (Courtesy of Clark, Martin, White, and Old, 1957.)

Fig. 4 (right).— Diagram of mid-thigh amputation performed for a soft tissue tumor below the knee. (Courtesy of Clark, Martin, White, and Old, 1957.)

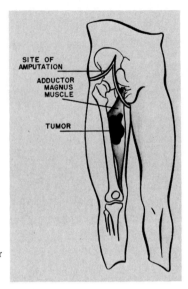

Fig. 5. – Diagram of hip disarticulation performed for a soft tissue tumor in the upper thigh. (Courtesy of Clark, Martin, White, and Old, 1957.)

fied hemipelvectomy requires the removal of the rami of the ilium; the symphysis is split in the midline and the ilium is resected at a line from the sciatic notch to the anterior superior spine (Fig. 6). If the lesion arises in the muscles of the pelvic wall, a total or "classic" hemipelvectomy is required, dividing the ilium at the symphysis and at the sacral iliac joint (Fig. 7). Lesions of the arm, which are often found above the elbow, necessitate amputation also, and for those lesions

Fig. 6. – Diagram of a modified hemipelvectomy performed for a soft tissue tumor protruding into the lower pelvis.

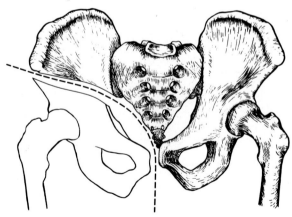

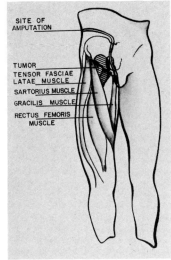

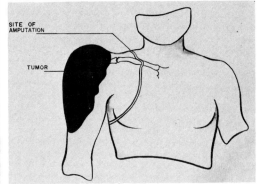

Fig. 7 (left).—Diagram of a total or "classic" hemipelvectomy performed for a soft tissue tumor in the muscles of the pelvic wall. (Courtesy of Clark, Martin, White, and Old, 1957.)

Fig. 8 (above).—Diagram of an intrascapulothoracic amputation for soft tissue tumors high in the upper arm or in the shoulder. (Courtesy of Clark, Martin, White and Old, 1957.)

high in the upper arm or in the shoulder an intrascapulothoracic amputation is required (Fig. 8).

Surgical resection in the head and neck area is, of course, limited, due to the nature of the soft tissue and bony structures, and radical resections are often impossible in this area. Soft tissue tumors arising in the retroperitoneal area usually surround, or are attached to, many of the organs in the abdomen, especially the kidney. Bowel resections often become necessary in order to remove these lesions. Recurrence rates for the head and neck area and the retroperitoneal area are very high (Martin, Butler, and Albores-Saavedra, 1965).

The surgical management discussed is required for all soft tissue sarcomas, regardless of histological diagnosis and grading, except: (1) congenital fibrosarcomas in infants (Balsaver, Butler, and Martin, 1967), (2) fibrosarcomas, Grade 1, desmoid type (Clark and Martin, 1970), and (3) dermatofibrosarcoma protuberans (Martin, 1976). This group of lesions is low-grade and, therefore, should be treated conservatively in the surgical management, using a less radical procedure for recurrence, if any, should it be local. A more conservative approach is the use of a wide local excision instead of amputation, even though the margins are not as wide as one would like; this is especially true of fibrosarcoma, Grade 1, desmoid type. To date, there has been no evidence of distant metastases in our series of 34 cases of desmoid tumors. However, in our series of 54 patients with dermatofibrosarcoma protuberans, we have had 4 cases of distant metastases (Martin, 1976). These lesions require wide excisions with margin checks of the skin, because these tumors tend to spread under the surface of the skin as plaques and surface as nodules at various intervals. If one is not careful, margins will be inadequate unless they are checked by frozen section specimens and, as stated earlier, this type of lesion usually requires skin grafting in order to close it properly (Martin, 1976).

Nodular fasciitis, although not a sarcoma, is frequently diagnosed as sarcoma, and too often is treated by radical resection, even amputation. On careful histological examination, this lesion should be differentiated from a true sarcoma. Nodular fasciitis is benign and usually arises fairly rapidly; it is most prominent in the upper extremities in the late teenager and young adult. Management of this lesion is by local excision (Clark and Martin, 1970).

Using only surgical management in the treatment of soft tissue sarcomas, the 5-year survival rate is approximately 40% (Martin, Butler, and Albores-Saavedra, 1965). Many patients referred to M. D. Anderson Hospital have had biopsy specimens taken previously in the form of excisional biopsies, very often enucleation. These patients are questioned carefully, therefore, to determine the size of the nodule in order that it might be compared with the length of the scar.

Patients with no palpable tumor present and who have had a wide excision of their scar have, in recent years, been treated with X-ray therapy. This procedure was initiated for those lesions excised near joints or in areas where a local resection was either impossible or would result in a useless limb requiring amputation. The purpose of treating these patients with X-ray therapy was to preserve a useful limb, and also to see if the local recurrence rate would be comparable to that of amputation and en bloc resection. This is more completely discussed by Lindberg (Lindberg, Martin, Romsdahl, and McMurtrey, 1977, see pages 289 to 298, this volume).

Summary

The role of surgical management of soft tissue sarcomas is based on the treatment emphasized by George Pack, that of amputation or wide en bloc resection whenever possible. These procedures often necessitate the removal of many of the surrounding muscles or amputation of a portion of, or all of the limb. The overall 5-year survival rate for such procedures is approximately 40%. The local recurrence rate for anything less than these procedures is approximately 72%. Numerous local excisions performed previous to referral to our institution are now managed by postoperative X-ray therapy to prevent amputation and preserve a useful limb. A small group of low-grade sarcomas, where local excision is adequate, have been discussed. These lesions should be histologically recognized, as should the benign lesion, nodular fasciitis, in order that amputation or radical resections may be prevented.

REFERENCES

Balsaver, A. M., Butler, J. J., and Martin, R. G.: Congenital fibrosarcoma. Cancer, 20:1607–1616, October 1967.

Clark, R. L., and Martin, R. G.: Fibrosarcoma: Management and end results. In *Sixth National Cancer Conference Proceedings.* Philadelphia, Pennsylvania, J. B. Lippincott Company, 1970, pp. 789–794.

Clark, R. L., Jr., Martin, R. G., and White, E. C.: A critical review of the management of soft-tissue sarcomas. The Journal-Lancet, 79:327–331, July 1959.

Clark, R. L., Jr., Martin, R. G., White, E. C., and Old, J. W.: Clinical aspects of soft-tissue tumors. Archives of Surgery, 74:859–870, June 1957.

Lindberg, R. D., Martin, R. G., Romsdahl, M. M., and McMurtrey, M. J.: Conservative surgery and radiation therapy for soft tissue sarcomas. In *Management of Bone and Soft Tissue Sarcomas* (The University of Texas System Cancer Center M. D. Anderson Hospital and Tumor Institute, 21st Annual Clinical Conference on Cancer). Chicago, Illinois, Year Book Medical Publishers, Inc., 1977, pp. 289 to 298.

Martin, R. G.: Dermatofibrosarcoma protuberans. In *Neoplasms of the Skin and Malignant Melanoma* (The University of Texas System Cancer Center M. D. Anderson Hospital and Tumor Institute, 20th Annual Clinical Conference on Cancer). Chicago, Illinois, Year Book Medical Publishers, Inc., 1976, pp. 243–250.

Martin, R. G., Butler, J. J., and Albores-Saavedra, J.: Soft tissue tumors: Surgical treatment and results. In *Tumors of Bone and Soft Tissue* (The University of Texas M. D. Anderson Hospital and Tumor Institute, 8th Annual Clinical Conference on Cancer). Chicago, Illinois, Year Book Medical Publishers, Inc., 1965, pp. 333–347.

Martin, R. G., Lindberg, R. D., Sinkovics, J. G., and Butler, J. J.: Soft-tissue sarcomas. In Clark, R. L., and Howe, C. D., Eds.: *Cancer Patient Care at M. D. Anderson Hospital and Tumor Institute.* Chicago, Illinois, Year Book Medical Publishers, Inc., 1976, pp. 473–483.

Pack, G. T., and Ariel, I. M.: Principles of treatment of tumors of the soft somatic tissues. In Pack, G. T., and Ariel, I. M., Eds.: *Treatment of Cancer and Allied Diseases, Tumors of the Soft Somatic Tissues and Bone.* 2nd edition. New York, New York, Hoeber Medical Division, Harper and Row, 1964, VIII, pp. 8–39.

Pack, G. T., Miller, T. R., and Ariel, I. M.: Hemipelvectomy (interilio-abdominal amputation). In Pack, G. T., and Ariel, I. M., Eds.: *Treatment of Cancer and Allied Diseases, Tumors of the Soft Somatic Tissues and Bone.* 2nd edition. New York, New York, Hoeber Medical Division, Harper and Row, 1964, VIII, pp. 284–302.

Conservative Surgery and Radiation Therapy for Soft Tissue Sarcomas

ROBERT D. LINDBERG, M.D.,* RICHARD G. MARTIN, M.D., MARVIN M. ROMSDAHL, M.D., Ph.D., and MARION J. McMURTREY, M.D.

Departments of Radiotherapy and Surgery, The University of Texas System Cancer Center M. D. Anderson Hospital and Tumor Institute, Houston, Texas*

UNTIL RECENTLY, THE TREATMENT OF CHOICE for soft tissue sarcomas has been surgical resection, and a wide variety of surgical techniques have been used. Experience has shown that the local recurrence rate after simple excision is 90% (Cadman, Soule, and Kelly, 1965; Shieber and Graham, 1962), after wide excision 39% (Shieber and Graham, 1962), after soft part resection 25% (Castro, Hajdu, and Fortner, 1973), and after amputation 18% (Cantin, McNeer, Chu, and Booker, 1968). The local recurrence rate after all forms of radical surgery is about 30% (Cantin, McNeer, Chu, and Booker, 1968; Martin, Butler, and Albores-Saavedra, 1965). The treatment of soft tissue sarcomas by radical radiation therapy alone is also unrewarding, with the local recurrence rate being 66% (Lindberg, 1973).

In an attempt to preserve a functional limb, a study was started of a select group of patients using a conservative surgical excision and postoperative radiation therapy. The purpose of this report is to update our previous publications (Lindberg, 1973; Lindberg, Fletcher, and Martin, 1975; Lindberg, Martin, and Romsdahl, 1975).

Case Material

The charts of all patients with soft tissue sarcomas treated with radiation therapy from 1963 through 1975 were reviewed in August 1976. Only those patients meeting the following criteria were included in the study: (1) 16 years of age or older, (2) no evidence of distant metastasis on admission, (3) tumor mass resected by conservative surgical excision, usually a simple "shelling out" or limited removal of only the gross tumor, and (4) immediate postoperative radiation therapy to the tumor bed (greater than 5,000 rads tumor dose in 5 weeks). Patients with tumors arising in organ sites, e.g., the uterus, were excluded. Two hundred and forty-five patients fulfilled the criteria; 166 of these were treated from 1963 through 1973 (minimum 2-year follow-up) and formed the basis of this study. During the period encompassed by this report, the histopathological material has been reviewed a number of times. The data are presented according to the current diagnosis (Table 1) rather than the diagnosis at the time of treatment.

The majority of the patients (102/166) were more than 40 years old, with a range of 16 to 81 years. The patient distribution by histopathologic type was independent of age except for those with rhabdomyosarcoma, in which case 10 of 16 patients were less than 30 years old. There was a slight preponderance of females (87 versus 79).

TABLE 1.–LOCAL RECURRENCE BY HISTOLOGY AND SITE
1963 THROUGH 1973
UNLIMITED FOLLOW-UP–MINIMUM 2 YEARS

DIAGNOSIS	HEAD AND NECK	TRUNK INTRA-ABDOMINAL[*]	OTHER	UPPER EXTREMITY	LOWER EXTREMITY	TOTAL
Liposarcoma	—	2/3	1/4	2/3	2/11	7/21
Fibrosarcoma	1/3	0/2	1/2	0/7	2/8	4/22
Rhabdomyosarcoma	2/4	1/1	1/4	0/4	1/3	5/16
Leiomyosarcoma	—	3/4	—	0/1	1/2	4/7
Neurofibrosarcoma	0/4	1/2	3/8	1/7	4/11	9/32
Synovial sarcoma	—	—	0/2	0/7	1/8	1/17
Malignant fibro-histiocytoma	—	0/2	1/3	4/9	4/15	9/29
Epithelioid sarcoma	0/1	—	—	0/2	2/3	2/6
Unclassified sarcoma	1/1	1/1	0/3	0/1	0/4	2/10
Miscellaneous sarcoma†	0/2	—	0/2	0/2	—	0/6
TOTAL	4/15	8/15	7/28	7/43	17/65	43/166

[*]Sarcomas arising in organs (e.g., uterus) are excluded.
†Angiosarcoma, 2; clear cell sarcoma, 2; dermatofibrosarcoma protuberans, 2.

Treatment

The majority of the patients were seen initially after incisional biopsy (16), simple excision (115), or gross tumor recurrence after simple excision (27). Patients with recurrence had a re-excision with a limited margin of normal tissue; therefore, there was no clinically detectable gross tumor at the start of radiation therapy.

In the early 1960's, patients with lesions arising in the distal portion of the extremity, for whom an amputation had been recommended, were irradiated under conditions of relative hypoxia by means of the tourniquet technique (Suit, 1965). Twenty-five patients were treated with the tourniquet technique, and the remaining 141 patients were irradiated with megavoltage external beam using conventional fractionation, i.e., 1,000 rads tumor dose per week in 5 fractions. Prior to 1971, most patients received 7,000 rads tumor dose in 7 weeks to 7,500 rads tumor dose in 7½ weeks, using a shrinking field technique after 5,000 rads. Since 1971, the total dose has been reduced to 6,000 rads tumor dose in 6 weeks to 6,500 rads tumor dose in 6½ weeks. The details of the radiotherapy technique have been previously published (Lindberg, Fletcher, and Martin, 1975).

Results

The status of the 166 patients at 2 years is shown in Table 2 according to the site of origin. Of the 166 patients, 87 have been followed at least 5 years, and their current status (unlimited follow-up, minimum 5 years) is shown in Table 3. A functional extremity was preserved in

TABLE 2.—SOFT TISSUE SARCOMA
1963 THROUGH 1973
STATUS AT 2 YEARS

SITE	TOTAL CASES	NED	CAUSE OF DEATH					
			P	P + DM	DM	UNK	ID	SP
Head and neck	15	10 (1)°	2	1	2			
Trunk { intra-abdominal	15	7	3	2	2	—	1	
{ other	28	14	3	3	8			
Upper extremity	43	33 (4)	—	—	9	—	—	1
Lower extremity	65	48 (8)	2	1	13	1		
TOTAL	166	112 (13)	10	7	34	1	1	1

°( )—Number of patients with recurrence at primary site, salvaged by surgery.
NED—Living, no evidence of disease; P—Primary failure; DM—Distant metastases; UNK—Unknown cause; ID—Intercurrent disease; SP—Secondary primary.

TABLE 3.—SOFT TISSUE SARCOMA
1963 THROUGH 1970
UNLIMITED FOLLOW-UP—MINIMUM 5 YEARS

SITE	TOTAL CASES	NED	CAUSE OF DEATH				
			P	P + DM	DM	ID	UNK
Head and neck	9	6 (1)°	2	1			
Trunk { intra-abdominal	9	3 (1)	2	2	2 (1)		
{ other	13	6	2	2	3		
Upper extremity	25	17 (3)			6 (1)	2	
Lower extremity	31	14 (3)	2	3	8 (1)	2	2
TOTAL	87	46 (8)	8	8	19 (3)	4†	2‡

°( ) Number of patients with recurrence at primary site, salvaged by surgery.
†Died at 33, 35, 60, and 62 months.
‡Died at 14 and 42 months.

81% (67/83) of the patients treated with conventional fractionation.

The recurrence time distribution for failure to control the primary lesion is shown in Figure 1. Seventy-two percent (31/43) of the recurrences are manifest by 2 years, but only 86% (37/43) were manifest by 5 years. The 6 recurrences at the primary site were noted at 62, 74, 78, 84, 90, and 120 months posttreatment. The frequency of local recurrence according to the location and histological type of the primary tumor is shown in Table 1. Although some differences are noted by histology, there are too few cases to be able to draw any conclusions. Table 4 shows the incidence of local recurrence according to the anatomical site within the trunk and extremities. Most of the failures in the extremities occur in primary tumors of the fleshy parts: 5 of 15 in the arm, 6 of 30 in the thigh, and 6 of 13 in the leg. The histopatho-

TABLE 4.—INCIDENCE OF LOCAL FAILURES
1963 THROUGH 1973
UNLIMITED FOLLOW-UP—MINIMUM 2 YEARS

TRUNK°		UPPER EXTREMITY		LOWER EXTREMITY	
Axilla and shoulder	1/6 (1)†	Arm	5/15 (1)	Thigh	6/30 (1)
Buttocks	2/14	Elbow	0/3	Knee	3/16 (3)
Single sites	4/8 (1)	Forearm	2/13	Leg	6/13 (3)
		Wrist	0/4	Ankle	1/3
		Hand	0/8	Foot	1/3
TOTAL	7/28 (2)		7/43 (1)		17/65 (7)

°Intra-abdominal primaries are excluded.
†( ) Number of geographical misses; recurrence outside irradiated volume.

TABLE 5.—SOFT TISSUE SARCOMAS
EXTREMITY LESIONS—
1963 THROUGH 1973

	LOCAL FAILURES	
Size of Primary	< 5 cm	≥ 5 cm
Grade 1	0/12	3/17 (17.7%)
Grades 2 and 3	7/37 (18.9%)	14/42 (33.3%)
	DISTANT METASTASIS	
Size of Primary	< 5 cm	≥ 5 cm
Grade 1	1/12 (8.3%)	1/17 (5.9%)
Grades 2 and 3	7/37 (18.9%)	22/42 (52.4%°)

°Patients with uncontrolled tumor at the primary site—18/38 (47.4%) were eliminated.

logical material of the extremity lesions was reviewed and graded. The frequency of local recurrence according to the grade and size of the initial lesion is shown in Table 5.

Of the 166 patients, 54 (32.5%) developed distant metastasis. The distant metastasis time distribution is shown in Figure 1. The distant metastasis appears somewhat earlier than recurrence at the primary site, i.e., 79.6% at 2 years and 98.2% at 4 years. The incidence of dis-

Fig. 1.—Local recurrence versus distant metastasis of soft tissue sarcoma from 1963 through 1973. Unlimited follow up, minimum 2 years.

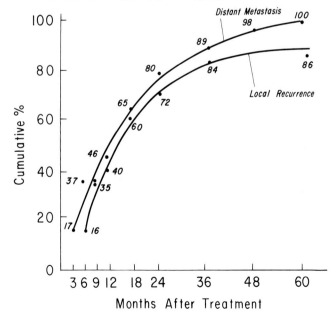

tant metastasis according to the histopathological diagnosis and site of the primary is shown in Table 6; however, there are too few cases to draw any meaningful conclusions. The most common initial site of distant metastasis was the lung (45/54 or 83%). The incidence of distant metastasis is related to the grade and size of the primary lesion (Table 5).

Occasionally patients will present with metastasis to the regional lymph nodes as the initial manifestation of spread. This occurred in 4% (7/166) of our patients: rhabdomyosarcoma, 2; neurofibrosarcoma, 2; synovial sarcoma, 1; leiomyosarcoma, 1; and epithelioid sarcoma, 1.

The incidence of significant complications in patients treated by conventional radiation therapy is low. Significant complications developed in only 8.4% (7/83) of the patients with lesions of the extremity. Two patients developed soft tissue necrosis. One patient with a fibrosarcoma of the forearm sustained thermal injury (cold) 26 months after treatment. A 2 × 2 cm area of necrosis appeared, which healed with conservative management after 36 months. The second patient was treated for liposarcoma of the posterior thigh with a 43 × 15 cm field including the buttocks. Forty-two months after treatment, necrosis developed in the gluteal fold which required an excision and

TABLE 6.—DISTANT METASTASIS BY HISTOLOGY AND SITE†
1963 THROUGH 1973
UNLIMITED FOLLOW-UP—MINIMUM 2 YEARS

| DIAGNOSIS | HEAD AND NECK | TRUNK | | UPPER EXTREMITY | LOWER EXTREMITY | TOTAL |
		INTRA-ABDOMINAL	OTHER			
Liposarcoma	—	1/3	3°/4	0/3	1°/11	5/21
Fibrosarcoma	2°/3	1/2	1°/2	0/7	3/8	7/22
Rhabdomyosarcoma	1/4	1/1	2°/4	3/4	2°/3	9/16
Leiomyosarcoma	—	3°°/4	—	1/1	1/2	5/7
Neurofibrosarcoma	1/4	0/2	2/8	0/7	4°/11	7/32
Synovial sarcoma	—	—	0/2	2/7	2/8	4/17
Malignant fibro-histiocytoma	—	0/2	1/3	3/9	4/15	8/29
Epithelioid sarcoma	0/1	—	—	0/2	1/3	1/6
Unclassified sarcoma	0/1	1°/1	2/3	0/1	4/4	7/10
Miscellaneous sarcoma‡	0/2	—	0/2	1/2	—	1/6
TOTAL	4/15	7/15	11/28	10/43	22/65	54/166

°Each asterisk indicates one patient had recurrence at the primary site also.
†Sarcomas arising in organs (e.g., uterus) are excluded.
‡Angiosarcoma, 2; clear cell sarcoma, 2; dermatofibrosarcoma protuberans, 2.

graft. Three patients experienced edema of the extremity distal to the irradiated volume; the entire cross section of the limb was irradiated in 1 patient and 90% of the limb was irradiated in the other 2 patients. The sixth complication occurred in a patient with neurofibrosarcoma of the anterior thigh. The scar extended into the inguinal region and required 37 × 16 cm fields. One year after treatment, there was marked fibrosis with limitation of hip movement. The last complication occurred in a 59-year-old female who had a Grade 2 epithelioid sarcoma on the dorsum of the foot excised 3 times prior to irradiation. Forty-one months after radiotherapy (6,500 rads tumor dose in 6½ weeks), a below-the-knee amputation was necessary because of necrosis. Histologic examination showed no tumor. The patient is living free of disease 10 months after amputation.

Discussion

The purpose of conservative surgery and postoperative radiation therapy in lesions of the extremities is to preserve a functional limb. In our series, a functional limb was preserved in 80% of the patients. By comparison, a recent surgical series (Simon and Enneking, 1976) reports that 53.7% (29/54) of the patients in the study were initially treated by amputation. The rationale for removing all gross tumor by conservative surgical excision is that the remaining subclinical disease can be destroyed by moderate doses of postoperative irradiation. This concept has been reported for carcinoma of the head and neck (Fletcher, 1972a) and breast (Fletcher, 1972b), i.e., 5,000 rads tumor dose in 5 weeks sterilizes more than 90% of the subclinical disease. This concept is also applicable to the soft tissue sarcomas. The survival rate free of disease in patients with lesions followed a minimum of 5 years (55.4%, 31/56) is similar to that of most surgical series. Further analysis shows that survival varies with histological grade, i.e., Grade 1, 66.7% (12/18); Grade 2, 60.9% (14/23); and Grade 3, 33.3% (5/15).

The local recurrence rate for primary lesions arising in the extremities is 22% (24/108). Nineteen of the 24 local recurrences (79%) were controlled by further surgery—15 amputations and 4 wide excisions. Most of the local failures were in the thigh, leg, or arm, where the tumors may have grown to 10 cm or more in diameter before they were detected. Lesions arising in the hand, foot, or around the joint are usually diagnosed when they are small, before they have had a chance to spread between the fascial planes. In spite of generous radiation fields, 8 of the 24 local recurrences were outside of the irradiated volume. Some recurrences were more than 10 cm beyond the treated volume, documenting the tendency of soft tissue sarcomas to spread for great distances along the fascial planes.

The radiotherapeutic techniques vary with the location of the primary tumor. Since the rate of local recurrence and distant metastasis is related to the grade and initial size of the primary tumor prior to excision, more generous fields are used in the large high-grade lesions. The current approach is to include the surgical field with a generous margin (5–7 cm). Parallel opposed ^{60}Co fields are used, usually encompassing one half of the cross-sectional plane of the extremity. A combination of open and wedge fields are used to deliver a homogeneous dose to the selected volume. After 5,000 rads tumor dose in 5 weeks, the scar area is boosted with an appositional electron beam field with a 3–4 cm margin. In Grade 1 lesions, an additional 1,000 rads tumor dose in 5 fractions is delivered to the entire depth of the scar. Usually the 90% isodose curve is used to compensate for the lower surface dose and it eliminates the need for bolus. In Grade 2 and Grade 3 tumors, the tumor dose is 6,500 rads in 6½ weeks. The last 500 rads are given through a field which includes only the scar (2 cm margin), because of the high probability that more than microscopic tumor has been left behind in that area.

Most complications can be avoided by careful planning. The entire circumference of an extremity must not be irradiated, since a severe constricting fibrosis may result with varying degrees of edema distal to the irradiated volume. The current technique is to leave a generous strip of unirradiated tissues, optimally one half of the cross section. In order to preserve function, the entire joint is irradiated only when absolutely necessary, e.g., the rare synovial sarcoma that penetrates the joint space. Patients presenting with primary lesions in the foot must be selected with great care since the foot is a weight-bearing structure and, therefore, prone to complications. Our only complication requiring an amputation occurred in a patient with a lesion on the dorsal aspect of the foot. If the toes, sole of the foot, and Achilles tendon must be included in the irradiated volume to insure adequate margin, a surgical ablation is the treatment of choice.

In 1973, a random study was started in patients with large high-grade lesions to test the efficacy of adjuvant chemotherapy. The preliminary results of this study are reported on pages 343–352 of this volume (Lindberg et al., 1977). Massive primary lesions in the extremities cannot be treated by this approach since conservative surgery is not possible. These patients receive preoperative irradiation and conservative excision if possible.

Conclusions

The role of radiotherapy is the treatment of soft tissue sarcomas has changed. Radiotherapy is not a substitute for surgery, but it is a valuable surgical adjuvant. A review of patients treated by conservative excision and postoperative radiotherapy shows:

(1) A functional limb can be preserved in 80% of patients.

(2) The local control rate for lesions of the extremities is 78% and depends upon histopathological grade, initial size, and location of the primary tumor.

(3) The incidence of distant metastasis is related to the grade and size of the primary tumor.

(4) Complications can be minimized if sufficient attention is given to the placement of the surgical scar and the radiotherapy technique, i.e., field reduction to include only the scar after 5,000 rads tumor dose. The incidence of significant complications is 8.4%.

REFERENCES

Cadman, N. L., Soule, E. H., and Kelly, P. J.: Synovial sarcoma; an analysis of 134 tumors. Cancer, 18:613–627, 1965.

Cantin, J., McNeer, G. P., Chu, F. C., and Booker, R. J.: The problem of local recurrence after treatment of soft tissue sarcoma. Annals of Surgery, 168: 47–53, July 1968.

Castro, E. B., Hajdu, S. I., and Fortner, J. G.: Surgical therapy of fibrosarcoma of extremities. Archives of Surgery, 107:284–291, August 1973.

Fletcher, G. H.: Elective irradiation of subclinical disease in cancers of the head and neck. Cancer, 29:1450–1454, June 1972a.

———: Local results of irradiation in the primary management of localized breast cancer. Cancer, 29:545–551, March 1972b.

Lindberg, R. D.: The role of radiation therapy in the treatment of soft tissue sarcoma in adults. *Proceedings of Seventh National Cancer Conference.* Philadelphia, Pennsylvania, J. B. Lippincott Co., 1973, pp. 883–888.

Lindberg, R. D. Fletcher, G. H., and Martin, R. G.: The management of soft tissue sarcomas in adults: Surgery and postoperative radiotherapy. Journal de Radiologie et d'Electrologie, 56:761–767, June 1975.

Lindberg, R. D., Martin, R. G., and Romsdahl, M. M.: Surgery and postoperative radiotherapy in the treatment of soft tissue sarcomas in adults. American Journal of Roentgenology, Radium Therapy, and Nuclear Medicine, 123:123–129, January 1975.

Lindberg, R. D., Murphy, W. K., Benjamin, R. S., Sinkovics, J. G., Martin, R. G., Romsdahl, M. M., Jesse, R. H., Jr., and Russell, W. O.: Adjuvant chemotherapy in the treatment of primary soft tissue sarcomas—A preliminary report. In *Management of Bone and Soft Tissue Tumors* (The University of Texas System Cancer Center M. D. Anderson Hospital and Tumor Institute, 21st Annual Clinical Conference on Cancer). Chicago, Illinois, Year Book Medical Publishers, Inc., 1977, pp. 343–352.

Martin, R. G., Butler, J. J., and Albores-Saavedra, J.: Soft tissue tumors: Surgical treatment and results. In *Tumors of Bone and Soft Tissue* (The University of Texas M. D. Anderson Hospital and Tumor Institute, 8th Annual Clinical Conference on Cancer). Chicago, Illinois, Year Book Medical Publishers, Inc., 1965, pp. 333–347.

Shieber, W., and Graham, P.: An experience with sarcoma of the soft tissues in adults. Surgery, 52:295–298, August 1962.

Simon, M. A., and Enneking, W. F.: The management of soft tissue sarcomas of the extremities. Journal of Bone and Joint Surgery, 58A:317–327, April 1976.

Suit, H. D.: Radiation therapy under conditions of local tissue hypoxia for bone and soft tissue sarcoma. In *Tumors of Bone and Soft Tissue* (The University of Texas M. D. Anderson Hospital and Tumor Institute, 8th Annual Clinical Conference on Cancer). Chicago, Illinois, Year Book Medical Publishers, Inc., 1965, pp. 143–163.

Preoperative Radiotherapy and Surgery in the Management of Soft Tissue Sarcoma

RICHARD G. MARTIN, M.D., ROBERT D. LINDBERG, M.D., and WILLIAM O. RUSSELL, M.D.

Departments of Surgery, Radiotherapy, and Pathology,
The University of Texas System Cancer Center
M. D. Anderson Hospital and Tumor Institute,
Houston, Texas

AT M. D. ANDERSON HOSPITAL, the idea of preoperative radiation for patients with large soft tissue sarcomas of the extremities which normally require amputation (Fig. 1) (Clark, Martin, White, and Old, 1957) was formulated quite by accident in 1971.

A 37-year-old white male presented with a large thigh lesion that had been biopsied previously. The lesion measured approximately 8 × 5 cm, and was diagnosed as malignant fibrohistiocytoma, Grade 2. Following biopsy, the patient developed a fever, and a chest X-ray film was reported as showing apparent pulmonary metastases. The patient was placed on antibiotics, and the apparent lung metastases cleared. The lesion was treated by radiotherapy. We delivered 7,000 rads tumor dose in 7 weeks in the routine manner; that is, we left a strip of normal tissue to prevent swelling distal to the radiation. Following radiotherapy, there was approximately 50% shrinkage of tumor; however, the remaining mass was quite tender. Therefore, a wide excision was done in March 1971, 3 months after completion of radiotherapy. The pathology reports showed no viable tumor cells, and the patient is living free of disease with good leg function at 5½ years postexcision (November 1976) (Figs. 2–5).

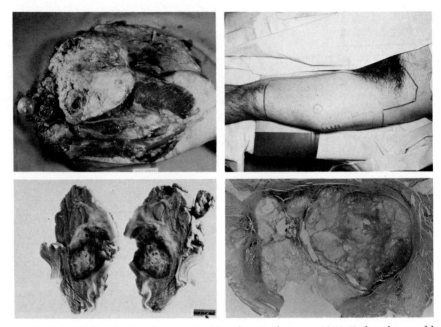

Fig. 1 (top left). — Lesion that required hip disarticulation in 1956. Today, this would be treated with preoperative radiation in an attempt to preserve a functional limb.

Fig. 2 (top right). — First case of preoperative radiation, showing area on left thigh marked for radiation.

Fig. 3 (bottom left). — First case of preoperative radiation, showing tumor specimen resected.

Fig. 4 (bottom right). — First case of preoperative radiation, showing whole organ specimen encapsulated with necrotic tissue removed from patient.

Approximately 1 year later, a 73-year-old white female was admitted with a high anterior thigh lesion diagnosed as a poorly differentiated unclassified sarcoma, Grade 3. Following preoperative radiotherapy totaling 6,250 rads tumor dose in 48 days, the tumor was excised in May 1972. At the time of surgery, the lesion revealed large encapsulation with marked necrosis. The pathology report showed a tumor measuring $7 \times 5 \times 4.5$ cm. Microscopically, very few tumor cells could be identified. The patient did well until December 1972, when she developed bilateral pulmonary metastases which were treated with chemotherapy. She died of necrotizing colitis in April 1973.

In October 1972, a 48-year-old white male presented with a large, painful lesion, measuring 15×20 cm, in the medial upper left thigh. The biopsy specimen revealed a liposarcoma, Grade 3. The patient received planned preoperative radiotherapy of 5,000 rads tumor dose in 5 weeks with ^{60}Co. Six weeks later, in January 1973, a wide local

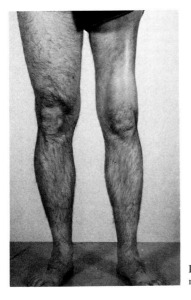

Fig. 5.—First case of preoperative radiation. Left leg of patient 2 years after preoperative radiation and excision.

excision was performed. Pathological review showed a 10 × 6 cm lesion with marked necrosis, but histologically viable tumor appeared to be present. This patient had a considerable amount of necrosis of the skin flaps which required skin grafting. He was last seen 47 months later (December 1976) with no evidence of recurrent disease.

These 3 cases gave us considerable reassurance. Therefore, it was agreed to see a 64-year-old white female with a posterior thigh mass measuring 20 cm that had been biopsied and diagnosed as unclassified high-grade sarcoma. The lesion had been treated with neutron beam. Because of a painful, ulcerated area in the posterior thigh, it was elected to excise this locally, and no viable tumor was found on pathological review. However, severe complications followed surgery, with inability of the wound to heal even with intravenous hyperalimentation. The patient died soon after returning home. This was not a planned case of preoperative radiation, but is included here only to show the complications that may arise from surgery following radiation and also to mention, again, that necrosis occurs in many cases of preoperative irradiation.

The next case of planned preoperative radiation was a 38-year-old white female who presented with a history of 4 × 3 cm mass removed by local excision from the posterior right thigh in February 1972. In August 1973, the patient presented at M. D. Anderson Hospital with a recurrent mass measuring 15 × 6 cm. More than 70% of these lesions will recur following such treatment (Clark, Martin, and White, 1959; Martin, Butler, and Albores-Saavedra, 1965). The diagnosis was malignant fibrohistiocytoma, Grade 2. The lesion was radiated in the usual manner, to a tumor dose of 5,000 rads in 5 weeks. On completion of radiation therapy, the patient developed severe hepatitis with alkaline phosphatase levels as high as 358 mU/ml. Two months later, a wide excision was performed to remove the tumor, which was easily excised; again, the tumor was found to be surrounded by a thick capsule, and fibrosis and necrosis were noted with no apparent viable tumor. Three years later, the patient is still without evidence of recurrent disease.

The second death in our series was that of a 19-year-old female with a neurofibrosarcoma in the upper left thigh. Preoperative radiation totaling 5,000 rads was given, and 2 months later it was followed by resection. Again, considerable reduction in tumor size was seen. The patient also received Adriamycin and DIC and 1½ years later, had a thoracotomy for metastatic disease. Four months later, due to recurrent right apically based disease, she received 3,000 rads followed by actinomycin-D, 5-FU, and Cytoxin. The patient died in October 1976, 2 years 8 months following the resection. At the time of death, there was no evidence of local recurrence of the primary lesion.

The next case in our series was that of a 75-year-old white female who had had an excision of a thigh mass before being referred to M. D. Anderson Hospital. At the time of referral, she was free of local and metastatic disease. She was placed on our VACAR program, however, because of marked bone depression and sepsis and a rapidly growing recurrent mass at the site of the previous excision; on biopsy examination, the mass proved to be recurrent disease, and she was switched to the preoperative radiation program followed by resection. The patient is now 1½ years without evidence of recurrent disease.

Three other patients have survived at least 1 year following surgical excision after preoperative radiation (Table 1). Of this group, 1 patient had an extremely large lesion of the upper thigh (over 20 cm in diameter). It was diagnosed as a low-grade leiomyosarcoma showing a considerable amount of necrosis, but with viable tumor present at the time of excision. The other 2 patients had lesions in areas other than the thigh. One, a 56-year-old white male with a large lesion of the posterior left shoulder was diagnosed as having neurofibrosarcoma, Grade 3. Preoperative radiation was given totaling 5,000 rads and was completed in May 1975. The tumor was excised along with the upper half of the scapula. Histologically, this tumor was a large necrotic mass. The patient is now 19 months postresection with no evidence of

TABLE 1.—PATIENTS TREATED WITH PLANNED PREOPERATIVE RADIATION AND SURGERY: MINIMUM 1-YEAR FOLLOW-UP

NO.	AGE	SEX	SITE	HISTOLOGY	TREATMENT	METASTASIS	LOCAL RECURRENCE	SURVIVAL (MONTHS)
1	37	M	Thigh	MFC, Grade 2	7,000 rads + Surgery	0	0	66 NED
2	73	F	Thigh	Unclassified sarcoma, Grade 3	6,250 rads + Surgery + Chemotherapy	Pulmonary	0	12 Expired
3	48	M	Thigh	Liposarcoma	5,000 rads + Surgery	0	0	47 NED
4	38	F	Thigh	MFC, Grade 2	5,000 rads + Surgery	0	0	36 NED
5	63	M	Thigh	MFC	6,000 rads + Surgery	0	0	24 NED
6	19	F	Thigh	Neurofibro-sarcoma	5,000 rads + Surgery + Chemotherapy	Pulmonary	0	32 Expired
7	75	F	Thigh	Unclassified	Chemotherapy + 5,000 rads + Surgery	0	0	18 NED
8	63	M	Thigh	Leiomyosarcoma, Grade 1	5,000 rads + Surgery	0	0	20 NED
9	56	M	Shoulder	Neurofibrosarcoma, Grade 3	5,000 rads + Surgery	0	0	19 NED
10	75	M	Axillary fold	MFC, Grade 3	5,000 rads + Surgery	0	0	16 NED

MFC Malignant fibrohistiocytoma.
NED No evidence of disease.

disease (Figs. 6–9). In treating this patient, it was learned that sutures should not be removed too readily if there is any tension, since these wounds heal slowly. The sutures are now routinely left in place for 14 days or more.

The second lesion was in the posterior axillary fold and was diagnosed as a malignant fibrohistiocytoma, Grade 3. This patient is now 16 months postresection with no evidence of recurrent disease.

Another tumor, in the popliteal area, was treated but not included in this series, because the patient had extensive pulmonary metastases. The tumor was treated by preoperative radiation, excision was performed, and chemotherapy was given for the pulmonary metastases. The patient developed metastases to liver and brain, and died 6 months after excision of the primary lesion. At the time of autopsy, it was noted that there were microscopic foci of tumor present in the primary site.

Fig. 6 (**top left**).—Case of shoulder lesion showing anterior radiation field.
Fig. 7 (**top right**).—Case of shoulder lesion showing posterior radiation field and unhealed biopsy scar.
Fig. 8 (**bottom left**).—Shoulder mass removed with upper portion of scapula.
Fig. 9 (**bottom right**).—Patient with shoulder lesion 1 year after preoperative radiation and excision with a good functional limb.

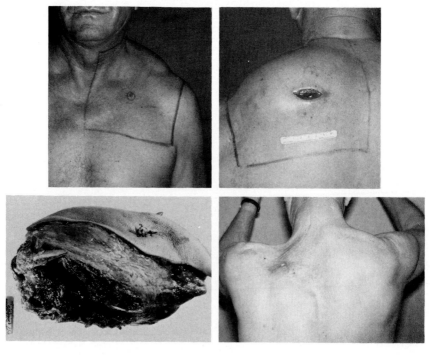

An additional group of 12 patients, all treated in 1976, is included in this series. Of these 12 patients, all are living. Two have pulmonary metastases, and these 2 have been placed on chemotherapy.

Discussion

These 22 patients presented with large, often deep-seated, lesions. Over 50 % of these lesions were located in the thigh (Table 2); other sites were the calf, shoulder, chest wall, buttocks, and arm. Lesions of the thigh lend themselves well to treatment by preoperative radiation followed by excision. It is difficult to excise large lesions located in the thigh before radiation, since they are often vascular, deep-seated, and close to major vessels and nerves.

Preoperative radiation seems to produce a thick capsule around the lesion, and the lesion itself becomes necrotic. Radiation appears to shrink the lesion, although it still remains sizable. Following preoperative radiation, the lesions are usually easily resected from adjacent nerves and vessels, whereas if this resection had been tried before radiation, it would have been impossible or, when rarely accomplished, would soon have resulted in local recurrence. It is gratifying to learn how many irradiated lesions can be resected from major vessels and nerves, thus preserving a functional limb.

Great care must be taken, however, in performing surgery in heavily irradiated areas. The tissue must be handled with care and the greatest possible blood supply preserved. Skin flips should be made as thick as possible and, in closing the wound, hemostasis must be meticulous. If dead spaces remain, suction catheters should be inserted in such a manner as to bring the catheter out through the skin away from the incision and out of the irradiated area whenever possible. The wound should be closed without tension and a mild pressure dressing applied. If the lesion is in the thigh, the entire limb should

TABLE 2. – LOCATION OF
SOFT TISSUE TUMORS

SITE	NUMBER
Thigh	15
Calf	3
Buttocks	1
Upper arm	1
Shoulder	1
Chest wall	1
Total:	22

be wrapped from the foot to the inguinal area in order to insure good venous circulation. The bandage must not be applied too tightly, because a tight bandage may produce pressure and ulceration of the wound. If there is any possible contamination, antibiotics should be given. When such a wound becomes infected, it will cause sloughing or open ulcers, and these are extremely difficult to heal.

After surgery, ambulation is encouraged and begins as soon as possible. Exercises are started in bed the day after surgery to keep all joints limber and to prevent contractions from developing; this is done especially in the calf. Once the wound is healed, full use of the extremity is encouraged. The patient is instructed that great care must be taken of the irradiated area and that it should not be subjected to long periods of bright sunlight or extremes in temperature. The patient must always guard against injury to this area, since scratches and cuts are difficult to heal.

Of the 10 patients who survived longer than 1 year, 2 have died, 1 due to disease and 1 due to complications involving chemotherapy (Table 1). In this group, there has been no failure due to recurrence. The only local recurrence was in the patient not included in this series because of the extensive disease at the time of treatment, and this recurrence was microscopic in nature.

This series is, of course, small and has not been followed long enough to assure that local recurrences will not appear; such local recurrences would necessitate amputation. Using preoperative radiation, it appears that local recurrences can be controlled to a point comparable to, if not better than, wide en bloc dissection or amputation alone; and, most importantly, a useful limb is preserved.

As previously stated, the recurrence rate for local excisions alone is over 70% (Clark, Martin, and White, 1959; Martin, Butler, and Albores-Saavedra, 1964). Soft tissue sarcomas occur in all age groups, and the amount of radiation given is not well-suited for the growing infant or child. The young adult who survives his disease may at a later date develop a tumor in the irradiated field due to the irradiation. This, of course, remains to be seen as these patients are followed over the ensuing years.

The majority of patients in this series have not had adjuvant chemotherapy, except for those who had pulmonary metastases or developed metastases following local treatment. This has been intentional in this series so that a comparison of the overall survival rate between wide en bloc resections and amputation alone can be made with preoperative radiation and local resection.

It has been found in this series using preoperative radiation that such radiation produces a capsule around a completely necrotic tumor mass. The tumor mass is frequently reduced in size; however, this may not be recognized until 4–5 weeks postradiation. A period of 4–5 weeks between radiation and the performance of resection is required so that the tissue in the radiated area can recover from the immediate effects of radiation.

Summary

Twenty-two patients have been presented who have undergone planned preoperative radiation, 10 of whom have survived at least 1 year. Of 10 patients who could have survived at least 1 year, 2 have died.

Preoperative radiation reduces the size of the tumor, and the tumor appears to become more encapsulated, often necrotic, and nonviable, thus making local excision easier. Local control, to date, has been most satisfactory and through this method of treatment, a good functional limb has been preserved.

In viewing the overall 80% survival rate, one must consider this a preliminary report which shows a series which has local recurrence rates and survival rates at least comparable to those series in which patients undergo amputations.

REFERENCES

Clark, R. Lee, Jr., Martin, R. G., and White, E. C.: A critical review of the management of soft tissue sarcomas. The Journal-Lancet, 79:327–331, July 1959.

Clark, R. Lee, Jr., Martin, R. G., White, E. C., and Old, J. W.: Clinical aspects of soft tissue tumors. Archives of Surgery, 74:859–870, June 1957.

Martin, R. G., Butler, J. J., and Albores-Saavedra, J.: Soft tissue tumors: Surgical treatment and results. In *Tumors of Bone and Soft Tissue* (The University of Texas M. D. Anderson Hospital and Tumor Institute, 8th Annual Clinical Conference on Cancer). Chicago, Illinois, Year Book Medical Publishers, Inc., 1965, pp. 333–347.

The Chemotherapy of Soft Tissue Sarcomas in Adults*

ROBERT S. BENJAMIN, M.D.†, LAURENCE H. BAKER,
D.O., VICTORIO RODRIGUEZ, M.D., THOMAS E.
MOON, Ph.D., ROBERT M. O'BRYAN, M.D., RONALD
L. STEPHENS, M.D., JOSEPH G. SINKOVICS, M.D.,
TATE THIGPEN, M.D., GERALD W. KING, M.D.,
RICHARD BOTTOMLEY, M.D., CARL W. GROPPE, Jr.,
M.D., GERALD P. BODEY, M.D., and JEFFREY A.
GOTTLIEB, M.D.‡

M. D. Anderson Hospital, Houston, Texas
Wayne State University School of Medicine, Detroit, Michigan
M. D. Anderson Hospital, Houston, Texas
M. D. Anderson Hospital, Houston, Texas
Henry Ford Hospital, Detroit, Michigan
University of Kansas Medical Center, Kansas City, Kansas
M. D. Anderson Hospital, Houston, Texas
University of Mississippi Medical Center, Jackson, Mississippi
Ohio State University Hospitals, Columbus, Ohio
Oklahoma Medical Research Foundation, Oklahoma City, Oklahoma
Cleveland Clinic, Cleveland, Ohio
M. D. Anderson Hospital, Houston, Texas
M. D. Anderson Hospital, Houston, Texas

PRIOR TO THE INTRODUCTION of Adriamycin into clinical trials in 1968, results in the chemotherapy of soft tissue sarcomas of adults

---

*All the authors of this manuscript are members of the Southwest Oncology Group, Kansas City, Kansas
†Junior Faculty Fellow of the American Cancer Society
‡Deceased

were extremely disappointing. The best results were obtained with a modification of the VAC regimen used for the treatment of childhood rhabdomyosarcoma. Although 3 of 5 patients with rhabdomyosarcoma had complete or partial (> 50% tumor regression) remissions, only 2 of 9 with other soft tissue sarcomas achieved partial remission (Jacobs, 1970). With Adriamycin, remissions were seen in 33%–40% of patients (O'Bryan *et al.*, 1973; Benjamin, Wiernik, and Bachur, 1975.) In addition, an important finding emerged from this dose-response study of Adriamycin carried out in the Southwest Oncology Group (SWOG). For patients with sarcomas, a clear trend toward increased response at higher doses was apparent, with 4 of 20 (20%) responding at 45 mg/M², 2 of 7 (29%) at 60 mg/M², and 12 of 33 (36%) at 75 mg/M² (Gottlieb *et al.*, 1975). Adriamycin thus became the primary drug used in the management of patients with soft tissue sarcomas.

The second most important drug used in the treatment of these tumors is DIC, a drug used primarily for malignant melanoma. In the broad Phase II trial of this agent by the SWOG, a 17% response rate was noted in 53 patients with sarcomas. If the highly responsive Kaposi's sarcoma is excluded, there are 71 patients with soft tissue sarcomas in the literature treated with DIC as a single agent with 1 complete remission (CR) and 11 partial remissions (PR) (15%) reported (Gottlieb *et al.*, 1976). The most responsive of the common soft tissue sarcomas to DIC is leiomyosarcoma (1 CR + 5 PR/24). In the other soft tissue sarcomas, the response rate (CR + PR) is only 11%.

In 1972, the late Dr. Jeffrey A. Gottlieb initiated a study by the SWOG, combining Adriamycin and DIC, which demonstrated an additive antitumor effect in terms of the response rate of 46% and the complete remission rate of 13% in 171 patients with soft tissue sarcomas (Gottlieb *et al.*, 1972, 1975, 1976). In addition, there was a marked improvement in survival from a median of 6 months on Adriamycin alone to 10 months for the combination. The survival of responding patients also increased from a median of 8 months to 15 months. The importance of DIC in the treatment of sarcomas has recently been reviewed (Gottlieb *et al.*, 1976).

Sequential additions of vincristine and cyclophosphamide were then made to the ADIC regimen (Gottlieb *et al.*, 1975). Although vincristine added little, it was retained pending final analysis, which demonstrated no reason for its inclusion in subsequent regimens. The CYVADIC pilot study resulted in a 59% response rate, including a 15% CR rate in 118 patients with soft tissue sarcomas.

Because of this encouraging result, CYVADIC was incorporated into the next SWOG study. Actinomycin-D had not been tried in earlier

SWOG studies because many patients had received it in prior therapy. As data with Adriamycin combinations accumulated, more patients were referred without prior therapy; therefore, the relative roles of DIC and actinomycin-D were compared by substituting actinomycin-D for DIC in a 4-drug combination (Benjamin, Gottlieb, Baker, and Sinkovics, 1976). Patients were randomized to receive either CYVADIC or CYVADACT; thus, all patients received cyclophosphamide, vincristine, and Adriamycin. Five hundred thirty-one eligible patients with sarcomas (including primary bone tumors) were registered in the study (Table 1). All patients who received protocol therapy and in whom data were available were considered evaluable. Patients dying early and those refusing further treatment or lost to follow-up were considered partially evaluable. The remainder, or fully evaluable group, is comparable to the evaluable patients in our earlier studies and represents a similar fraction of the eligible patients. The complete-plus-partial remission rates for patients with soft tissue sarcomas receiving CYVADIC, 44% of those eligible, 45% of those evaluable, and 52% of those fully evaluable, were significantly higher than the rates of those patients treated with CYVADACT, where corresponding response rates were 35%, 36%, and 40%, respectively (Table 2). The most responsive tumor was synovial sarcoma, in which the response rates (of fully evaluable patients) were 67% (CYVADIC) and 64% (CYVADACT). The superiority of the CYVADIC regimen in response rate was apparent at the 10% probability level in patients with fibrosarcoma, leiomyosarcoma, mesothelioma, and undifferentiated sarcoma. CYVADACT was similar to CYVADIC in the other tumors.

Remission duration was longer for patients receiving CYVADIC than for those receiving CYVADACT (p = 0.03). For complete responders to CYVADIC, the duration has not been reached but it is

TABLE 1.—CYVADIC vs CYVADACT:
EVALUABLE PATIENTS

	CYVADIC	CYVADACT
Eligible	270	261
Not Evaluable	10	12
Inadequate data	2	5
Major protocol violation	4	6
Intercurrent disease	4	1
Partially Evaluable	39	25
Early death	19	11
Lost to follow-up	10	10
Refused further treatment	10	4
Fully Evaluable	221	224

TABLE 2. — CYVADIC vs CYVADACT
RESPONSE OF SOFT TISSUE SARCOMAS

	NUMBER OF PATIENTS	PERCENT WITH: CR	CR + PR
Eligible			
CYVADIC	238	11	44 ⎫ p = 0.04
CYVADACT	234	11	35 ⎭
Evaluable			
CYVADIC	229	12	45 ⎫ p = 0.04
CYVADACT	224	11	36 ⎭
Fully Evaluable			
CYVADIC	193	14	52 ⎫ p = 0.02
CYVADACT	199	12	40 ⎭

projected to be 14 months and cannot be shorter than 7 months, as contrasted with 5.5 months for CYVADACT. Similarly, for partial responders, the current median durations are 5 months for patients receiving CYVADIC and 4 months for those receiving CYVADACT, and these values can increase by no more than 1 month each.

Survival of patients with sarcomas of soft tissue and bone who received CYVADIC was also superior to survival of those who received CYVADACT, particularly when only responding patients are considered (p = 0.006) (Fig. 1, Table 3). Survival on CYVADIC was not sig-

Fig. 1 (left). — Survival of responding patients with sarcomas in sequential SWOG studies.
Fig. 2 (right). — Survival of all sarcoma patients in sequential SWOG studies.

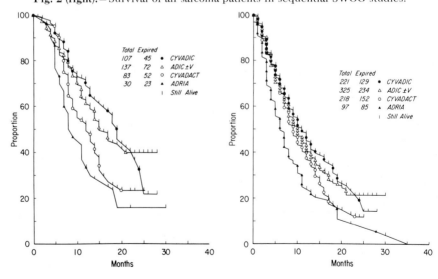

TABLE 3.—MEDIAN SURVIVAL: SEQUENTIAL SWOG
SARCOMA STUDIES

REGIMEN	NUMBER OF PATIENTS	MEDIAN SURVIVAL IN MONTHS	
		All Patients	Responders
Adriamycin	97	6	8
CYVADACT	225	9	12
ADIC ($\pm$V)	325	10	15
CYVADIC	221	11	19

nificantly superior to survival with ADIC $\pm$ V (p = 0.24), which was also superior to survival with CYVADACT (p = 0.07). The combinations were all superior to Adriamycin, with p values of 0.10 for CYVADACT, 0.008 for ADIC $\pm$ V, and 0.002 for CYVADIC. For all patients (Fig. 2, Table 3), survival was correspondingly shorter and the differences between regimens less marked. The combination regimens were all significantly superior to Adriamycin alone (p < 0.005).

One reason for the success of these programs may be the vigorous approach to chemotherapy employed. The protocol called for escalation in the dose of chemotherapy until the lowest recorded granulocyte count was $1,000/\mu$l. Despite this requirement, only 16% of patients required hospitalization for fever in the presence of neutropenia, 12% had documented infection, and 4% suffered drug-related death. This toxicity is acceptable for patients with advanced disease, particularly considering the fact that less aggressive use of similar regimens has resulted in substantially inferior response rates.

An alternative approach to CYVADIC chemotherapy has been to escalate the doses of chemotherapy without regard for hematologic toxicity in the absence of documented infection. Such an approach has been utilized in a pilot study, in the Department of Developmental Therapeutics at M. D. Anderson Hospital, which randomizes patients as follows: one group is in a standard single hospital room and the other is in a protected environment laminar air flow room and given nonabsorbable oral prophylactic antibiotics (PEPA) (Rodriquez, Bodey, and Freireich, in press). The CYVADIC regimen was used, starting 20% above the standard doses and escalating myelosuppressive agents approximately 20% per course in the absence of severe infection. As might be expected, there were fewer severe infections, 1/14 vs 6/12 for patients treated in the PEPA group. All PE patients received subsequent dose escalations, compared with 9 of 12 treated outside the PE. The preliminary analysis of this study suggests that treatment in the PE with dosage escalation results in a higher CR rate, overall response rate, and survival rate than does treatment outside the PE,

TABLE 4.—CYVADIC—PEPA AND SWOG

	SWOG	NO PE	PE
Number of Patients	221	11	14
% CR	14	9	29
% CR + PR	50	45	79
Median duration of response (months)	6	6	10
Median survival (months)	11	9	22

which is similar to our standard therapy (Table 4). Particularly impressive is the median survival of 22 months, which is longer than the survival of responding patients on our standard CYVADIC program.

Table 5 summarizes the response of over 1,000 patients with sarcomas treated with Adriamycin alone or in combination. Our best results are in the 707 patients treated with Adriamycin and DIC, with or without other drugs, in which almost 50% have achieved remission. Our future studies will further define the roles of cyclophosphamide and actinomycin-D in combination with Adriamycin and DIC, evaluate immunotherapy with this chemotherapy, continue treatment in the protected environment, and move ADIC chemotherapy into the adjuvant setting in an attempt to increase the cure rate of patients with prognostically poor sarcomas.

Abbreviations

VAC	vincristine, actinomycin-D, and cyclophosphamide
SWOG	Southwest Oncology Group
DIC	Dimethyl triazeno imidazole carboxamide (Dacarbazine)
CR	Complete remission
PR	Partial remission
ADIC	Adriamycin and DIC

TABLE 5.—RESPONSE OF SARCOMAS TO ADRIAMYCIN ALONE AND IN COMBINATION (MDAH AND SWOG)

REGIMENS	NO. EVALUABLE PATIENTS	% CR	% CR + PR
Adriamycin	97	3	31
Adriamycin combinations	932	12	46
ADIC combinations	(707)	13	48
Total no. evaluable patients	1029	12	46

CYVADIC Cyclophosphamide, vincristine, Adriamycin, and DIC
CYVADACT Cyclophosphamide, vincristine, Adriamycin, and
            actinomycin-D
V   Vincristine
PEPA   Protected environment, prophylactic antibiotics
PE   Protected environment

Acknowledgments

This work was supported in part by U.S. Public Health Service grants #CA-10379, CA-14028, CA-12014, CA-04915, CA-16943, CA-12644, CA-16385, CA-04920, CA-16957, and CA-04919 and by contract NO1-CM-53832.

REFERENCES

Benjamin, R. S., Gottlieb, J. A., Baker, L. O., and Sinkovics, J. G.: CYVADIC vs CYVADACT—A randomized trial of cyclophosphamide (Cy), vincristine (V) and Adriamycin (A), plus either dacarbazine (DIC) or actinomycin-D (DACT) in metastatic sarcomas. (Abstract) Proceedings of the American Association of Cancer Research and American Society of Clinical Oncology, 17:256, 1976.

Benjamin, R. S., Wiernik, P. H., and Bachur, N. R.: Adriamycin: A new effective agent in the therapy of disseminated sarcomas. Medical and Pediatric Oncology, 1:63–76, 1975.

Gottlieb, J. A., Baker, L. H., O'Bryan, R. M. et al.: Adriamycin (NSC 123127) used alone and in combination for soft tissue and bony sarcomas. Cancer Chemotherapy Reports, (Part 3) 6:271–282, 1975.

Gottlieb, J. A., Baker, L. H., Quagliana, J. M., Luce, J. K., Whitecar, J. P., Jr., Sinkovics, J. G., Rivkin, S. E., Brownlee, R., and Frei, E., III: Chemotherapy of sarcomas with a combination of Adriamycin and dimethyl triazeno imidazole carboxamide. Cancer, 30:1632–1638, December 1972.

Gottlieb, J. A., Benjamin, R. S., Baker, L. O., O'Bryan, R. M., Sinkovics, J. G., Hoogstraten, B., Quagliana, J. M., Rivkin, S. E., Bodey, G. P. Sr., Rodriguez, V., Blumenschein, G. R., Saiki, J. H., Coltman, C., Jr., Burgess, M. A., Sullivan, P., Thigpen, T., Bottomley, R., Balcerzak, S., and Moon, R. E.: Role of DTIC (NSC-45388) in the chemotherapy of sarcomas. Cancer Treatment Reports, 60:199–203, February 1976.

Jacobs, E. M.: Combination chemotherapy of metastatic testicular germinal cell tumors and soft part sarcomas. Cancer, 25:324–332, 1970.

O'Bryan, R. M., Luce, J. K., Talley, R. W., Gottlieb, J. A., Baker, L. H., and Bonadonna, G.: Phase II evaluation of Adriamycin in human neoplasia. Cancer, 32:1-8, July 1973.

Rodriguez, V., Bodey, G. P., and Freireich, E. J: Increased remission rate and prolongation of survival in patients with soft-tissue sarcomas treated with intensive chemotherapy on protected environment prophylactic antibiotic program (PEPA). Proceedings of the American Assocation of Cancer Research and American Society of Clinical Oncology 17, 1977. (In press.)

Preliminary Results of the Intergroup Rhabdomyosarcoma Study (IRS)*

HAROLD M. MAURER, M.D., THOMAS MOON, Ph.D., M.D., MILTON DONALDSON, M.D., CARLOS FERNANDEZ, M.D., EDMUND A. GEHAN, Ph.D., DENMAN HAMMOND, M.D., DANIEL M. HAYS, M.D., WALTER LAWRENCE, Jr., M.D., WILLIAM NEWTON, Jr., M.D., ABDELSALAM RAGAB, M.D., BEVERLY RANEY, M.D., EDWARD H. SOULE, M.D., W. W. SUTOW, M.D., and MELVIN TEFFT, M.D.

Medical College of Virginia, Richmond, Virginia
M. D. Anderson Hospital, Houston, Texas
Fox Chase Cancer Center, Philadelphia, Pennsylvania
M. D. Anderson Hospital, Houston, Texas
M. D. Anderson Hospital, Houston, Texas
University of Southern California School of Medicine,
Los Angeles, California
Children's Hospital of Los Angeles, Los Angeles, California
Medical College of Virginia, Richmond, Virginia
The Children's Hospital, Columbus, Ohio
Emory University, Atlanta, Georgia
Children's Hospital, Philadelphia, Pennsylvania
Mayo Clinic, Rochester, Minnesota
M. D. Anderson Hospital, Houston, Texas
Brown University, Providence, Rhode Island

---

*Representing Cancer and Acute Leukemia Group B, Children's Cancer Study Group, and Southwest Oncology Group

In 1972, ACUTE LEUKEMIA GROUP B, Children's Cancer Study Group, and Southwest Oncology Group combined their resources and initiated a prospective intergroup study of childhood rhabdomyosarcoma (RMS) (Maurer, 1976 a, b). The primary objectives of the study are:

(1) To determine if local radiation is a necessary adjunct to combined chemotherapy (vincristine, VCR; dactinomycin, AMD; and cyclophosphamide, CYC) for local disease control in patients who have had (pathologically confirmed) complete excision of a localized tumor.
(2) To compare the length of remission produced by a regimen of VCR and AMD versus that produced by VCR, AMD, and CYC in patients with grossly resected regional disease but with microscopic residual tumor at the margin of resection, all of whom receive local radiation.
(3) To compare the response rates and duration of response from intensive therapy with VCR, AMD, and CYC as opposed to the same drug combination plus Adriamycin (ADR), in patients with gross residual disease following surgery or with metastatic disease at diagnosis.
(4) To collect a large enough group of cases to permit characterization of the disease more thoroughly than was previously possible, and to relate multiple factors including age, histologic cell type, site of tumor origin, and extent of disease to treatment responses and prognosis.

Although the study is still in progress, findings of considerable clinical interest already have emerged. The purpose of this report is to present these initial results, focusing particularly on the response rate, duration of response, and survival produced thus far by each treatment regimen.

Methods

PATHOLOGICAL FINDINGS

The pathology subcommittee reviewed the histologic material submitted for each patient registered in the study to determine patient eligibility. The eligibility requirement was that the material be interpreted as being 1 of or a mixture of the 4 recognized subtypes of RMS; namely, embryonal, alveolar, botryoid, and pleomorphic. Three additional tumor types were recognized and are also included. These subtypes were coded as special undifferentiated; Type I and Type II; and undifferentiated, type indeterminate.

CLINICAL GROUPING CLASSIFICATION

Since the therapeutic questions posed required a clinical grouping (staging) classification, a system based on the extent of disease and the type of surgery performed was established for all patients, and treatment regimens were randomly assigned to each patient according to clinical group. The clinical grouping classification is as follows:

Group I: Localized disease, completely resected. Regional nodes not involved
(a) Confined to muscle or organ of origin.
(b) Contiguous involvement—infiltration outside the muscle or organ of origin, as through fascial planes.
Notation: This includes both gross inspection and microscopic confirmation of complete resection.

Group II: (a) Grossly resected tumor with microscopic residual disease. No evidence of gross residual tumor. No clinical or microscopic evidence of regional node involvement.
(b) Regional disease, completely resected. Regional nodes involved and/or extension of tumor into an adjacent organ. All tumor completely resected with no microscopic residual disease.
(c) Regional disease with involved nodes grossly resected, but with evidence of microscopic residual disease.

Group III: Incomplete resection or biopsy with gross residual disease.

Group IV: Metastatic disease present at onset.

STUDY DESIGN

The study design and treatment schedules are illustrated in Figure 1. Previously untreated patients under 21 years of age are eligible.

Fig. 1.— Treatment schedules for the Intergroup Rhabdomyosarcoma Study.

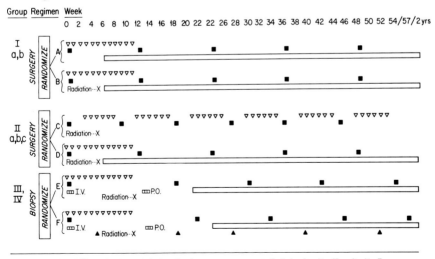

∇ Vincristine, 2 mg/m², I.V. (Maximum single dose, 2mg)

■ Dactinomycin, 0.015mg/kg/d, I.V. (Maximum single dose, 0.5mg) x5

▢ Cyclophosphamide, 2.5 mg/kg/d, P.O.

▥ Cyclophosphamide, 10 mg/kg/d x7

▲ Adriamycin, 60 mg/m², I.V.

Patients in Group I are randomized between 2 treatment regimens: (A) – VCR (2 mg/m² i.v. weekly × 12); AMD (0.015 mg/kg/day i.v. ×5; course repeated × 4 in 48 weeks); and CYC (2.5 mg/kg/day p.o. from day 42 up to 24 months); or (B) – VCR, AMD, and CYC in the same schedule as regimen A, plus postoperative irradiation to the primary tumor site.

Patients in Group II all receive radiation to the local tumor site following surgery. In addition, they receive treatment regimen (C) – VCR (2 mg/m² i.v. weekly × 6; 6 courses over a 48-week period) plus AMD (0.015 mg/kg/day i.v. × 5; course repeated × 5 in 45 weeks); or regimen (D) – VCR, AMD, and CYC in the same schedule as in regimen (B) in Group I above.

Patients in Groups III and IV are randomized between treatment regimen (E) – VCR (2 mg/m² i.v. weekly × 12); AMD (0.015 mg/kg/day i.v. × 5; course repeated × 4 in 54 weeks); and CYC (10 mg/kg/day i.v. days 1 – 7, course repeated orally days 84 – 90, then 2.5 mg/kg/day p.o. from day 140 to 24 months, "pulse" VAC); or regimen (F) – the same drug combination plus Adriamycin (ADR) (60 mg/m² i.v. × 5 in 51 weeks). The first dose of ADR is reduced to 30 mg/m² if significant bone marrow volume is to be irradiated, e.g., the whole retroperitoneum and whole pelvis. In Group III patients, the primary tumor site is radiated after 6 weeks of chemotherapy. Only Group IV patients with lung metastases receive radiation to the primary site and to the lungs. Surgery may be performed subsequently, particularly if nonoperative treatment has been effective in shrinking the primary lesion.

The radiation therapy employed in this study has been standardized as much as possible. Recommendations include delivering 5,000 to 6,000 rads in 5 to 6 weeks to the primary site of tumor origin. Radiation to clinically uninvolved regional nodes has not been advised. It has been advised that children under 3 years of age should not receive more than 4,000 rads. Radiation is to be delivered at the rate of 900 to 1,200 rads per week with supervoltage. Normal tissue such as lung, liver, kidney, and nervous system tissue requires shielding so as not to exceed tolerance. When metastatic disease is confined to the lung, bilateral pulmonary radiation is given simultaneously with radiation of primary site. The dose should not exceed 1,800 rads in 9 equal fractions. Radiation is to be administered even when there is total regression of all demonstrable lesions from the initial chemotherapy.

Major deviations in chemotherapy are judged to exist if any of the following apply: failure to begin therapy by the 21st day following the definitive operative procedure or within 42 days following the initial operative procedure; use of chemotherapy not specified by the assigned regimen; failure to administer appropriate dose or schedule of drugs as specified by protocol unless omission or reduction in dosage is necessitated by toxicity or acceptable clinical reason.

A major radiotherapy deviation exists if any of the following apply: less than 85% of the prescribed dose is administered; the volume of radiation is too limited for the known extent of the disease; the rate of delivery of radiation is prolonged excessively; or radiation is begun prior to the prescribed time without evidence of local tumor progression during the initial chemotherapy.

EVALUATION PROCESS

Each patient is thoroughly evaluated by members of the multidisciplinary steering committee, from the standpoints of pathological findings, staging, and treatment received. Patients are classified as evaluable or nonevaluable, depending on the degree of variance from the recommendations prescribed in the protocol. Evaluability requires review of pathology, surgery, radiotherapy, and chemotherapy data by members of the committee for documentation of compliance with the recommendations prescribed in the protocol. Nonevaluability status is assigned to patients who have major protocol deviations in chemotherapy or radiotherapy.

Response to all treatments received is described as complete remission (CR) or partial remission (PR). In the latter category, at least a 50% reduction of gross disease is required. Other designations of response include: (1) no measurable disease (considered a partial response)—the site of involvement precludes definite measurement of disease extent except where gross residual disease is known to exist at the start of chemotherapy but regresses either partially or completely with treatment; (2) mixed response (MR)—regression and progression of disease are noted simultaneously at different sites; (3) no response (NR); and (4) progressive disease (PD). Additional terms used are as follows: complete remission—absence of any demonstrable tumor; continuous response—maintenance of the CR, PR status, or continued regression of disease in patients in PR status.

At least 6 weeks of treatment according to protocol is considered an adequate trial. Deaths occurring within 6 weeks of registration are considered "early deaths." Reappearance or progression of disease at any site or the appearance of disease at new sites is considered a relapse, and the patient is eliminated from the study.

Statistical analyses of survival and disease-free periods have been performed using the Kaplan-Meier method for calculating and project-

TABLE 1.—INTERGROUP
RHABDOMYOSARCOMA STUDY

PATIENT STATUS	NUMBER
Total Registered	423
Not Eligible	33 (8%)
Too Early to Evaluate	82 (19%)
Eligible	308 (73%)
Evaluable	278
Not Evaluable	30

ing curves. This method incorporates all of the follow-up information for each patient who has died or relapsed as well as for those patients who are still alive or in remission. Each patient's follow-up information influences the curve only up to the point of his last contact date, or death or relapse. The statistical significance of the differences among curves has been evaluated by the modified Wilcoxon statistic (Gehan, 1965).

Results

A total of 423 patients were randomized for study between November 21, 1972, and March 8, 1976 (Table 1). Thirty-three (8%) are not eligible, 82 (19%) are considered too early to evaluate because of insufficient data, and 308 (73%) are eligible.

CLINICAL GROUP

Table 2 shows the distribution of eligible patients according to clinical group. The group with the largest number of patients (36%) consists of those with gross residual disease (Group III); together Groups III and IV (those with metastatic disease) make up 56% of the total num-

TABLE 2.—INTERGROUP
RHABDOMYOSARCOMA STUDY.
DISTRIBUTION OF ELIGIBLE
PATIENTS BY CLINICAL GROUP

CLINICAL GROUP	NO. (%)
I	50 (16)
II	85 (28)
III	111 (36)
IV	62 (20)
Total	308 (100)

ber of evaluable patients. Disease has been localized and completely resected in only 16% of patients.

TREATMENT RESULTS

Of the 308 eligible patients, 278 (90%) are evaluable for this analysis and 30 (10%) are not evaluable because of major protocol violations in radiotherapy (7 patients) or chemotherapy (10 patients), early death (8 patients), and incorrect clinical grouping (5 patients). Of the 8 early deaths, 6 were due to toxicity, 1 was due to a probable brain hemorrhage, and 1 occurred because of advanced metastatic disease. Thirteen patients are not included in the tabulation of evaluable patients because they were incorrectly grouped at the time of the randomization, based on later review of all the data.

CLINICAL GROUP I (DISEASE LOCALIZED AND COMPLETELY RESECTED)

Figure 2 illustrates the duration of disease-free interval and survival for Group I patients. By definition, these patients are considered to be in complete remission from the date they were entered in the study, since the only known disease was resected completely. Two of the 24

Fig. 2.—Duration of complete response (CR) *(upper graph)* and survival *(lower graph)* by regimen for clinical Group I patients.

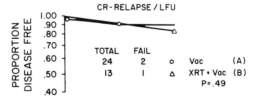

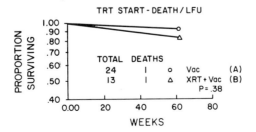

patients (8%) who received no postoperative irradiation of the primary site have relapsed, with disease at the local site, and 1 of them has died. One of the 13 patients (8%) who received postoperative irradiation developed metastatic disease and died. By actuarial analysis, at least 80% of the patients in each treatment group are expected to remain disease-free at 60 weeks. Local recurrence rates (8%) and duration of disease-free interval in the irradiated and nonirradiated groups are not statistically different at this time (p values > .49). There is also no significant difference in survival from the start of chemotherapy (p = .38).

Five patients in Group I (5/42) had amputations performed for primary lesions involving an extremity or the paratesticular area and were assigned treatment regimen A, omitting postoperative irradiation to the tumor bed. From the standpoint of the study, these patients are evaluated separately and are not included with the patients in Figure 2. All 5 patients in this group continue in complete remission from 49 to 136 weeks.

CLINICAL GROUP II (REGIONAL DISEASE—RESECTED)

The duration of disease-free interval and survival for Group II patients is illustrated in Figure 3. Group II patients are also considered

Fig. 3.—Duration of complete response *(upper graph)* and survival *(lower graph)* by regimen for clinical Group II patients.

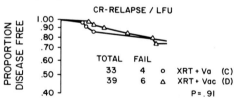

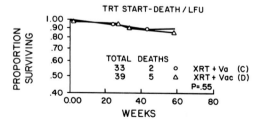

to be in complete remission from the date they begin chemotherapy. Four of 33 (12%) patients who received VCR and AMD for 1 year have relapsed, (1 local, 3 metastatic), while 6 of 39 (15%) who received VCR, AMD, and CYC for 2 years have relapsed (4 local, 2 metastatic). The difference in relapse rates is not significant (p = .48), nor is there a significant difference in disease-free interval or survival (p values > .55). At least 75% of patients in each treatment group are expected to remain disease-free at 60 weeks, and the projected survival is greater than 80% for the same time period.

Although the number in each subgroup is still small, no significant differences in relapse rate among the clinical Group II subgroups (IIa, IIb, and IIc, i.e., regional resections with or without microscopic residual or nodal involvement) have emerged as yet.

CLINICAL GROUP III (LOCALIZED DISEASE—NOT COMPLETELY RESECTED)

The response to regimens E and F in Group III patients is shown in Table 3. Twenty-five of 48 patients (52%) receiving regimen E ("pulse" VAC) have achieved a complete remission and 14/48 (29%) have achieved a PR. For those receiving regimen F ("pulse" VAC plus ADR), 22/47 (47%) have achieved a complete remission and 16/47 (34%) have had a PR. Thus, 81% (77/95) of the patients on regimens E and F have responded favorably. The median time to complete remission is almost the same for both regimens (8 weeks for regimen E and 7 weeks for regimen F); 28% and 32% of complete remissions have been achieved at 6 weeks, prior to the start of radiation in regimens E and F, respectively. After obtaining a complete remission, 5/25 (20%) patients in regimen E and 7/22 (32%) in regimen F have relapsed. This difference is not statistically significant (p = .33). Five of 14 (36%) and 7/16 (44%) patients in partial response in regimens E and F, respectively, have relapsed. This difference is not statistically significant (p = .28).

Nine of 10 relapses in regimen E involved local recurrences or extension into adjacent sites; 1 was due to distant metastases. In contrast, relapses in regimen F have been essentially evenly divided, with metastases in 8/14 patients and local recurrence or adjacent extension in 6/14 patients.

As yet, there is no significant difference in either length of complete remission (p = .18) or survival between regimen E and F (Fig. 4). Sev-

TABLE 3.—INTERGROUP RHABDOMYOSARCOMA STUDY
RESPONSE DURATION BY CLINICAL GROUP AND TREATMENT FOR EVALUABLE
GROUP III PATIENTS (CLINICAL GROUP DETERMINED BY INSTITUTION)

CLINICAL GROUP TREATMENT	NUMBER EVALUATED	NO. CR (%)	NO. STILL IN CR (%)	DURATION OF CR (WKS) RANGE	NO. PR (%)	NO. STILL IN PR (%)	DURATION OF PR (WKS)	WEEKS TO CR, MEDIAN (RANGE)
III-E	48	25 (52)	20 (80)	0–139	14 (29)	9 (64)	3–71	8 (0–34)
III-F	47	22 (47)	15 (68)	20–125	16 (34)	9 (56)	0–56	7 (0–22)
Total	95	47	35		30	18		
		P = .33		P = .18	P = .28		P = .38	P = .78

CR = complete response; PR = partial response.

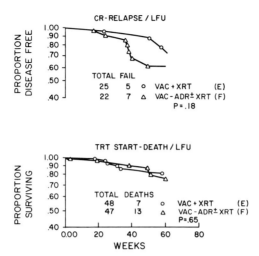

Fig. 4.—Duration of complete response *(upper graph)* and survival *(lower graph)* by regimen for clinical Group III patients.

en of 48 patients (15%) in regimen E and 13/47 (28%) in regimen F have died (p = .65).

CLINICAL GROUP IV (METASTATIC DISEASE PRESENT AT DIAGNOSIS)

Clinical Group IV patients' responses are shown in Table 4. Thirteen of 26 (50%) patients who received regimen E ("pulse" VAC) have achieved a complete remission and 8/26 (31%) have obtained a PR. Thirteen of 30 patients (43%) obtained a complete remission with regimen F ("pulse" VAC plus ADR) and 12/30 (40%) have obtained a PR. Thus, 81% and 83% of patients with metastatic disease at diagnosis have responded favorably to regimens E and F, respectively. These differences are not statistically significant (p values > .25). Although patients who achieve a complete remission on "pulse" VAC plus ADR have done so earlier than those achieving complete remission on "pulse" VAC alone (medians: 5 versus 11 weeks), this difference is not statistically significant (p = .33). As in Group III patients, 23% and 31% of complete remissions, respectively, have occurred prior to the start of radiation to the primary site.

There is no statistically significant difference in relapse rates between regimens: 9/13 (69%) receiving regimen E and 7/13 (54%) receiving regimen F have relapsed after obtaining a complete remission (p = .39). All 8 patients who obtained a PR with regimen E have re-

TABLE 4.—INTERGROUP RHABDOMYOSARCOMA STUDY
RESPONSE DURATION BY CLINICAL GROUP AND TREATMENT
FOR EVALUABLE GROUP IV PATIENTS
(CLINICAL GROUP DETERMINED BY INSTITUTION)

CLINICAL GROUP TREATMENT	NUMBER EVALUATED	NO. CR (%)	NO. STILL IN CR (%)	DURATION OF CR (WKS) RANGE	NO. PR (%)	NO. STILL IN PR (%)	DURATION OF PR (WKS)	WEEKS TO CR, MEDIAN (RANGE)
IV–E	26	13 (50)	4 (31)	4–127	8 (31)	0 (0)	4–40	11 (1–26)
IV–F	30	13 (43)	6 (46)	1–113	12 (40)	6 (50)	6–74	5 (0–100)
Total	56	26	10		20	6		
		P = .34		P = .75	P = .25		P = .21	P = .33

CR = complete response; PR = partial response.

lapsed, whereas only half (6/12) of the patients with PR in regimen F have relapsed.

As in Group III, better local disease control is obtained with regimen F than with regimen E. Four of 13 patients (31%) receiving regimen F have had local recurrences, 8/13 (62%) had metastases, and 1/13 (8%) had both local recurrence and metastases. In regimen E, the disease of 8/17 patients (47%) has recurred locally, 8/17 (47%) distantly, and 1/17 (6%) both locally and distantly.

So far, there is no significant difference in either length of complete remission or survival between regimens E and F (Fig. 5). Sixteen of 26 patients (62%) who received regimen E and 12/30 (40%) who received regimen F have died (p = .54).

Lengths of survival from the time of disease recurrence for each clinical group are shown in Figure 6. The median length of survival after disease recurrence is surprisingly similar for clinical Groups II through IV; it is 12 weeks for Group II, 17 weeks for Group III, and 16 weeks for Group IV. Even though the number of patients in Groups

Fig. 5. – Duration of complete response *(upper graph)* and survival *(lower graph)* by regimen for clinical Group IV patients.

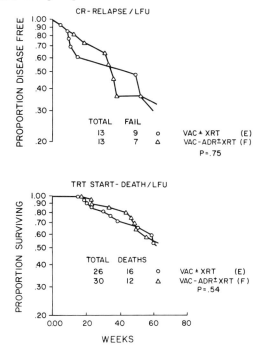

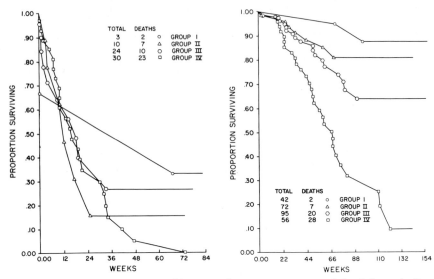

Fig. 6 (left). – The time interval between disease recurrence and death for each clinical group of patients.

Fig. 7 (right). – Comparison of the survival duration for each clinical group of patients. (Survival duration equals the interval between treatment start and death or last follow-up date.)

I and II who have relapsed is still small, the data currently suggest that recurrent disease is generally resistant to treatment.

The validity of the clinical grouping classification for RMS employed in this study is substantiated by the curves shown in Figure 7. The projected survival curve for all patients of each clinical group is shown and compared. There is a statistically significant difference in survival between each pair of curves (all p values < .05), except that between Groups II and III. These data clearly indicate that survival decreases substantially as the clinical group progresses from I through IV.

TOXICITIES

The majority of toxicities have occurred with regimens E and F, during the first week of treatment. Complications have included leukopenia and sepsis, and 5 toxic deaths have been reported. No toxic deaths have occurred since the initial course of CYC has been reduced by protocol modification from 7 to 5 doses (May 1, 1975).

Discussion

The preservation of maximum function is an important aim of therapy. Each modality has its own undesirable sequelae. The IRS addressed itself to refining therapy for Group I patients (Maurer, 1976). We assessed the need for postoperative local irradiation as an adjunct to chemotherapy in patients free of any known residual disease. Thus far, 92% of patients in both irradiated and nonirradiated groups remain disease-free at 60 + weeks, and local disease recurrence rates are not significantly different as yet. Thus, radiation therapy does not seem to influence local disease control when patients received VCR, AMD, and CYC. However, more time is needed for accrual and follow-up of Group I patients before a statistically valid conclusion can be reached and we can recommend that local irradiation be deleted from the treatment plan for this category of patients.

For Group II patients, there is no indication as yet that the 3-drug regimen, which includes CYC administered over a 2-year period, is superior to the 1-year intensive 2-drug regimen consisting of VCR and AMD. Eighty-five percent or more of patients remain disease-free in both groups, and over 87% are still alive. However, we believe that further patient accrual and follow-up are required to support these early findings.

Groups III and IV patients are randomized to receive either the more intensive "pulse" VAC or "pulse" VAC plus ADR regimens. Both combinations are remarkably effective in inducing remission of gross disease — producing favorable responses in over 80% of patients. Complete regression of disease has been observed in approximately half of the patients in these 2 groups and in over one-fourth even before the start of regional radiation therapy (Tefft, Fernandez, and Moon, in press). This gives some encouragement to the future use of chemotherapy as the initial treatment method for a broader range of lesions. There is still no indication that within clinical Groups III and IV, one chemotherapy treatment program is superior to the other.

Seventy-five of 95 (79%) patients in Group III are alive and 53/95 (56%) remain in continuous response (CR, PR). These 53 patients in continuous response represent 69% (53/77) of the total number of responders in this group.

Twenty-eight of 56 (50%) patients in Group IV are alive and 16/56 (29%) continue to maintain their response status (CR, PR). Of the total number of Group IV patients who responded (46/56), 16/46 (35%) remain in response.

Significant therapeutic problems continue for Groups III and IV patients. Although "cure" is now possible for patients with localized gross residual or metastatic disease, control fails in a substantial proportion and they die. Delineation of high risk factors may allow for identification of these individuals and permit the early use of other therapeutic programs of greater intensity.

When all clinical groups are considered together, 208 of 265 (79%) evaluable patients are alive and 170 of 237 (72%) remain in continuous response. Although no significant difference between treatment options for each of the 4 clinical groups has emerged as yet, the overall follow-up period is still short. Differences may emerge later as the follow-up period increases.

Abbreviations

ADR — adriamycin
AMD — dactinomycin
CR — complete response
CYC — cyclophosphamide
IRS — Intergroup Rhabdomyosarcoma Study
PR — partial response
VAC — vincristine, dactinomycin, cyclophosphamide
VCR — vincristine

Acknowledgment

This study was supported by grants CA 03735, CA 04646, CA 12014, CA 16943, CA 13539, and CA 16118 from the National Institutes of Health, U. S. Public Health Service.

REFERENCES

Gehan, E.: A generalized Wilcoxon test for comparing arbitrarily singly-censored samples. Biometrika 52:203–224, 1965.

Maurer, H. M., for the I. R. S. Committee: Intergroup Rhabdomyosarcoma Study (I.R.S.): Progress report. (Abstract) Proceedings American Society of Clinical Oncology, Toronto, May 4–5, 1976, p. 24.

Maurer, H. M.: Rhabdomyosarcoma in children: Progress and problems. In Sinks, L. F., and Godden, J. O. Eds.: Conflicts in Childhood Cancer. New York, Alan R. Liss, Inc., 1975a, pp. 345–357.

Maurer, H. M.: The Intergroup Rhabdomyosarcoma Study (N.I.H.) objectives and clinical staging classification. Journal of Pediatric Surgery, 10:977–978, 1975b.

Tefft, M., Fernandez, C. H., and Moon, T. E.: Rhabdomyosarcoma: Response with chemotherapy prior to radiation in patients with gross residual disease. Cancer (In press.)

Palliative Neurosurgical Procedures

MILAM E. LEAVENS, M.D.

Department of Surgery, Section of Neurosurgery,
The University of Texas System Cancer Center
M. D. Anderson Hospital and Tumor Institute,
Houston, Texas

SARCOMAS OF BONE AND SOFT TISSUE produce intractable pain as they infiltrate and compress tissue containing nerve pain fibers or nerve endings such as those in periosteum, fascia, tendons, skin, dura, air sinus, and mucous membrane, as well as nerve roots, plexuses, and peripheral nerves. The pain is usually intermittent in the beginning but will become constant unless effective surgery, radiation, or chemotherapy is given. The pain is described as aching, grabbing, boring, sharp, or burning. The location of the pain is generally in the region of the primary tumor or a metastasis. Thumb pressure on the tumor or the involved bone usually aggravates the pain. In the case of a primary or metastatic vertebral tumor, the spine pain is aggravated many times when the patient is in bed.

Pain remote from the site of the tumor is present in many patients. This may be true nerve origin pain, which radiates in an extremity superficially in the distribution of a nerve root or peripheral nerve, or it may be referred pain which is deep or diffuse in an extremity. Complaints of numbness, tingling, sensory loss, or dysesthesias, when in peripheral nerve distribution, and appropriate muscle weakness and deep tendon reflex reduction indicate involvement of nerve roots, plexus, or peripheral nerve. Some patients will have a central lesion with long tract motor and sensory spinal cord symptoms and signs as well as spine and root pain; this indicates a double neurologic problem to be solved, namely that of pain and impending paraplegia.

There may be obvious physical evidence of a mass lesion accounting for the neurologic symptoms and signs, e.g., a subcutaneous chest wall tumor involving ribs and intercostal nerves or a posterior thigh mass involving the sciatic nerve. Plain X-ray examination or tomographic X-ray examination, isotope bone scan, i.v. pyelogram, lymphangiogram, arterial and venous angiography, ultrasound studies, and myelography are some of the studies useful in determining the location of sarcomas and their relation to adjacent organs, blood vessels, and nervous structures. Some tumors, because of their small size and failure to destroy, alter, or distort adjacent bony or soft tissue structures in the retroperitoneal area, may not be detectable by the above-mentioned tests even though pain and neurologic signs indicate a lesion in that location. Computerized tomographic body scanning has aided in detecting these hidden neoplasms.

Pain due to sarcoma, as with pain from other cancers, may become incapacitating and interfere with a patient's ability to work, walk, sit, enjoy life, or even to lie still under a radiotherapy treatment machine.

Generally, early neurosurgical intervention is indicated only in those patients who have impending paraplegia due to spinal cord compression as a result of vertebral and epidural tumor. In such cases; laminectomy with excision of spinal canal tumor can be combined with dorsal root rhizotomy to relieve pain and preserve spinal cord function. Patients with intractable pain due to sarcoma in the spine or paraspinal region, but not in the intraspinal region or the calvarium, trunk, or extremities, are not usually considered for neurosurgical pain-relieving procedures until after the results of local surgery, radiotherapy, or chemotherapy of the tumor are known. Increasing amounts of analgesics and narcotics are required as these patients have tumor recurrence or fail to respond to treatment. A noninvasive form of therapy for patients needing pain relief is available through the Department of Rehabilitation Medicine at M. D. Anderson Hospital. Doctors R. Villanueva and N. Lawson and their staff currently are treating patients by cutaneous electrical stimulation therapy and evaluating this treatment. Another pain-relieving procedure, percutaneous subarachnoid alcohol block of the dorsal spinal cord sensory roots, is used by Dr. Win Chu of the Department of Anesthesiology for patients who have localized pain coming from structures innervated by a few spinal nerve roots.

Neurosurgical pain-relieving procedures usually are considered when pain relief has not been adequate following treatment of the patient's disease, when increasing amounts of analgesics and narcotics are required, and when one or both of the above-mentioned pain relieving procedures no longer provide relief. Open dorsal or sensory root rhizotomy and percutaneous and open cordotomy are the invasive neurosurgical procedures we use in relieving pain in these patients.

Dorsal sensory root rhizotomy is a division of posterior roots in the spinal canal (Fig. 1) through hemilaminectomy or full laminectomy. It is most useful in the case of unilateral localized disease causing pain and sometimes is useful in bilateral pain in the thorax; it is generally not useful in the case of disseminated metastatic tumor causing bilateral pain at multiple sites. A determination of the roots involved in the pain processes is made by calculating those roots which innervate the anatomical structures which are painful. The neurological examination which may reveal sensory dysesthesias related to root, plexus, or peripheral nerve involvement is helpful in determining the involved nerve roots. One or 2 dorsal roots cephalic and caudal to the involved roots in the painful process are divided along with the involved roots to better insure that the pain will be relieved and that this relief will last for a reasonable period of time.

One advantage of dorsal root rhizotomy is that the resulting anesthesia endures and is well-tolerated by the patient. Pain relief can be expected to last until the tumor spreads beyond the anatomic struc-

Fig. 1.— Dorsal aspect of the spinal cord, the dentate ligament, and the filaments of a sensory root before rhizotomy division.

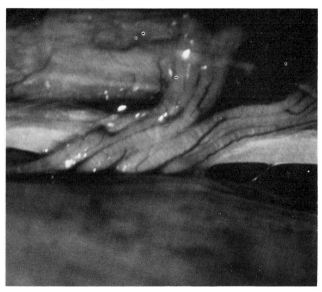

tures made anesthetic by the rhizotomy. Rarely, pain will not be relieved by rhizotomy; this is due either to an incomplete rhizotomy or a poorly understood central nervous system mechanism perpetuating the pain. A disadvantage of dorsal root rhizotomy is that it results in loss of all modalities of sensation and is therefore limited in treating a painful but functioning and useful extremity. However, if tumor has rendered an arm or a leg permanently useless, multiple root rhizotomy would be appropriate to relieve pain in that extremity. Unilateral pain due to tumor involving the chest or abdominal wall can be dealt with quite well by multiple thoracic dorsal root rhizotomies. Midline pain in the perineum, anus, and vagina due to tumors in the pelvis or mid or lower sacrum is relieved by laminectomy and selective bilateral sacral root rhizotomy. Cervical dorsal rhizotomy is combined with a cranial nerve sensory rhizotomy when there is unilateral pain due to tumor involving the head and neck.

Lateral spinothalamic tractotomy is a well-known invasive spinal cord operation in which analgesia, but not touch sensory reduction, can be produced over many dermatomes on the opposite side of the body. There are 2 advantages of this operation over dorsal root rhizotomy. First, a painful but functioning extremity made analgesic continues to function; second, it is possible to make many dermatomes analgesic with a cordotomy, whereas, from the practical standpoint, the number of roots divided by a rhizotomy is limited. Two disadvantages of cordotomy are that the maximum area of analgesia and sensory level seen immediately after the procedure is not enduring; the sensory level tends to fall. This is especially true a year or more after cervical cordotomy, and this may result in pain recurrence. The other risk or disadvantage is that postoperatively, in a small group of patients, an annoying, painful dysesthesia occurs in the area which should be without pain. Another disadvantage of cordotomy is the risk of the procedure to the corticospinal tract adjacent to the spinothalamic tract. After a cordotomy there may be extremity monoparesis, hemiparesis, or impairment of control of the bowel and bladder. These latter neurologic problems are generally few and temporary. They are more likely to be seen when bilateral cordotomies are done at the same time. Respiratory paralysis, especially during sleep, may occur in patients who have had bilateral upper cervical cordotomies.

Two methods are commonly used in performing lateral spinothalamic cordotomy. One is incising the appropriate site in the spinal cord under direct vision through a laminectomy exposure (Fig. 2). The other is a percutaneous electrode radiofrequency method of producing a lesion under X-ray control at the level of C_1 and C_2 (Fig. 3) or

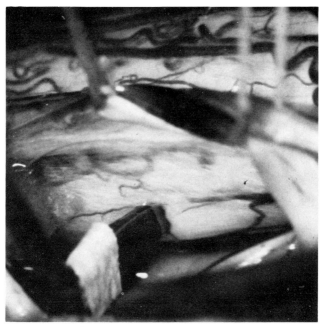

Fig. 2.—An operative view of the spinal cord during an open cordotomy. The cordotomy knife is entering the anterior lateral quadrant of the spinal cord just anterior to the dentate ligament attachment to the cord.

lower. The open method requires a patient who is in good enough general condition to tolerate a major operation. It is a useful procedure for patients with bilateral pain below the waist as well as those with unilateral pain in the trunk, upper extemity, or lower extremity. The percutaneous method requires a cooperative patient who can be tested neurologically during the procedure and is most useful in the control of unilateral upper extremity, trunk, or lower extremity pain.

Because of the risks to respiratory function, we do not perform bilateral upper cervical cordotomies in patients with bilateral pain. Cancer patients with disseminated disease causing bilateral upper thoracic and upper extremity pain are generally poor-risk patients with limited life expectancy, and we believe such patients are not suitable for cordotomies or rhizotomies, but are best treated with narcotics and a trial of cutaneous electrical stimulation.

Rosomoff and co-workers (Rosomoff, Carroll, Brown, and Sheptak, 1966; Rosomoff, Sheptak, and Carroll, 1966) and Lin and co-workers (Lin, Gildenberg, and Polakoff, 1966) have described the technique and results of upper and lower cervical percutaneous cordotomies.

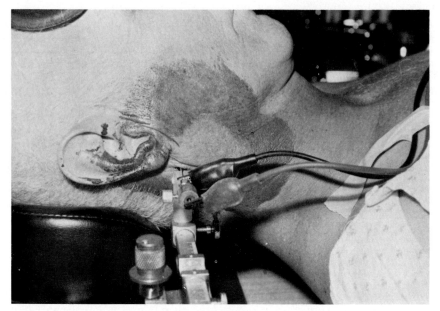

Fig. 3.—This patient, with an electrode in the spinal cord at the level between C_1 and C_2, is in position for a percutaneous cordotomy.

The immediate good results for pain relief can be as high as 90%. In chronic long-term surviving patients, 50% have a return of pain, according to Mullen as quoted by White and Sweet (1969).

Dorsal rhizotomy, reported by Barrash and Leavens (1973), resulted in satisfactory relief of pain in 50 of 71 patients. Two thirds of 33 patients who had rhizotomies for head and neck cancer had satisfactory pain relief, as reported by Leavens and Barrash (1974). The pain relief lasted an average of 14 months.

The case histories of 3 patients who had intractable pain due to sarcoma are presented in order to demonstrate the usefulness of and problems associated with cordotomy and rhizotomy.

CASE 1. — This patient, a 35-year-old woman, had a 3-year history of pain in her right hip and groin. An osteogenic sarcoma of the right ischium was treated by partial resection and 2 courses of radiotherapy. Eight months after radiotherapy, there was recurrence of tumor with excruciating pain in the right pelvis, hip, and perineum. Her pain was so severe that examination to test sensation and motor strength in her right lower extremity was inadequate. She was taking 1/32 grains of Dilaudid or 100 mg of Demerol every 3 to 4 hours, but pain relief was inadequate.

An open second thoracic lateral spinalothalamic cordotomy on the left side was done, resulting in analgesia below the ninth thoracic dermatome on the right side. There was a transient left ankle clonus, no Babinsky sign, mild weakness of the left lower extremity, and a Foley catheter was required. She was pain-free, and remained without pain, but died of metastatic tumor 5 weeks later.

Comment. — This patient's pain was adequately controlled by cordotomy during the remaining period of her life. It is unlikely in her case that a percutaneous cordotomy would have been successful because of the severity of her pain and her inability to cooperate during an operative procedure under local anesthesia. As in her case, bladder control may be deficient and a Foley catheter required after a unilateral cordotomy in patients with pelvic tumors who have bladder or sacral plexus involvement by tumor.

CASE 2. — A 28-year-old man was referred in February 1972 with a history of a mass in the left lower quadrant of the abdomen. Biopsy had been done of a retroperitoneal mass which was firmly fixed in the region of the fourth and fifth lumbar vertebra and the iliac vessels. The pathologic diagnosis was "poorly differentiated Grade 2 sarcoma suggestive of neurofibrosarcoma." On examination, the only abnormal finding was a mass, measuring approximately $11 \times 12 \times 7$ cm, in the left lower quadrant adjacent to the pelvic rim. Consultations by members of the Departments of Surgery and Radiotherapy determined that the tumor was considered unresectable and unresponsive to radiotherapy; chemotherapy consisting of vincristine, Cytoxan, and actinomycin-D was begun.

In May 1972, the patient developed pain in the lumbar paraspinal region, lower abdomen, pelvis, and hip on the left side. By July 1972, his pain had become severe and constant. Neurological examination was normal, except for findings referable to the left lower extremity. There was weakness of hamstring muscles, flexor, and extensor muscles of the foot and toes, and the left ankle reflex was absent. There was hyperesthesia to pin stick and reduced touch sense in the first sacral root distribution. Straight leg raising was limited and painful, and the patient limped when he walked. He was taking 20 mg of morphine sulphate by intramuscular injection every 6 hours for pain.

In July 1972, a right cervical C 6–7 percutaneous cordotomy was done with the following results: Pain on his left side was gone. He was analgesic on the left side in the fourth thoracic through the fifth sacral dermatomes (Fig. 4). There was slight weakness of the right lower and upper extremities. The patient had some difficulty voiding which the urologist said was due to a neurogenic bladder and distor-

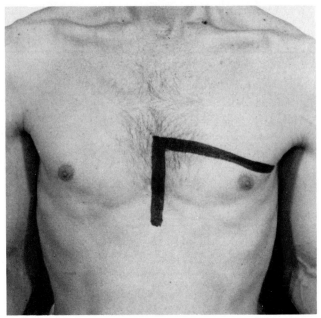

Fig. 4.—Postcordotomy anterior trunk view of the patient described in Case 2, which shows a satisfactory analgesic level at the fourth thoracic dermatome on the left.

tion of the bladder neck by tumor compression. He was dismissed to the care of his home physician 11 days after the cordotomy. He did take Tylenol for hip pain on the right side which appeared after the cordotomy; however, he was free from pain on his left side.

Pain relief was satisfactory for about 3 months. In October 1972, he returned to his doctor with increasing pain. He was given transfusions for severe anemia. Narcotics were required. He died at the end of October 1972.

Comment.—This patient had a large retroperitoneal mass causing severe unilateral pain which repressed awareness of the pain in the opposite side. Many other patients with similar bilateral tumors complain of pain in a previously nonsymptomatic side almost immediately after being relieved of the original pain by cordotomy. If the pain is severe enough, a second cordotomy may relieve the new pain.

CASE 3.—A 21-year-old man with a 5-month history of painful swelling and numbness of his right cheek was first seen in September 1965. An embryonal rhabdomyosarcoma of the maxilla was excised. The tumor had invaded the infraorbital nerve. During the next 2 years, recurrent tumor in the antrum and orbit was excised several times. The orbit was exenterated, and the patient received radiotherapy and infusions of methotrexate and actinomycin-D. Pain was lessened by this treatment for a number of months.

However, in May 1968 he again had severe pain in the region of the right orbital roof and frontal sinus. Neurological examination was normal except for a reduction in sensation in the distribution of the ophthalmic and maxillary divisions of the fifth cranial nerve. Because of the severity of the pain confined to the distribution of the trigeminal nerve, a complete posterior root sectioning of that nerve was done for pain relief.

The patient's pain was completely relieved for 3 months, when he developed pain in a different location. There was pain, swelling, and tumor recurrence in the right temporal region; this was treated by radiotherapy and incomplete removal of a right anterior middle fossa metastasis plus chemotherapy consisting of vincristine and Cytoxan.

He subsequently had progressive intense pain, requiring morphine, in the right side of his head, face, and neck. In March 1969, his pain became so severe that additional attempts to surgically relieve it were believed warranted. The anesthesia of the previous trigeminal rhizotomy was added to by sectioning the nervus intermedius, the glossopharyngeal nerve, the upper fibers of the vagus nerve, and the dorsal second and third cervical roots. Postoperatively, the patient had satisfactory relief of most of his pain for 2 months; he did require mild analgesics for some residual aching in the right orbit. During the third month after rhizotomy, severe pain in the entire right side of his head returned, requiring frequent injections of Demerol. He died 2 months later.

*Comment.—*Trigeminal rhizotomy for unilateral pain in the face and head due to cancer which seems to be confined to structures innervated by the first and second divisions of the fifth cranial nerve can be of value in some patients. It was of value in this patient for 3 months. However, patients treated in this manner eventually will experience pain recurrence if their tumor progresses and involves anatomical structures innervated by other cranial and cervical nerves. When the pain returns, a more extensive rhizotomy may be required. In other patients it will be obvious that the pain is in areas, such as the ear, pharynx, jaw, and neck, which have dual or multiple cranial and cervical nerve innervation. In these cases, a more extensive rhizotomy procedure is required rather than the simpler trigeminal rhizotomy.

The use of cordotomy and rhizotomy in the treatment of pain due to sarcomas and other types of cancer is of benefit in properly selected cases. However, a high percentage of patients treated will eventually develop intractable pain again if they live long enough and if their cancer progresses locally or at distant sites.

REFERENCES

Barrash, J. M., and Leavens, M. E.: Dorsal rhizotomy for the relief of intractable pain of malignant tumor origin. Journal of Neurosurgery, 38:755–757, June 1973.

Leavens, M. E.: Pain control in cancer patients. The Cancer Bulletin, 21: 51–55, May–June 1969.

Leavens, M. E., and Barrash, J. M.: Sensory rhizotomy (cranial and spinal) and Gasserian ganglionectomy in pain of the head and neck resulting from cancer. In Neoplasia of Head and Neck (The University of Texas System Cancer Center M. D. Anderson Hospital and Tumor Institute, 17th Annual Clinical Conference on Cancer). Chicago, Illinois, Year Book Medical Publishers, Inc., 1974, pp 261–272.

Lin, P. M., Gildenberg, P. L., and Polakoff, P. P.: An anterior approach to percutaneous lower cervical cordotomy. Journal of Neurosurgery, 25:553–560, November 1966.

Rosomoff, H. L., Carroll, F., Brown, J., and Sheptak, P.: Percutaneous radiofrequency cervical chordotomy. Journal of Neurosurgery, 23:639–644, December 1966.

Rosomoff, H. L., Sheptak, P., and Carroll, F.: Modern pain relief: Percutaneous chordotomy. Journal of the American Medical Association, 196: 482–486, May 9, 1966.

White, J. C., and Sweet, W. H.: *Pain and the Neurosurgeon. A Forty-Year Experience.* Springfield, Illinois, Charles C Thomas, Publisher, 1969, 1,000 pp.

Adjuvant Chemotherapy in the Treatment of Primary Soft Tissue Sarcomas: A Preliminary Report

ROBERT D. LINDBERG, M.D.,* WILLIAM K. MURPHY, M.D.,† ROBERT S. BENJAMIN, M.D.,† JOSEPH G. SINKOVICS, M.D.,‡ RICHARD G. MARTIN, M.D.,§ MARVIN M. ROMSDAHL, M.D., Ph.D.,§ RICHARD H. JESSE, JR., M.D.,§ and WILLIAM O. RUSSELL, M.D.#

Departments of Radiotherapy, Developmental Therapeutics,†
Medicine,‡ Surgery,§ and Pathology,#
The University of Texas System Cancer Center M. D.
Anderson Hospital and Tumor Institute, Houston, Texas*

UNTIL RECENTLY, THE USE OF CHEMOTHERAPY in the management of soft tissue sarcomas has been restricted to patients with metastatic disease. The purpose of this report is to give the preliminary results of adjuvant chemotherapy in the treatment of localized soft tissue sarcomas in adults.

In the early 1960s, a study was started using conservative surgery and postoperative radiation therapy in an attempt to preserve a functional limb. The latest results of this study are reported on pages 289–298 of this volume (Lindberg, Martin, Romsdahl, and McMurtrey, 1977). A review of these data showed that the incidence of local recurrence and distant metastasis was influenced by the grade and the initial size of the primary lesion. In Grade 1 lesions of the ex-

343

tremities, the incidence of local recurrence was 10% (3/29). In Grade 2 and Grade 3 lesions less than 5 cm in diameter, the incidence was 18.9% (7/37), whereas in high-grade lesions 5 cm or larger, the incidence was 35% (14/40). In head and neck lesions, the local recurrence was 4/9 and in intra-abdominal lesions, it was 6/9. The rate of distant metastasis followed the same pattern as local recurrence rates: In Grade 1 lesions of the extremities, the incidence was 6.9% (2/29), in Grade 2 and Grade 3 lesions less than 5 cm, 18.9% (7/37), and in Grade 2 and Grade 3 lesions larger than 5 cm, 52.4% (22/42). The disease-free survival at 5 years was 66.7% (12/18) for Grade 1 lesions, 60.9% (14/23) for Grade 2 lesions, and 33.3% (5/15) for Grade 3 lesions. Since we were able to define a high-risk patient, for whom the present therapy of conservative excision and postoperative radiation therapy was inadequate, adjuvant chemotherapy (VACAR) (in addition to surgery and radiotherapy) was started in this high-risk group.

Study Protocol

All adult patients (more than 15 years old) with extremity and trunk soft tissue sarcomas (except those with intra-abdominal lesions) who were in the high-risk group, i.e., with lesions equal to or greater than 5 cm in diameter and Grade 2 or Grade 3 histological type, received adjuvant chemotherapy on a randomized basis in addition to surgery and radiotherapy. All patients with head and neck and abdominal lesions received adjuvant chemotherapy (not randomized), since the local recurrence rate is high with surgery and radiotherapy alone. Also, there are too few cases in these latter sites to make a random study feasible. The reasons for exclusion were: (1) palpable gross tumor after surgery; (2) prior radiation therapy; (3) prior exposure to any chemotherapeutic agents; (4) distant metastasis; (5) uncontrolled other primary cancers; (6) medical contraindications, i.e., patients must have had an absolute granulocyte count of $2,000/mm^3$ or greater and a platelet count of $100,000/mm^3$ or greater, reasonable liver function (bilirubin less than 2.0 mg/100ml), and renal function (blood urea nitrogen less than 30 mg/100ml); and (7) arbitrary elimination for nonmedical reasons, not to exceed 10% of the eligible cases.

The randomization was stratified according to histological type. In both the control and chemotherapy groups, the gross tumor was removed by conservative surgical excision. Postoperative radiation therapy was initiated as soon as healing was complete. In general, the tumor dose was 6,500 rads in 6½ weeks, using the shrinking field technique after 5,000 rads. In the abdomen, the dose ranged from 5,000 rads in 5 weeks to 5,500 rads tumor dose in 5½ weeks. The details of the radiotherapy technique have been published previously (Lindberg, Fletcher, and Martin, 1975).

All patients receiving chemotherapy were treated with the following drug regimen:

(1) Vincristine – 1.5 mg/m² (top dose limit 2 mg/dose) i.v. on day 1. Day 1 of the chemotherapy coincided with day 1 of the radiotherapy. Vincristine was continued weekly for 9 weeks, and then on day 1 of each chemotherapy cycle.

(2) Adriamycin – 60 mg/m² i.v. on day 2 and repeated every 4 weeks for 7 doses (total dose limit 420 mg/m²).

(3) Cyclophosphamide – 200 mg/m² orally on days 3, 4, and 5 of each cycle. Cyclophosphamide was repeated every 4 weeks with Adriamycin and every 8 weeks while actinomycin-D was being given.

(4) Actinomycin-D – substituted for Adriamycin after the dose limitation had been reached. The dose of actinomycin-D was 0.3 mg/m² (top dose limit was 0.5 mg/dose) given on days 1 through 5 of each cycle every 8 weeks. Six courses of actinomycin-D were given over a period of 1 year. The total time of chemotherapy was 18 months.

Adjustments of the chemotherapy were anticipated in the following situations: (1) For patients developing serious infection or hemorrhage, the dose of Adriamycin and/or cyclophosphamide would be reduced by 25% in subsequent courses. No dose escalation was intended. A dose adjustment of Adriamycin and/or actinomycin-D might be required for severe skin or mucous membrane reactions. (2) For patients with severe skin reactions or myelosuppression, it might be necessary to delay the second course of chemotherapy. (3) For patients whose radiotherapy field covered more than 35% of the active bone marrow, chemotherapy followed radiotherapy because of the myelosuppression anticipated if they were given concomitantly.

Case Material and Results

From October 1973 to September 1976, 75 patients were seen who met the requirements to enter this study. Four patients were excluded: 3 patients refused chemotherapy and 1 patient wanted chemotherapy. Fifty-nine of the 71 patients in this study received radiation therapy before January 1976 and form the basis of this preliminary report. All patients have had a minimum 9-month follow-up. The location of the primary lesion of these 59 patients is as follows: head and neck, 8; abdomen, 4; trunk, 13; upper extremity, 6; and lower extremi-

TABLE 1.—CURRENT STATUS OF VACAR-TREATED PATIENTS
OCTOBER 1973 THROUGH DECEMBER 1975
FOLLOW-UP—9 TO 34 MONTHS

			CAUSE OF FAILURE		
SITE	TOTAL PATIENTS	NED	P ± DM	DM	COMP
Head and neck	8	4	1	2	1
Intra-abdominal	4	3	1		
Trunk and extremity					
Chemotherapy	27	18		9	
Control	20	17 (2)°		3	

°( ) Number of patients with recurrence at primary site salvaged by surgery.
NED—No evidence of disease; P—Primary failure; DM—Distant metastases;
Comp—Complications.

ty, 28. In addition to the 12 patients with head and neck and abdominal primary lesions, 27 of the 47 patients with primary lesions of the
trunk and extremities were randomized to receive adjuvant chemotherapy in addition to surgery and postoperative irradiation. The remaining 20 patients were in the control group (they received only
conservative surgery and postoperative irradiation).

The overall survival free of disease is 71% (42/59); the current status of patients is shown in Table 1. In patients with trunk and extremity lesions, the survival rate is 66.7% (18/27) for the chemotherapy
group and 85% (17/20) for the control group. In the control group,
however, 2 patients have developed local recurrences. In 1 patient the recurrence was outside the previously irradiated volume

TABLE 2.—LOCAL RECURRENCE BY HISTOLOGICAL TYPE
AND SITE: VACAR-TREATED PATIENTS
OCTOBER 1973 THROUGH DECEMBER 1975

	HEAD AND		TRUNK AND EXTREMITIES	
HISTOLOGY	NECK	ABDOMEN	CHEMOTHERAPY	CONTROL
Liposarcoma		1/2	0/5	0/3
Fibrosarcoma	1/1		0/1	0/2
Rhabdomyosarcoma	0/4		0/3	0/1
Leiomyosarcoma		0/1		
Neurofibrosarcoma	0/2		0/4	2/5†
Synovial sarcoma			0/5	0/2
Malignant fibrohistiocytoma	0/1		0/6	0/4
Unclassified sarcoma			0/1	0/2
Epithelioid sarcoma			0/1	0/1
Miscellaneous°		0/1	0/1	
TOTAL	1/8	1/4	0/27	2/20

°One malignant mesenchymoma and 1 neuroepithelioma.
†One recurrence outside of irradiated volume.

TABLE 3.—DISTANT METASTASES BY HISTOLOGICAL TYPE
AND SITE: VACAR-TREATED PATIENTS
OCTOBER 1973 THROUGH DECEMBER 1975

HISTOLOGY	HEAD AND NECK	ABDOMEN	TRUNK AND EXTREMITIES CHEMOTHERAPY	CONTROL
Liposarcoma		0/2	0/5	0/3
Fibrosarcoma	1/1		0/1	0/2
Rhabdomyosarcoma	2/4		0/3	1/1
Leiomyosarcoma		0/1		
Neurofibrosarcoma	0/2		2/4	1/5
Synovial sarcoma			3/5	0/2
Malignant fibrohistiocytoma	0/1		2/6	0/4
Unclassified sarcoma			1/1	1/2
Epithelioid sarcoma			1/1	0/1
Miscellaneous°		0/1	0/1	
TOTAL	3/8	0/4	9/27	3/20

°One malignant mesenchymoma and 1 neuroepithelioma.

(geographical miss), and this patient was treated by conservative excision and radiation therapy. The second patient had a recurrence within the irradiated volume and was treated by conservative excision. Both patients are living free of disease. There have been no local recurrences in the chemotherapy group.

The incidence of local recurrence and distant metastasis according to the primary site and histological type is shown in Tables 2 and 3, respectively. Only 1 patient (with fibrosarcoma of the head and neck region) has developed both a local recurrence and a distant metastasis. The highest incidence of failure (local recurrence and distant metastasis) occurred in patients with neurofibrosarcoma (5/11). Since the randomization of lesions of the trunk and extremities was not stratified by grade (Grade 2 versus Grade 3) or by size (5 cm to 8 cm versus greater than 8 cm), there are some differences between the chemotherapy and the control groups (Table 4). In the chemotherapy group,

TABLE 4.—DISTANT METASTASES BY SIZE AND GRADE OF
RANDOMIZED LESIONS OF THE TRUNK AND EXTREMITIES:
VACAR-TREATED PATIENTS
OCTOBER 1973 THROUGH DECEMBER 1975

	≥ 5 CM and < 8 CM		≥ 8 CM	
	CHEMOTHERAPY	CONTROL	CHEMOTHERAPY	CONTROL
Grade 2	1/4	1/9°	5/12	0/7
Grade 3	0/2	1/2	3/9	1/2

°Two additional patients had local recurrences; no local recurrences in chemotherapy group.

16 of 27 patients had Grade 2 lesions, whereas 16 of 20 patients had Grade 2 lesions in the control group. Also, the majority of patients (21/27) in the chemotherapy group had lesions 8 cm or greater, as compared to 9 of 20 in the control group. The incidence of distant metastasis in the chemotherapy group is highest in patients with Grade 2 lesions 8 cm or larger (5/12), whereas in the control group the incidence is 0/7 (p > .10).

Complications

The reactions of the patients in the control group treated by radiation therapy alone were minimal. A moist desquamation was noted in the irradiated fields, primarily in the skin folds, in 4 patients. Myelosuppression was negligible; the lowest recorded white blood count was 3,900/mm^3. So far, there have been no significant delayed reactions.

The toxic reactions of the patients in the chemotherapy group (excluding head and neck patients) differed according to the 2 phases. In the vincristine, Adriamycin, Cytoxan phase of the chemotherapy, the toxic reaction was considerable. The majority of the patients (nearly 100%) experienced nausea, vomiting, and alopecia. The skin reactions within the irradiated fields were augmented with an increased incidence of moist desquamation (44%, 12/27). Due to severe reactions, the radiotherapy was interrupted in 3 patients and stopped after 5,000 rads tumor dose in 2 additional patients. Thrombocytopenia was negligible; median platelet count was 182,000/mm^3 (range 90,000 to 405,000). There were no bleeding episodes, and platelet transfusions were not necessary. The median white blood cell count was 1,540/mm^3 (range 600 to 3,200). The median granulocyte count was 400/mm^3, with a range of 0 to 2,100/mm^3, and 24 of 27 patients (88.9%) below 1,000/mm^3. Three patients were hospitalized due to granulocytopenia; 1 was hospitalized twice for cellulitis, and 2 were hospitalized for fever of undetermined origin. There were 3 episodes of congestive heart failure: 1 not related to Adriamycin, 1 probably related, and 1 possibly related. All were easily controlled by routine therapy. Parasthesia from vincristine occurred in 16 of 27 patients (59.3%), but significant weakness occurred in only 4, and a foot drop in only 1. Hemorrhagic cystitis occurred in 1 patient as a secondary reaction to Cytoxan and radiation therapy (bladder included in the field).

The actinomycin-D, Cytoxan, vincristine phase of the chemotherapy was fairly well-tolerated, but the data are minimal. Significant toxic reactions were encountered, however, including myelosuppression, severe nausea and vomiting, glossitis, phlebitis, and infiltration with local necrosis and ulceration.

Head and neck patients receiving simultaneous radiation therapy and chemotherapy are discussed as a separate group because of the marked toxicity of this therapy. All patients experienced nausea, vomiting, and myelosuppression. Five patients required hospitalization and 4 had life-threatening toxic reactions (sepsis). There was 1 fatal complication in a patient who had an orbital rhabdomyosarcoma. This patient received 6,000 rads tumor dose in 6 weeks with concomitant chemotherapy and had no particular problems during treatment. Five months after completion of treatment, a craniotomy was performed because of suspected tumor. At the time of surgery, frontal lobe necrosis was noted without evidence of tumor. The patient died 19 months after the beginning of radiotherapy of central nervous system complications.

After the first 4 patients were treated, it became obvious that the toxic reactions in head and neck patients receiving simultaneous irradiation and chemotherapy were unacceptable. Therefore, the protocol was altered so that the treatment modalities were sequential rather than simultaneous. Three patients received chemotherapy after the completion of radiation therapy. One patient with rhabdomyosarcoma of the upper gum was placed on 2 courses of chemotherapy followed by a local resection and then radiation therapy. This patient developed pulmonary metastasis during the fifth week of radiotherapy.

Discussion

These data must be considered preliminary since the minimum follow-up is only 9 months. The local recurrence rate in the control group is low: 1 failure within the irradiated volume and 1 geographical miss. There are no local recurrences in the chemotherapy group. Since the minimum follow-up is only 9 months, and many of the patients are still receiving chemotherapy, local recurrence may be only displaced in time.

Comparing the rates of distant metastasis, the incidence in the chemotherapy group is more than double that of the control group, 9 of 27 and 3 of 20, respectively. The difference is not statistically significant ($p > .30$). This trend, however, is disturbing, since it may indicate that the adjunctive chemotherapy is adversely affecting the immune mechanism, with a resultant increase in the incidence of distant metastasis.

As a matter of interest, the 47 patients in the random study were compared with 53 patients treated between 1963 and Ocotber 1973 (historical group). All patients in the historical group had Grade 2 or 3 lesions 5 cm or larger in diameter, located in either the trunk (excluding the abdomen) or the extremities, and all had been treated by conservative surgery and postoperative radiotherapy. The survival rate free of disease without relapse (local recurrence and/or distant metastasis) for the 3 groups is shown in Table 5. The disease-free survival rate appears to be improved in both arms of the VACAR study as compared to the historical study, i.e. at 18 months the survival rates are 76.2% (16/21), 83.3% (10/12), and 45.3% (24/53) for chemotherapy, control, and historical groups, respectively. The survival rates at 18 months of all patients in the VACAR study (26/33) are significantly better than those of the historical group (24/53, with $p < .005$). The improved survival rate in the random study was due to better local control, e.g., 94% (31/33) at 18 months versus 75.5% (40/53) for the historical group. The incidence of distant metastasis is similar (30.3% or 10 of 33 for the random study and 30.2% or 16 of 53 for the historical group). The improved local control rate in the control group is due to refinement of the radiotherapeutic techniques (Lindberg, Fletcher, and Martin, 1975).

It is clear that VACAR was unsuccessful in preventing pulmonary metastases. The VACAR chemotherapy regimen was designed based on evidence suggesting the value of cyclophosphamide, vincristine, and actinomycin-D in the treatment of patients with sarcomas. It is now apparent, however, that DIC is a more important addition to Adriamycin in the treatment of metastatic sarcomas than all 3 of these agents (Benjamin *et al.*, 1977, see pages 309–315, this volume).

TABLE 5.—SURVIVAL FREE OF DISEASE WITHOUT RELAPSE: VACAR-TREATED PATIENTS OCTOBER 1973 THROUGH DECEMBER 1975

TIME IN MONTHS	VACAR° CHEMOTHERAPY	VACAR° CONTROL	HISTORICAL[†] GROUP
3	24/27	19/20	50/53
6	23/27	18/20	42/53
9	20/27	18/20	38/53
12	17/24	15/18	36/53
15	16/21	13/16	29/53
18	16/21	10/12	24/53
24	7/9	5/6	19/53
30	2/5	3/3	18/53

°Follow-up 9 to 34 months.
†Minimum follow-up 30 months.

A critical review has shown that the toxic reactions secondary to the chemotherapy used in this study have been excessive. The severity of skin reactions during radiation therapy has been increased, resulting in the cessation or interruption of radiotherapy in 5 patients. Severe myelosuppression occurred in the vincristine, Adriamycin, and Cytoxan phase, with 24 of 27 patients having a granulocyte count below 1,000/mm³ (median 400). In patients with soft tissue sarcomas of the head and neck, the toxicity of combined treatment was totally unacceptable, with 1 fatal complication. The design of an adjuvant chemotherapy trial in patients with localized disease is difficult. The dilemma is to deliver an adequate dose of chemotherapy for maximum antitumor effect without undue toxicity. The acceptable levels of toxicity in this study were clearly exceeded.

Conclusions

The preliminary results of this randomized trial to test the efficacy of adjuvant chemotherapy (vincristine, Adriamycin, Cytoxan and actinomycin-D) in adult patients with localized soft tissue sarcomas has shown the following:

(1) The survival rate free of disease of patients in both arms of the study is similar (76% for the chemotherapy group and 83% for the control group) at 18 months follow-up.
(2) The incidence of distant metastasis is not decreased by this adjuvant chemotherapy (VACAR).
(3) There are too few local recurrences to provide meaningful data.
(4) The toxicity of the adjuvant VACAR chemotherapy was excessive, especially in patients with head and neck lesions.

Acknowledgment

This investigation was supported in part by grants # CA-06294 and CA-05654, awarded by the National Cancer Institute, Department of Health, Education and Welfare.

Robert S. Benjamin is a Junior Faculty Fellow of the American Cancer Society.

REFERENCES

Benjamin, R. S., Baker, L. H. Rodriquez, V., Moon, T. E., O'Bryan, R., Stephens, R. L., Sinkovics, J. G., Thigpen, T., King, G. W., Bottomley, R., Groppe, C. W., Jr., Bodey, G. P., and Gottlieb, J. A.: Chemotherapy of adult soft tissue sarcomas. In *Management of Bone and Soft Tissue Tumors* (The

University of Texas System Cancer Center M. D. Anderson Hospital and Tumor Institute, 21st Annual Clinical Conference on Cancer). Chicago, Illinois, Year Book Medical Publishers, Inc., 1977, pp. 309–315.

Lindberg, R. D., Fletcher, G. H., and Martin, R. G.: The management of soft tissue sarcomas in adults: Surgery and postoperative radiotherapy. *Journal de Radiologie et d'Electrologie,* 56:761–767, June 1975.

Lindberg, R. D., Martin, R. G., Romsdahl, M. M., and McMurtrey, M. J.: Conservative surgery and radiation therapy for soft tissue sarcomas. In *Management of Bone and Soft Tissue Tumors* (The University of Texas System Cancer Center M. D. Anderson Hospital and Tumor Institute, 21st Annual Clinical Conference on Cancer). Chicago, Illinois, Year Book Medical Publishers, Inc., 1977, pp. 289–298.

Regional Chemotherapy for Soft Tissue Sarcomas

CHARLES M. McBRIDE, M.D.

Department of Surgery, The University of Texas System Cancer Center
M. D. Anderson Hospital and Tumor Institute,
Houston, Texas

THE SUCCESSES OF CHEMOTHERAPY in the treatment of soft tissue sarcomas were rather limited until the team at Tulane, headed by Creech, demonstrated the technique of isolation-perfusion in 1957 (Ryan, Winblad, Krementz, and Creech, 1958). This technique of regional chemotherapy was designed to deliver a high dose of anticancer agents directly to a tumor-bearing area, in either a region or organ of the body, and it demonstrated that these high doses of drugs could cause the death of tumor cells. Although well-standardized (McBride, 1975) and used in many centers, the technique is still controversial because of the problems encountered by surgeons who do only occasional perfusions.

Between January 1960 and June 1976, 89 perfusions were performed at M. D. Anderson Hospital on 85 patients with soft tissue sarcomas of the limbs, in an effort to reduce the necessity for major amputation. In most instances, the chemotherapeutic agents used were 1-phenylalanine mustard and actinomycin-D, and the perfusion was followed by a local excision of the lesion 6 weeks later. The distribution of the patients by sex and involved limb is given in Table 1. Of the patients perfused, 28% had liposarcoma, 19% unclassified sarcoma, 13% fibrosarcoma, 11% synovial sarcoma, 8% angiosarcoma, 6% neurofibrosarcoma, 5% giant cell sarcoma of tendon sheaths, 3% malignant fibrous histiocytoma, and 7% other sarcomas such as rhabdomyosarcoma, leiomyosarcoma, extraosseous osteogenic sarcoma, extraos-

TABLE 1.—SARCOMA PATIENT DISTRIBUTION
BY SEX AND LIMBS INVOLVED

	MALES 60%	FEMALES 40%
Arm	24%	26%
Leg	76%	74%

seous chondrosarcoma, and epithelioid sarcoma. Only 16% of the sarcomas were graded histologically; 3 were Grade 1, 8 Grade 2, and 3
Grade 3. Table 2 shows the raw survival statistics for these patients
with different types of sarcomas, as related to lesion size—either
greater than or equal to 5 cm in diameter or less than 5 cm in diameter.
The distribution by age and sex of the patients with sarcomas of the
limbs is given in Figure 1.

The selection of drug dosage used depended on 3 factors: local tis-

Fig. 1.—Distribution by age and sex of 85 patients with sarcomas of the limbs.

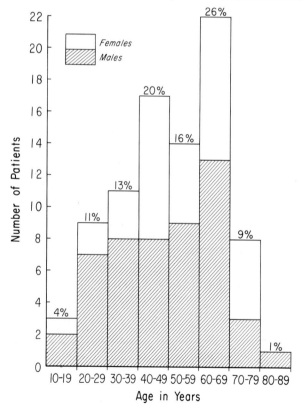

TABLE 2.—SURVIVAL RATES BY TISSUE TYPES FOR PATIENTS WITH SARCOMAS OF THE LIMBS TREATED BY ISOLATION-PERFUSION

TYPE	1-YEAR SURVIVAL		5-YEAR SURVIVAL		10-YEAR SURVIVAL	
	< 5 CM	> 5 CM	< 5 CM	> 5 CM	< 5 CM	> 5 CM
Liposarcoma	4/4	9/20	3/3	9/15	2/2	7/13
Unclassified sarcoma	4/5	10/11	3/5	6/10	3/5	2/5
Fibrosarcoma	7/7	4/4	7/7	2/2	5/5	1/3
Synovial sarcoma	4/4	5/5	3/4	2/4	2/3	2/4
Angiosarcoma	4/5	1/2	2/5	1/2	1/4	0/2
Neurofibrosarcoma	3/3	1/2	2/2	1/1	1/1	—
Giant cell sarcoma of tendon sheath	4/4	—	4/4	—	—	—
Malignant fibrous histiocytoma	1/1	2/2	1/1	—	—	—
Other soft tissue sarcomas*	—	6/6	—	1/4	—	1/3

*Rhabdomyosarcomas, leiomyosarcomas, extraosseous osteogenic sarcomas, extraosseous chondrosarcomas, and epithelioid sarcomas.

sue tolerance (i.e. a person with fair skin will not tolerate as high a dose of drug as a person with dark skin), leak of the drug into the systemic circulation, and size of the patient. In the series of patients reported here, the median dose used in the leg was 1-phenylalanine mustard, 1.3 mg/kg and actinomycin-D, 0.03 mg/kg. In the arm, the median dosage of 1-phenylalanine mustard was 0.7 mg/kg, and of actinomycin-D it was 0.02 mg/kg. Both drugs were given sequentially at the beginning of the perfusion, which normally lasted for 1 hour. Iliac dissections were performed on 46% of the patients, 25% had axillary perfusions, 17% had femoral perfusions, and 12% had popliteal perfusions.

The leakage of drug into the systemic circulation was monitored by placing a scintillation counter over the ventricular blood mass, injecting radioiodinated serum albumin into the pump circuit, and monitoring for appearance of this isotope in the systemic circulation (Stehlin, Clark, and Dewey, 1961). The dissection was checked and the tourniquet adjusted until the rate of leakage from the perfusion circuit was such that it would not exceed 15% during the 1-hour period. When this was established, the drugs were injected into the isolation-perfusion circuit.

The survival curves for the 85 sarcoma patients, uncorrected for age at diagnosis or the cause of death, are given in Figure 2. Of the pa-

Fig. 2.—Raw survival curve for 85 patients with soft tissue sarcomas of the limbs.

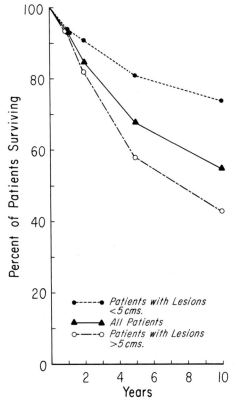

TABLE 3.—STATUS AT 5 YEARS OF 72
PATIENTS WITH SOFT TISSUE
SARCOMAS OF THE LIMBS

Alive, no evidence of disease	45	(62%)
Dead, documented intercurrent disease	4	(6%)
Lost to follow-up	2	(3%)
Dead of disease	21	(29%)
Determinant cases at 5 years	66	(92%)

tients with soft tissue sarcoma of the limbs, 72 had at least a 5-year follow-up, and the status of their disease at that time is given in Table 3.
The regional recurrence rate for these patients with a 5-year follow-up
was 20%, and a further 18% had developed systemic metastasis by
that time (Table 4). Of the patients who experienced regional recurrence during the 5 years following isolation-perfusion, 20% were salvaged by retreatment using such modalities as local reexcision, major
amputation, radiation therapy, or a combination of these.

The high doses of drugs necessary to obtain local control of soft tissue sarcomas in the limbs may result in complications. As seen in Table 5, 11% of the patients subsequently required amputation, either
secondary to recurrent disease (6 patients) or from complications of
the perfusion itself (3 patients). Only 1 patient in this series died within 30 days of the perfusion, and this death resulted from a pulmonary
embolus.

Of the patients followed 5 years, 69 were thought to have localized
tumors only, and of these, 39 were treated for the initial primary tumor, while 28 had locally recurrent tumor that had been treated pre-

TABLE 4.—SARCOMAS OF THE LIMBS
IN PATIENTS FOLLOWED 5 YEARS:
FIRST RECURRENCE AFTER TREATMENT
AND EFFECTS OF RETREATMENT

		RETREATMENT	
SITES	PATIENTS	NED	DOD
REGIONAL			
Local recurrence	10 (15%)	4 (16%)	6 (24%)
In the limbs	0 (0%)	0 (0%)	0 (0%)
Regional lymph nodes	3 (5%)	1 (4%)	2 (8%)
SYSTEMIC			
Disseminated metastasis	12 (18%)	0 (0%)	12 (48%)
DETERMINATE CASES (%)	25 (38%)	5 (8%)	20 (30%)

NED—No evidence of disease; DOD—Died of disease.

TABLE 5.—COMPLICATIONS RESULTING FROM 89
PERFUSIONS IN 85 PATIENTS

Death (Pulmonary Embolus)	1 (1%)
Subsequent amputation	9 (11%)
Edema of limb	4 (5%)
Major skin slough	1 (1%)
Major wound infection	1 (1%)

viously and had recurred up to a maximum of 6 times. No significant difference was detected between the survival of these 2 groups of patients following treatment. The survival of the 31 patients whose tumor masses were less than 5 cm in diameter, however, was significantly better than that for the 38 patients whose tumors were greater than or equal to 5 cm in diameter (p =0.04).

Since most soft tissue sarcomas grow with a compression capsule, it is easy for a surgeon who rarely treats this disease to "shell out" the tumor. The frequency of this form of inadequate initial treatment of the primary sarcoma makes these tumors among the most difficult to control. The point made, that the time to gain local control of sarcomas is at the time of initial therapy, is certainly a most important one (Clark, Martin, White, and Old, 1957). In the series reported here, the regional recurrence rate of 20% after initial therapy compares favorably with reports from this institution using other modalities (Suit, Martin, and Russell, 1975), the 29% reported in another series (Cantin, McNeer, Chu, and Booher, 1968), and the 39% reported earlier (Pack and Ariel, 1958). These earlier series were treated by radical surgical therapy; some patients were included, however, whose primary site of origin of disease was not in the limbs. Although the series of patients reported here is small, the results suggest that survival rates for recurrent sarcoma of the limbs when treated by isolation-perfusion may be equal to that for patients treated for the first time.

Differences in numerical distribution of the various histological types of sarcomas in various series of patients may affect the reported control rates. As suggested previously, however, (McBride, 1974; Suit and Russell, 1975), the histological type of sarcoma may not be as important as other considerations, such as the size of the tumor mass, which appears to be most important. The age of the patient at the time of treatment for a soft tissue sarcoma may have an effect on the survival unless corrections are made, which was not done for the series of patients reported here. The age distribution of the patients treated by isolation-perfusion for soft tissue sarcomas of the limbs is similar to that in a series reported from this institution (Clark, Martin, White, and Old, 1957) and also in a series reported in 1962 (Shieber and Graham, 1962). As this is a retrospective study without a true control group available, it is impossible to state that factors other than treatment may have contributed to the overall 10-year survival rate of 55%, which is slightly better than that previously reported (Martin, Butler, and Albores-Saavedra, 1965; Pack and Ariel, 1958; Shieber and Graham, 1962).

The fact that 20% of patients who failed initial therapy were salvaged by retreatment suggests that even when initial control is not obtained by regional chemotherapy the tumor may be modified to the extent that it may respond to an alternative type of treatment. Although the group of patients reported here had an 11% amputation rate, this again compares favorably with most reported series for soft tissue sarcomas of the limbs. The surgical mortality of 1% is what would be expected of any group of patients having operations of a similar magnitude.

A regional recurrence rate of 75% following excisional surgery, or 70% following X-ray therapy alone, clearly indicates that radical surgical resection, or a combination of these therapies, is the minimal treatment for soft tissue sarcoma of the limbs. Although a major amputation is not the treatment of choice for primary soft tissue sarcomas, the decision to amputate must take into account the anatomic structures involved by the sarcoma and any signs of increased aggression of the tumor with each local recurrence. The fact that the patients with recurrent sarcomas did as well as the patients with intact primary sarcomas, when treated by isolation-perfusion, is a more encouraging result than suggested previously (Ryan, Winblad, Krementz, and Creech, 1958).

No absolute guidelines have been established by this study as to the best form of therapy for soft tissue sarcomas of the limbs. Constant reevaluation of anticancer techniques and agents is necessary to ensure the best form of treatment for patients. Adjuvant chemotherapy by isolation-perfusion treats all of the tissues involved primarily by soft tissue sarcomas arising in the limbs and makes it possible to reduce the extent of surgical resection necessary to obtain control of the disease. It is a safe procedure and has been used on patients ranging in age from 11 to 80 years. Isolation-perfusion with 1-phenylalanine mustard and actinomyocin-D provides an acceptable rate of regional control for patients with soft tissue sarcomas of the limbs, and it is not associated with a higher incidence of systemic metastasis.

REFERENCES

Cantin, J., McNeer, G. P., Chu, F. C., and Booher, R. J.: The problem of local recurrence after treatment of soft tissue sarcoma. Annals of Surgery, 168: 47–53, 1968.

Clark, R. L., Martin, R. G., White, E. C., and Old, J. W.: Clinical aspects of soft tissue tumors. Archives of Surgery, 74:859–870, June 1957.

Martin, R. G., Butler, J. J., and Albores-Saavedra, J.: Soft tissue tumors: Surgical treatment and results. In *Tumors of Bone and Soft Tissue* The University of Texas M. D. Anderson Hospital, 8th Annual Clinical Conference on Cancer, Chicago, Illinois, Year Book Medical Publishers, Inc., 1965, pp. 333–347.

McBride, C. M.: Sarcomas of the limbs: Results of adjuvant chemotherapy using isolation-perfusion. Archives of Surgery, 109:304–308, 1974.

————.: Regional chemotherapy. In *Cancer Chemotherapy–Fundamental Concepts and Recent Advances* (The University of Texas System Cancer Center M. D. Anderson Hospital and Tumor Institute, 19th Annual Clinical Conference on Cancer) Chicago, Illinois, Year Book Medical Publishers, Inc., 1975, pp. 369–384.

Pack, G. T., and Ariel, I.: End results in the treatment of sarcoma of the soft somatic tissues. In Pack, G. T. and Ariel, I. M. Eds.: *Tumors of the Soft Somatic Tissues: A Clinical Treatise,* New York, New York, Paul B. Hoeber, Inc., 1958, pp. 779–796.

Ryan, R. F., Winblad, J. N., Krementz, E. T., and Creech, O. Jr.: Treatment of malignant neoplasms with chemotherapeutic agents utilizing a pump-oxygenator: Techniques and early results. Bulletin of the Tulane Medical Faculty, 17:133–143, 1958.

Shieber, W., and Graham, P.: An experience with sarcomas of the soft tissues in adults. Surgery, 52:295–298, 1962.

Stehlin, J. S., Jr., Clark, R. L., and Dewey, W. C.: Continuous monitoring of leakage during regional perfusion. Archives of Surgery, 83:943–949, 1961.

Suit, H. D., Martin, R. G., and Russell, W. O.: Sarcoma of soft tissue: Clinical and histopathological parameters and response to treatment. Cancer, 35: 1478–1483, April 1975.

Suit, H. D., and Russell, W. O.: Radiation therapy of soft tissue sarcomas. Cancer, 36:759–764, 1975.

Immunotherapy of Human Sarcomas

JOSEPH G. SINKOVICS, M.D., CARL PLAGER, M.D.
MARION J. McMURTREY, M.D., JIMMY J. ROMERO,
B.S., and MARVIN M. ROMSDAHL, M.D., Ph.D.
Section of Clinical Tumor Virology and Immunology,
Department of Medicine and Department of Surgery,
The University of Texas System Cancer Center
M. D. Anderson Hospital and Tumor Institute,
Houston, Texas

The Immunology of Patients with Sarcoma

GENERAL IMMUNE STATUS

PATIENTS WITH ADVANCED MALIGNANT TUMORS often show profoundly compromised reactions to recall antigens and fail to respond to primary antigenic stimuli. In certain tumor categories these immune defects are severe and are either present at the time of diagnosis when the tumor burden is relatively small or persist even after the elimination of all apparent tumors. In the first category are patients with bronchogenic carcinoma; in the second category are patients cured by radiotherapy of squamous carcinoma of the head and neck (Holmes, 1976a; Tarpley, Potvin, and Chretien, 1975).

It is not entirely clear whether these patients suffer from intrinsic defects of macrophages and lymphocytes or whether they circulate serum factors that inhibit cell-mediated immune reactions. When inhibitory serum factors could be demonstrated, these belonged to the class of $\alpha 2$ globulins (Glasgow, *et. al.*, 1974; McLaughlin and Brooks, 1974).

361

Patients with brain tumors displayed compromised lymphocyte blastogenesis to phytohemagglutinin and to autologous or allogeneic tumor cell membranes. Reactivity to recall antigens and sensitization to the primary antigen dinitrochlorobenzene were also deficient. These patients circulated a serum factor inhibitory to lymphocyte-mediated immune reactions (Brooks, Roszman, and Rogers, 1976; Young, 1976).

IMMUNE ASSESSMENT OF PATIENTS WITH SARCOMAS. — Patients with sarcoma and malignant melanoma often preserve normal reaction patterns. These tumors commonly afflict young or middle-aged persons in the prime of their health. Often, no immune defects are detectable, and patients with advanced tumors respond well to recall antigens or to primary sensitization with dinitrochlorobenzene (Pinsky *et al.*, 1974).

Differences in general immune assessment of patients with different tumor types are shown in Table 1. Patients with sarcomas occupy an intermediate position. Many patients with carcinomas failed to restore their immunocompetence in the tumor-free clinical state, whereas patients with melanoma or sarcoma readily regained immunocompetence in the tumor-free clinical state (Golub, O'Connel, and Morton, 1974;Twomey, Catalona, and Chretien, 1974)

Recent studies at the Mayo Clinic have established that patients with nonprogressive sarcomas or tumor-free patients with sarcomas did not differ from healthy controls in their skin test reactivity to recall antigens, but patients with progressive sarcomas produced weaker reactions (Pritchard, Ivins, and Ritts, 1976).

TABLE 1.—DIFFERENCES IN ASSESSMENT OF GENERAL IMMUNE STATUS ACCORDING TO TUMOR TYPE

TESTS	CARCINOMAS	SARCOMAS	MELANOMAS
DHS skin tests	decreased	intermediate	retained
PHA blastogenesis in vitro	retained	intermediate	decreased
DNCB sensitization	negative early	may remain positive late	may remain positive late
	becomes negative with increasing tumor burden		
Immunocompetence in tumor-free patients	remains compromised	restored	restored

DHS—delayed hypersensitivity; PHA—phytohemagglutinin; DNCB—dinitrochlorobenzene.
Data based on reports by Golub, O'Connel, and Morton, 1974; Holmes, 1976; Kotz, Rella, and Salzer, 1976; Pinsky *et al.*, 1974; Twomey, Catalona, and Chretien, 1974.

However, the healthy controls' lymphocytes responded better in blastogenesis assays to concanavalin A, phytohemagglutinin, and pokeweed mitogen than did the lymphocytes of patients with sarcomas. The lymphocyte response to concanavalin A reflected clinical state in that it was decreased in patients with progressive sarcomas; however, responses to phytohemagglutinin and pokeweed mitogen were not different in various stages of the disease.

Another evaluation of the general immune status of patients with sarcomas was conducted in Vienna, Austria. Reactions to the primary antigen dinitrochlorobenzene were positive in 7 of 12 tumor-free patients and negative in 5 patients. Of 10 patients with metastases and advancing disease, 6 had positive reactions and 4 had negative reactions. In the follow-up studies of 9 patients with positive reactions, 5 patients achieved disease-free status and 4 developed metastases. Of 13 patients with negative reactions, 4 later had positive reactions; 2 of these achieved disease-free clinical status and 2 developed metastases. Nine patients remained negative; 5 of these patients achieved disease-free clinical status and 4 developed metastases. Therefore, this test was of little, if any, prognostic value for patients with sarcomas (Kotz, Rella, and Salzer, 1976).

According to a trial done in Los Angeles, California (Eilber, Nizze, and Morton, 1975; Holmes, 1976a), 11 of 13 patients with stage I, 5 of 8 patients with stage II, and 7 of 19 patients with stage III sarcomas had positive reactions in the DNCB primary skin sensitization test; thus, in early disease, there were more positive responders (85%) than in late disease (37%).

Of 25 patients displaying initially positive reactions to recall skin antigens, 22 remained positive, but only 10 of these patients achieved tumor-free status; 12 patients with positive reactions developed metastases. Of 6 initially negative reactors, 5 became positive; 4 of these were disease-free and 1 positive reactor developed metastases. The sixth patient who remained negative succumbed to metastatic disease (Kotz, Rella, and Salzer, 1976).

The blastogenic response of lymphocytes to phytohemagglutinin was of dubious prognostic value. For example, of 7 patients reacting strongly in this assay, 3 were of disease-free status and 4 had metastases. Of 8 weak reactors, 3 were disease-free and 5 had metastases (Kotz, Rella, and Salzer, 1976).

TUMOR-SPECIFIC IMMUNITY

THE INFLUENCE OF ETIOLOGY ON THE ANTIGENICITY OF TUMORS. — In the animal world, virally induced tumors share common antigens, whereas physicochemically induced tumors express individually specific antigens. The etiology of human sarcomas is unknown. Trauma has often been suspected but seldom, if ever, could be proved as an important etiologic factor (Sinkovics and Mackay, 1977). Accidental and therapeutic irradiation causes sarcomas in man (Armine and Sugar, 1976; Glicksman and Toker, 1976; Gonzalez-Vitale, Slavin, and McQueen, 1976; Paik and Wilkinson, 1976). Among the chemically induced sarcomas, angiosarcoma of the liver in vinyl chloride workers appears to be one of the best-documented examples (Makk et al., 1976; Waxweiler, et al., 1976). Association of sarcomagenesis with genetically determined diseases and with the so-called degenerative diseases is also conspicuous. Neurofibrosarcoma develops in 5 to 10% of patients with the mendelian dominant neurofibromatosis of von Recklinghausen. In Gardner's syndrome, also with mendelian dominant inheritance, the retroperitoneal fibrosis is often interpreted to be a low-grade fibrosarcoma. In the enchondromatosis of Ollier, or in the Maffucci-Ollier syndrome, more than 10% of the patients develop chrondrosarcomas. In patients with Paget's osteitis deformans, the development of osteogenic sarcoma is estimated to be between 3 to 15% (Sinkovics and Mackay, in press). Patients with phacomatosis tuberous sclerosis, or Bourneville disease, often develop liposarcomas of the kidney (Williams and Savage, 1958). Increased sarcomagenesis has been observed in basal cell nevus syndrome and in Wermer's syndrome or adult progeria (Haynes and Fitzpatrick, 1974).

Kaposi's sarcoma has been shown to be associated with immune defects of the host. Immunosuppressed organ transplant recipients or patients receiving immunosuppressive therapy for systemic lupus erythematosus developed this tumor, and clinical tumor regression occurred upon discontinuation of the immunosuppressive medication (Hardy, et al., 1976; Myers, et al., 1974).

Human sarcomas may express cross-reacting Forssman-type and embryonic antigens (Hirshaut, et al., 1974; Mukherji and Hirshaut, 1973). These antigens probably do not function as rejection antigens, i.e. immune reactions directed toward these antigens, even if detectable, do not result in tumor rejection. Some sarcoma-associated antigens appear to be expressed best in the G_1 phase of the cell cycle (Burk, Drewinko, Lichtiger, and Trujillo, 1976).

Human sarcomas express cell membrane, cytoplasmic, and soluble antigens detectable by immunofluorescence (Fig. 1), complement fixation, and lymphocyte-mediated cytotoxicity (Giraldo et al., 1971; Morton, Malmgren, Hall, and Schidlovsky, 1969; Sinkovics et al., 1975b). These antigens cross-react between different tissue subtypes

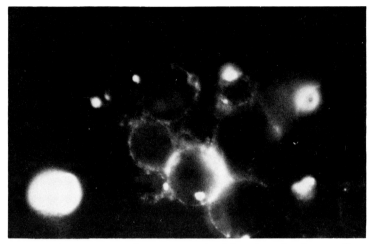

Fig. 1.—Membrane immunofluorescence of viable cultured malignant fibrous histiocytoma sarcoma cells (culture #2291) with autologous serum.

of sarcomas and thus suggest viral etiology. It is not known whether there is any difference in the antigenic expression of sarcomas of various etiology: "spontaneous" sarcomas, those developing in traumatized areas, radiation or chemically induced sarcomas, or those developing in patients with genetic or degenerative diseases.

THE POSSIBILITY OF VIRAL ETIOLOGY.—Avian, murine, feline, and simian sarcomas were shown to be caused by type C oncornaviruses (for review, see Sinkovics, 1976b). There is no established oncogenic virus strain isolated from human sarcomas (or from other human tumors). The following arguments suggest that human sarcomas may be caused by oncornaviruses:

1. The phenomenon of antigenic conversion which consists of the synthesis of new, sarcoma-specific antigens by human fetal cells after inoculation of cultured human fetal fibroblasts with cell-free filtrates of sarcomatous tumors or of cultured sarcoma cells (Giraldo *et al.*, 1971; Morton, Malmgren, Hall, and Schidlovsky, 1969; Sinkovics *et al.*, 1974b). Table 2 summarizes our experience with the study of antigenic conversion.

2. The phenomenon of focus formation (Fig. 2) which consists of the changed growth pattern of cultured human fetal fibroblasts after inoculation of cultured fetal fibroblasts with cell-free filtrates of sarcomatous tumors or of cultured sarcoma cells (Giraldo, *et al.*, 1971; Morton, Malmgren, Hall, and Schidlovsky, 1969; Sinkovics and Harris, 1976). This changed growth pattern of human embryonic fibro-

TABLE 2.—ANTIGENIC CONVERSION: EXPRESSION OF
ANTIGENS DETECTABLE BY INDIRECT IMMUNO-
FLUORESCENCE IN HUMAN EMBRYONIC FIBROBLASTS AFTER
INOCULATION WITH CELL-FREE FLUID FROM CULTURED
SARCOMA CELLS

SARCOMA CULTURE FLUIDS TESTED FROM ESTABLISHED CELL LINES		POSITIVE IMMUNOFLUORESCENCE[†] OF FETAL HUMAN FIBROBLASTS AFTER INOCULATION OF SARCOMA CULTURE FILTRATES		
TISSUE CULTURE	SARCOMA SUBTYPE	CULTURE ESTABLISHED BY	NUMBER OF TESTS	% POSITIVE
1459	Chondrosarcoma	SCTVI[°]	3/15	60
2089	Rhabdomyosarcoma	McAllister	14/65	21.5
2178	Giant cell tumor, bone	SCTVI[°]	7/41	17
2291	Malignant fibrous histiocytoma	SCTVI[°]	6/36	16
2117	Neurofibrosarcoma	Trujillo	7/45	15
3406	Fibrosarcoma	SCTVI[°]	5/44	11.4
1846	Ewing's sarcoma	SCTVI[°]	5/49	10.2
3370	Synovial sarcoma	SCTVI[°]	4/41	9.7
		TOTAL	51/336	15.6

[°]Established by one of the authors (J.G.S.) at the Section of Clinical Tumor Virology and Immunology (SCTVI), Department of Medicine, M. D. Anderson Hospital.

[†]Tested with heat-inactivated human sera from patients with sarcomas that were positive on indirect immunofluorescence assay against autologous acetone-fixed printed or cultured sarcoma cells.

These data were published previously only in part (Gonzalez *et al.*, 1974; Sinkovics *et al.*, 1971).

blasts is that of cells without contact inhibition: the cells assume a round shape and pile up on top of one another. Occasionally, type C virus particles appear in the transformed cultures. The transformed cultures express the sarcoma-associated antigens, but cells undergoing antigenic conversion do not necessarily undergo morphological transformation.

3. The presence of oncornaviral genomes or genome fragments in human sarcoma cells cross-hybridizing with those of animal oncornaviruses (Kufe, Hehlman, and Spiegelman, 1972).

4. The induction of oncornaviral particles in cultured human sarcoma cells (Stewart, Kasnic, and Draycott, 1972).

5. The expression of human osteosarcoma antigens in hamster osteosarcomas induced in vivo by cell-free filtrates of human osteosarcomas (Pritchard, Reilly, Finkel, and Ivins, 1974).

Viruses other than those of the oncornavirus class that may be involved in the induction of human tumors are herpes viruses which are possibly responsible for the etiology of Burkitt's lymphoma and squamous cell carcinomas, among them carcinoma of the uterine cervix and nasopharyngeal carcinoma. Herpes viruses appeared in primary

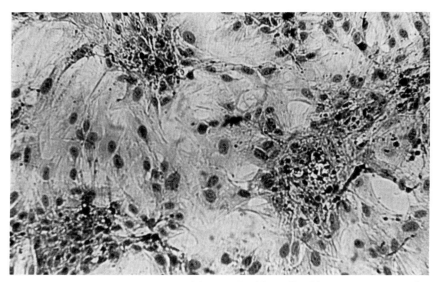

Fig. 2.—Wistar Institute 38 normal human fetal lung fibroblasts growing in multi-layered foci with central cell death after inoculation with filtrate from chondrosar-coma culture #1459.

cultures of Kaposi's sarcomas, but it was the lymphocytes infiltrating the tumor and not the sarcoma cells that carried herpes virus particles (Wang *et al.*, 1975).

Papovaviruses appearing in multifocal leukoencephalopathy and in cultured human lymphocytes are potentially oncogenic. Human malignant melanoma cells occasionally expressed papovavirus antigens (Soriano, Shelburn, and Gökcen, 1974). In connection with sarcomas, inclusions resembling subviral structures (papova-, myxo-, or oncornaviruses) were sighted in the cells of Paget's osteitis deformans (Rebel, 1975), a condition in which an increased incidence of osteogenic sarcomas occurs.

In cultured cells of human sarcomas derived from children, no virus particles could be demonstrated (McAllister *et al.*, 1975).

TISSUE CULTURES FOR IMMUNOLOGICAL STUDIES.—Sarcoma-associated antigens have been demonstrated best in cultured sarcoma cells. Table 3 lists established cell lines of human sarcomas developed by one of us (J.G.S.) at the Section of Clinical Tumor Virology and Immunology (Figs. 3–8). Patients with sarcomas express more frequent and stronger cell- and antibody-mediated immune reactions toward cultured sarcoma cells than toward cultured carcinoma cells (Sinkovics, Kay, and Thota, 1976). However, healthy donors also fre-

TABLE 3.—TISSUE CULTURE CELL LINES OF HUMAN SARCOMAS ESTABLISHED AT THE SECTION OF CLINICAL TUMOR VIROLOGY AND IMMUNOLOGY

TISSUE CULTURE #	DATE OF INITIATION OF CULTURE	HIGHEST PASSAGE CARRIED	CHARACTERISTICS OF CULTURE (REFERENCE)	PATIENT'S INITIALS, MDAH #, GENDER, RACE, BIRTHDATE, BLOOD GROUP	VERIFIED TISSUE DIAGNOSIS OF TUMOR FROM WHICH CULTURE WAS ESTABLISHED
778	5–19–66	136	Round, elongated, and giant cells. Used for immunotherapy of malignant lymphomas (Sinkovics et al., 1976).	H.F., #54537 male, black 11–11–04 O+	Lymphocytic lymphoma (lymph node)
1846	3–10–70	53	Small, round cells with large, dense nucleus and narrow rim of cytoplasm (Sinkovics et al., 1975b). Available as viral oncolysate.	E.G., #79610 female, white 8–22–60 O+	Ewing's sarcoma (tibia)
2178	3–24–71	95	Elongated cells, occasional giant cell.	T.L., #84231 male, white 8–20–45 O–	Giant cell tumor of bone (femur)
2291	6–11–71	105	Large, "epithelioid" cells with features of fibroblasts. Available as viral oncolysate (Sinkovics et al., 1975b).	C.H., #85890 male, white 8–15–99 A+	Undifferentiated sarcoma (widely metastatic)
2322	6–30–71	101	Pleomorph, elongated cells growing in haphazard multilayers. Available as viral oncolysate.	B.L., #86191 female, white 7–21–06 O+	Chondroblastic osteosarcoma (hip)
2454	9–14–71	143	Elongated cells growing in irregular multilayers. Available for immunotherapy as viral oncolysate.	G.B. #87288 male, white 3–29–96 A+	Chondrosarcoma (humerus, scapula)

3123	6–2–72	63	Elongated cells with extremely long, slender cytoplasmic protusions. Available as viral oncolysate.	H.E., #89355 male, white 11–22–35 A+	Neurofibrosarcoma (widely disseminated)
3370	10–04–72	48	Elongated cells growing in multilayers and "foci" (Sinkovics *et al.*, 1975a). Available as viral oncolysate.	C.H., #84788 female, white 7–27–51 A+	Synovial sarcoma (foot; widely metastatic including brain)
3743	2–27–73	72	Elongated cells with phagocytized lipid growing in multilayers. Available as viral oncolysate.	M.G., #95749 female, white 11–18–21 O+	Malignant cystosarcoma phylloides (breast)
4052	6–21–73	8	"Epithelioid" cells with numerous, short protrusions of cytoplasm growing poorly in small colonies (Sinkovics and Mackay, 1977).	H.T., #86301 male, white 11–21–14 O−	Angiosarcoma (head and neck)
4929	2–15–74	22	Small round cells and large elongated multinuclear cells with myofibrils (Sinkovics and Mackay, 1977). Available as viral oncolysate.	L.H., #95042 female, white 12–24–52 A+	Clear cell sarcoma of tendon sheath (hand; widely metastatic). Revised: Rhabdomyosarcoma
5005	3–27–74	33	Plump elongated cells and large "foci" and multilayers. Cytoplasmic myofibrils occasionally occur.	M.D.C., #99077 female, white 4–20–57 A+	Alveolar rhabdomyosarcoma (metastatic to lung and pleura)
5469	11–13–74	26	Large foci of small round cells on top of multilayered elongated cells.	T.B., #106227 female, white 7–11–61 A+	Sarcoma, type uncertain

TABLE 3.—*Continued*

TISSUE CULTURE #	DATE OF INITIATION OF CULTURE	HIGHEST PASSAGE CARRIED	CHARACTERISTICS OF CULTURE (REFERENCE)	PATIENT'S INITIALS, MDAH #, GENDER, RACE, BIRTHDATE, BLOOD GROUP	VERIFIED TISSUE DIAGNOSIS OF TUMOR FROM WHICH CULTURE WAS ESTABLISHED
5659	1–21–75	75	Plump elongated cells growing rapidly in large "foci" and thick multilayers; elongated cells contain myofibrils (Sinkovics and Mackay, 1977).	B.C. #100798 male, white 9–11–49 A+	Rhabdomyosarcoma (hand; metastastic to lung and pleura)
5958	3–24–75	23	Plump and large elongated (often multinucleated) cells growing in multilayers; elongated cells contain myofibrils.	J.P. #108434 male, white 12–12–51 O+	Alveolar rhabdomyosarcoma (maxillary sinus)
6096	9–2–75	25	Large elongated cells growing in multilayers; "foci" of large "epithelioid" cells.	J.D.H. #103941 male, white 5–23–65 O+	Malignant fibrous histiocytoma
6097 7004	9–2–75 9–11–75	22	Elongated cells growing in multilayers and large "foci" (Sinkovics and Mackay, 1977).	H.S. #108588 female, white 8–12–43 AB+	Monophasic synovial sarcoma (metastastic to lungs and pleura)
8021	3–19–76	13	Slender elongated cells growing in multilayers.	L.R.L. #112129 male, white 9–19–55 O+	Malignant neoplasm consistent with sarcoma (metastastic to lungs and pleura)

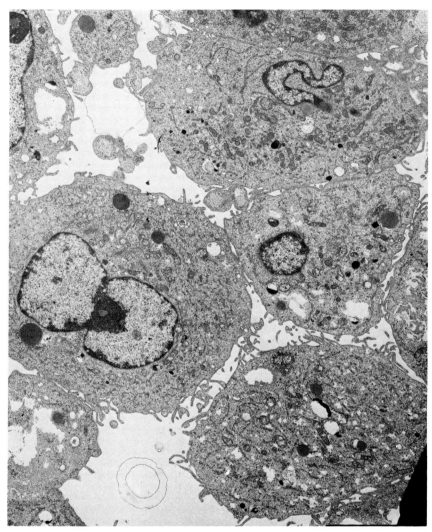

Fig. 3.—Electron microscopic view of cell line #2291 established by the senior author and derived from a patient (MDAH #85890) with undifferentiated sarcoma, probably malignant fibrous histiocytoma. Reduced from magnification ×15,000. (Courtesy of Dr. Bruce Mackay, Department of Pathology, M.D. Anderson Hospital.)

quently yield lymphocytes which are more cytotoxic toward cultured sarcoma cells than toward cultured carcinoma cells (Kay, Thota, and Sinkovics, 1976). This can be interpreted to mean that cultured sarcoma cells, for reasons other than immunological, are more susceptible to lymphocyte-mediated cytotoxicity than are cultured carcinoma

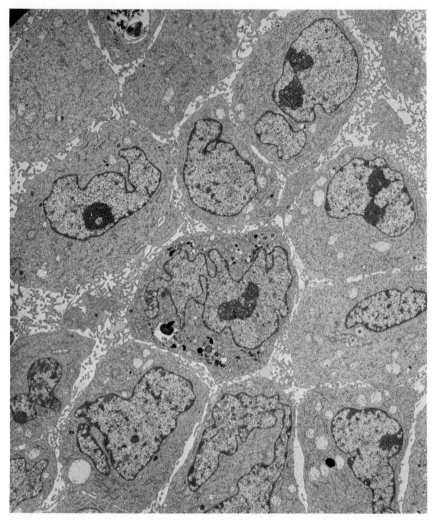

Fig. 4.—Electron microscopic view of cell line #2454 established by the senior author and derived from a patient with chondrosarcoma (MDAH #87288). Reduced from magnification ×15,000. (Courtesy of Dr. Bruce Mackay, Department of Pathology, M. D. Anderson Hospital.)

cells; however, it is also possible that human sarcomas are caused by ubiquitous oncornaviruses and that sarcoma-specific immunity is widespread in the healthy human population (Kay, Thota, and Sinkovics, 1976). This latter possibility is supported by the detection of sarcoma-directed antibody- and lymphocyte-mediated immune reactions

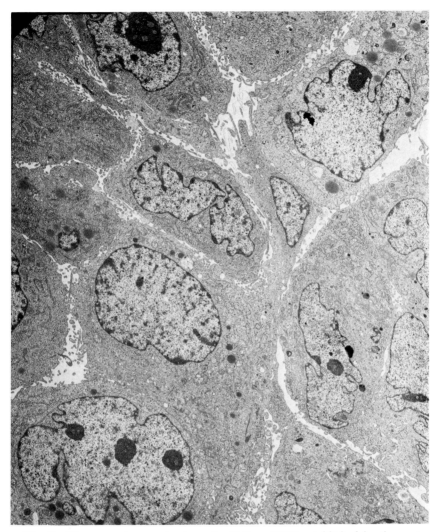

Fig. 5.—Electron microscopic view of cell line #3123 established by the senior author and derived from a patient (MDAH #89355) with von Recklinghausen's neurofibromatosis and neurofibrosarcomas. Reduced from magnification ×20,000. (Courtesy of Dr. Bruce Mackay, Department of Pathology, M. D. Anderson Hospital.)

in close contacts of patients with sarcomas (Byers, Levin, Hackett, and Fudenberg, 1975).

Cultured sarcoma cells permit the study of cell kinetics. The taxonomy of poorly understood sarcomas such as epithelioid sarcoma, clear cell sarcoma, cystosarcoma phylloides, bimodal synovial sarcoma,

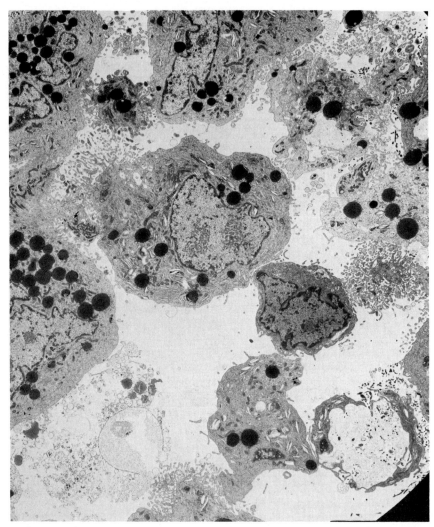

Fig. 6.—Electron microscopic view of cell line #4052 established by the senior author and derived from a patient (MDAH #86301) with angiosarcoma. Reduced from magnification ×22,000. (Courtesy of Dr. Bruce Mackay, Department of Pathology, M. D. Anderson Hospital.)

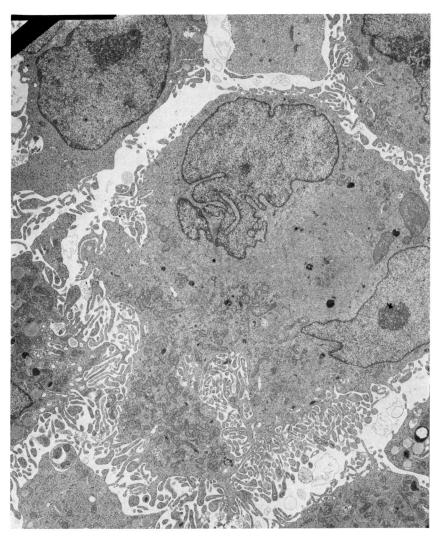

Fig. 7. — Electron microscopic view of cell line #5469 established by the senior author and derived from a child with probable malignant fibrous histiocytoma (MDAH #106227). Reduction from magnification ×20,000. (Courtesy of Dr. Bruce Mackay, Department of Pathology, M. D. Anderson Hospital.)

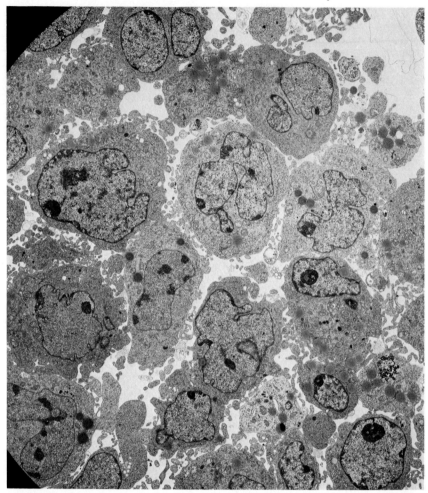

Fig. 8.—Electron microscopic view of a cell line #6097 established by the senior author from the pleural effusion of a patient with metastatic synovial sarcoma (MDAH #108588). Reduced from magnification ×12,000. (Courtesy of Dr. Bruce Mackay, Department of Pathology, M. D. Anderson Hospital.)

Ewing's sarcoma, and Kaposi's sarcoma could be better understood. Cultured sarcoma cells may serve not only as target cells in immune reactions, but also as immunizing antigens for immunotherapy.

Correlations of Immune Reactions with Clinical Course

LYMPHOCYTE-MEDIATED CYTOTOXICITY, MIGRATION INHIBITION, AND CYTOLYTIC ANTIBODIES

In an early study, it was estimated that the clinical course of about 70% of the patients with sarcomas correlated with an in vitro assay measuring lymphocyte-mediated cytotoxicity and serum factors antagonistic to or synergistic with lymphocytes cytotoxic to cultured sarcoma cells (Campos *et al.*, 1974; Sinkovics *et al.*, 1974a), but patients whose clinical courses were contradictory to the assay were also recognized (Sinkovics, *et al.*, 1975a). There were patients whose lymphocyte-mediated cytotoxicity remained intact after chemotherapy while serum factors blocking this reaction disappeared; however, tumor growth continued in some of these patients (Sinkovics, Cabiness, and Shullenberger, 1972).

Lymphocyte-mediated cytotoxicity directed toward allogeneic cultured sarcoma cell lines was claimed to correlate fairly well with the clinical course in one recent study (Kotz, Rella, and Salzer, 1976). Of 7 patients with initially positive cytotoxicity, 4 remained tumor-free; 3 patients became negative in the cytotoxicity assay; 1 of these patients was found to be tumor-free, whereas 2 developed metastases. Of 12 initially cytotoxicity negative patients, 4 later became positive, and 3 of these remained tumor-free, while 1 developed metastases. Of the 8 patients who remained negative in the cytotoxicity assay, only 3 stayed tumor-free while 5 succumbed to metastases.

The lymphocyte-mediated cytotoxicity of patients with osteosarcoma is especially controversial. According to a study, approximately 60% of healthy individuals expressed some degree of lymphocyte-mediated cytotoxicity to cultured osteosarcoma cells. Accepting this as "normal cytotoxicity," 95% of patients with osteogenic sarcoma expressed stronger than normal cytotoxicity. Highly significant ($P < 0.002$) cytotoxicity was expressed by 86% of patients with osteogenic sarcoma, 45% of patients with carcinoma, 15% of patients with nonneoplastic bone diseases, and 14% of healthy individuals (Gangal, Agasho, Nair, and Rao, 1973). In contrast, other studies found the lymphocytes of immunologically competent osteosarcoma patients poorly reactive to autologous tumor cells (McMaster, Ferguson, Weinert, and Dickens, 1974). Of 15 patients with primary osteosarcoma, 80% showed depressed lymphocyte blastogenesis to PHA (Twomey, and Chretien, 1975); in the same assay, patients with soft tissue sarcomas did not differ from healthy controls. A recently introduced lymphocyte proliferation assay in which lymphocytes of osteosarcoma patients proliferate upon exposure of soluble osteosarcoma antigen suggests that the osteosarcoma antigen does not cross-react with soft tissue sarcoma antigens (Gainor, Forbes, Enneking, and Smith, 1976).

According to the recently introduced leukocyte migration assay in agarose, the leukocytes of 66% of 27 patients with sarcomas were inhibited upon exposure to solubilized sarcoma antigens; reactivity to nonsarcomatous tumor antigens was low. In spite of its tumor-specificity, this assay did not correlate with stage of disease (Boddie, *et al.*, 1976).

The role of antibodies in human tumor immunology should not be underestimated. Patients with sarcomas circulate antibodies that are capable of lysing sarcoma cells in the presence of complement (Wood and Morton, 1971; Romero, Campos, and Sinkovics, 1976). The cell line established by one of us (J.G.S.) from a patient with malignant fibrous histiocytoma (culture #2291) appears to express antigens reactive in the cytolytic antibody test (Table 4). These antibodies occur more frequently and in higher titers in patients with localized sarcomas than in patients with metastatic sarcomas (Table 4) (Romero, Campos, and Sinkovics, 1976).

TABLE 4.—COMPLEMENT-FIXING
CYTOLYTIC ANTIBODIES DIRECTED TO
CULTURED SARCOMA CELLS°

>30% TARGET CELL° GROWTH REDUCTION	PATIENTS TESTED
	18/40 with sarcomas
	0/20 with melanomas
	0/8 with carcinomas
	0/26 healthy
1:4 serum dilution of patients with sarcomas tested	Averaged target cell° reduction
14 patients with metastases	19%
21 patients with primary or regional tumor	38%
	P < .003

°Target sarcoma cells: Established malignant fibrous histiocytoma cell line #2291.

IMMUNOLOGICALLY DEFINED GROUPS OF PATIENTS WITH SARCOMAS

Estimates based on 75 patients tested in vitro in lymphocyte-mediated cytotoxicity assay against a battery of cultured sarcoma, carcinoma, and melanoma cells and skin-tested with recall antigens permit a tentative subdivision of these patients into 4 groups (Table 5). The first group consists of immunologically compromised patients whose disease advances to death. The second group includes patients whose reactions vary widely during their clinical course. This is a heterogenous group of patients and it is not clear whether it will be possible to correlate the patient's clinical course with the immunological assays; however, most patients with a favorable clinical course were reactive and did not circulate serum factors blocking lymphocyte-mediated cytotoxicity. The third group of patients is the most paradoxical. This group of patients is highly immunoreactive but succumbs to advancing tumors. The lymphocytes of some of these patients could be tested for cytotoxicity against autologous and allogeneic cultured sarcoma cells. It was conspicuous that lymphocyte-mediated cytotoxicity was strong toward allogeneic cell lines but was absent toward autologous cell lines. Furthermore, these patients were characterized by the lack of serum factors blocking lymphocyte-mediated cytotoxicity (Sinkovics, *et al.*, 1976). This is in sharp contrast to patients succumbing to metastatic sarcomas in groups 1 and 2. The interpretation offered for group 3 patients is that the sarcomas of these immunocompetent patients grow without expressing sarcoma-specific target antigens (Sinkovics, *et al.*, 1976). Thus, these sarcomas are "immunoresistant" because of lack of "rejection antigens." This interpretation still requires direct proof.

In the fourth group are the patients apparently cured of metastatic sarcomas. These patients, even without immunotherapy, or before immunotherapy, have expressed strong, apparently sarcoma-specific, immune reactions. The abbreviated case histories of some of these remarkable patients attended by one of us (J.G.S.) at the Solid Tumor Service, Department of Medicine, are given below.

CASE 1. – A 48-year-old man (MDAH #74215) developed, in 1968, a large unclassified rhabdomyosarcoma in the left upper abdomen, recurrent after surgery and invading the bone marrow. The primary site was irradiated with 3,000 rads X-ray. Treatment with cyclophosphamide, vincristine, and actinomycin D resulted in complete remission which was still maintained in mid-1976. This patient tolerated un-

TABLE 5.—IMMUNE STATUS OF PATIENTS* WITH METASTATIC
(OR LOCALLY DESTRUCTIVE) SARCOMAS RECEIVING THERAPY†

TUMOR STATUS	OCCURRENCE %	DELAYED HYPERSENSITIVITY	LYMPHOCYTE-MEDIATED CYTOTOXICITY	SERUM FACTORS‡
Advancing rapidly to death	approx. 10–15	Decreased	Decreased	Blocking No blocking
CR, PR, St and relapse	approx. 50–70	Retained Decreased	Retained Decreased	Blocking No blocking
Advancing to death	approx. 10–25	Retained	Strong, selective or nonselective. Reactivity to allogeneic cells stronger than to autologous cells§	No blocking Potentiating
Long CR > 3 yr Cure > 5 yr	< 5	Retained	Strong, selective or nonselective	No blocking Unblocking Potentiating

*Estimates based on 75 patients tested repeatedly.
†Surgery; intermittent, combination chemotherapy; radiotherapy as indicated.
‡Blocking of lymphocyte-mediated cytotoxicity; unblocking of blocking effect; potentiating lymphocyte-mediated cytotoxicity. In 35 patients, cytolytic antibody titer tested against sarcoma cell line #2291 correlated with stage of disease.
   CR—complete remission; PR—partial remission; St—stable.
§Tested only occasionally, because autologous cells were seldom available in established cultures.

usually high doses of chemotherapy; until August 1973, cyclophosphamide, 87 gm; vincristine, 118 mg; and actinomycin D, 7.5 mg were administered. The patient yielded sarcoma-distinctively cytotoxic lymphocytes and unblocking serum factors (Sinkovics, *et al.*, 1974b). In 1973, he received further chemotherapy with cyclophosphamide, vincristine, and actinomycin D, but all chemotherapy was discontinued in 1974. He remains in complete remission in mid-1976.

CASE 2. — A 22-year-old man (MDAH #77650) developed embryonal rhabdomyosarcoma in the right paranasal sinus in 1969, recurrent after extensive surgery (Caldwell-Luc) and radiotherapy with 6,000 rads. Invasion of the left ethmoid and sphenoid bones took place. Chemotherapy with cyclophosphamide, vincristine, and actinomycin D was begun in early 1970. The patient continued to receive chemotherapy until early 1975 and remains in complete remission in July 1976.

CASE 3. — A 48-year-old man (MDAH #89868) developed a pleomorphic rhabdomyosarcoma of the left buttock in 1971. After excision, 5,040 rads ^{60}Co radiotherapy was given. During treatment, biopsy-proven metastasis in the right pectoralis muscle appeared. The patient received chemotherapy with cyclophosphamide, vincristine, and actinomycin D and remains clinically free of tumors at the end of 1976.

CASE 4. — A 69-year-old man (MDAH #92046) developed a large, poorly differentiated sarcoma (liposarcoma?) of the left thigh which recurred after excision. A second excision was followed by radiotherapy with 5,022 rads, but after the completion of this regimen, a metastatic poorly differentiated sarcoma was removed from the right orbit. For 1 year the patient received chemotherapy with vincristine, doxorubicin (Adriamycin), and dimethyl triazeno imidazole carboxamide (DTIC), and thereafter for 2 years with actinomycin D and DTIC. He is clinically tumor-free in 1976, 4½ years after the excision of the primary tumor and 3½ years after the removal of the metastasis.

CASE 5. — A 19-year-old girl (MDAH #99800) developed a large, retroperitoneal neurofibrosarcoma attached to the vertebral column and sacrum; this tumor was only partly excised. For the treatment of residual retroperitoneal tumors, the patient received vincristine, cyclophosphamide, doxorubicin (Adriamycin), and DTIC in 9 courses and continued on this regimen with actinomycin D replacing doxorubicin for an additional year (DTIC was omitted; total duration of chemotherapy was 23 months). In addition, immunotherapy with BCG scarifications and intracutaneous inoculations of viral oncolysates were given between courses of chemotherapy. These viral oncolysates (see later) were prepared from our neurofibrosarcoma cell line #3123, established from a patient with von Recklinghausen's disease and multiple neurofibrosarcomas. This patient (MDAH #99800), with palpable retroperitoneal tumors after surgery, remains clinically tumor-free 3½ years after surgery and 1 year after cessation of all therapy.

CASE 6.—A 47-year-old woman (MDAH #93403) developed a pleomorphic, poorly differentiated sarcoma of the left breast metastatic to both lungs in 1972. She received chemotherapy with vincristine, Adriamycin, and DTIC from October 1972 to July 1973 in 10 courses; from August 1973 to May 1974, she received 16 courses of vincristine, actinomycin D, and DTIC. She rapidly achieved complete remission status (Figs. 9–11). In 1974–1975 she received immunotherapy with scarified Chicago BCG and sarcoma viral oncolysates (see later) prepared from our cell line #3743 established from another patient with cystosarcoma phylloides. The patient (MDAH #93403) remains in complete remission at the end of 1976 without any further treatment.

These patients with metastatic or locally destructive sarcomas

Fig. 9 (left).—Large, bilateral pulmonary metastases of pleomorphic sarcoma of the left breast after mastectomy.

Fig. 10 (right).—Complete remission achieved by combination chemotherapy and maintained 4 years later.

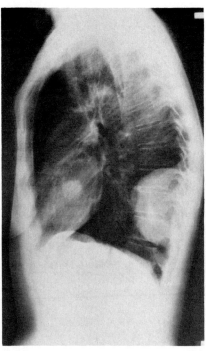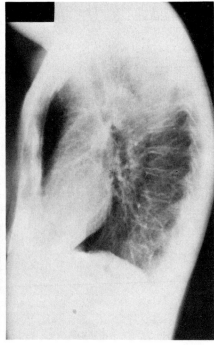

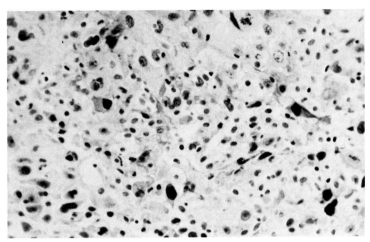

Fig. 11.—Pleomorphic sarcoma from biopsy of pleural-based tumor shown in Figure 9. (Courtesy of Dr. Steven Gallager, Department of Pathology, M. D. Anderson Hospital.)

showed a high level of immune reactivity toward cultured sarcoma (and occasionally carcinoma) cells. They circulated serum factors potentiating lymphocyte-mediated cytotoxicity that were present even before immunotherapy; some patients cured of metastatic sarcomas in this group never received any immunotherapy.

In comparing this unique group of patients with the previous group, immunocompetence is evident in both groups, including lymphocytes cytotoxic to various cultured sarcoma (and occasionally carcinoma) cells and serum factors potentiating this effect. Yet patients in the previous group, as documented elsewhere (Sinkovics, *et al.*, 1976) succumbed to advancing sarcomas, whereas patients in the last group survived tumor-free. The immunological assays are not refined enough to distinguish these 2 groups of patients; we theorize that the advancing tumors of immunocompetent patients fail to express tumor antigens, whereas the tumors of surviving immunocompetent patients remain highly antigenic.

Immunotherapy

IMMUNOTHERAPEUTIC PRINCIPLES AND MODALITIES

Immunotherapy of human tumors is a highly investigational attempt at the improvement of results achieved by conventional means (surgery, radiotherapy, and chemotherapy) of treatment. After initial claims of sensational success of immunotherapy (nonspecific immunostimulation in most cases with live bacteria or bacterial vaccines)in practically every tumor category in which it was used, a great deal of retreat and moderation permeates the field now. At best, nonspecific immunostimulation adds approximately 5–20% improvement to conventional treatment modalities in terms of remission maintenance but not in terms of remission induction. This marginal effect is seldom significant in randomized, prospective clinical trials, but can be recognized as a trend only. In clinical trials analyzed against so-called "matched historical controls," this difference may be of borderline significance, but the influence of human bias in selecting the matched controls cannot be dismissed. Further, the marginal effects of nonspecific immune stimulation can possibly be explained by better supportive care extended to the patients receiving immunotherapy versus those patients who receive only conventional therapy. Finally, what is thought to be nonspecific immunostimulation may be tumor-specific active immunotherapy in the sense that some bacterial surface antigens cross-react with surface antigens of certain tumor cells. Thus, recent clinical trials have failed to demonstrate the decisive effect of nonspecific immunostimulation in acute lymphoblastic leukemia (Kay, in press; Otten, in press); Burkitt's lymphoma (Magrath and Ziegler, 1976); malignant melanoma (Costanzi, in press; Cunningham, *et al.*, in press; Mastrangelo, Bellet, and Berd, in press; and Pinsky *et al.*, in press); and colorectal carcinoma (Engstrom *et al.*, in press; and Moertel, *et al.*, in press). The trend toward some clinical benefit, such as prolonged remission maintenance and survival, however, could be observed in acute myelogenous leukemia, (Cuttner, Glidewell, and Holland, in press; Hewlett, Balcerzak, and Gutterman, in press; and Vogler *et al.*, in press), and non-Hodgkin's lymphoma (Jones, Salmon, Moon, and Butler, in press) even though this beneficial clinical effect remains an insignificant trend only, in most of the randomized prospective trials. Also, only clinical trials evaluated against the so-called matched historical controls claim small but significant benefits in acute myelogenous leukemia, malignant melanoma, colorectal carcinoma, and breast carcinoma, i.e. in all disease categories in which such immunostimulation was applied (Gutterman *et al.*, 1976).

It appears that the combination of appropriate active tumor-specific immunization with nonspecific immunostimulation increases the effectiveness of some treatment regimens. In mouse mammary carcinoma, nonspecific immunostimulation enhanced tumor growth, but the combined administration of nonspecific immunostimulation with tumor-specific active immunization resulted in tumor rejection (Jacobs and Kripke, 1974).

In acute and chronic myelogenous leukemia, the combined administration of allogeneic (or autologous) leukemia cells and immunostimulation with BCG resulted in significant prolongation of chemotherapy-induced remissions (Bekesi, Roboz, and Holland, 1976; Powles, *et al.*, in press; Sokal, Aungst, Snyderman, and Gomez, 1976). In malignant melanoma, 1 clinical trial with chemotherapy, immunostimulation with BCG, and tumor-specific immunization with X-irradiated melanoma cells resulted in a most impressive remission rate of more than 50% of patients with metastatic disease (Currie and McElwain, 1975), but without improved survival (Newlands *et al.*, 1976). In 2 other trials, the combination of tumor-specific immunization with nonspecific immunostimulation failed to improve the benefits for patients with regional lymph node metastases of malignant melanoma that were claimed to have been achieved by immunostimulation alone against historical controls (Eilber *et al.*, 1976); or no difference in the median duration of remission between patients receiving chemotherapy (MeCCNU and vincristine) only, or chemoimmunotherapy (MeCCNU, vincristine, BCG, and X-irradiated allogeneic melanoma cells) was observed. However, 10 of 24 patients in the chemoimmunotherapy group were alive, in contrast to 5 of the 26 patients in the chemotherapy group (Mastrangelo, Bellet, and Berd, in press).

Presuming that future clinical trials of human tumor immunotherapy will be freed from sensationalism and human bias (and the urge to produce positive results in return for a continuing flow of large funds invested), one may foresee modest but clinically beneficial effects from the use of well-standardized microbial vaccines or products in combination with active tumor-specific immunization and from the administration of instructive-adoptive modalities of immunotherapy such as transfer factor and immune RNA. Chemicals (levamisole) and hormones (thymosine) that appear to restore defective T lymphocyte-mediated immune reactivity to normal will also require well-controlled clinical trials in the near future.

NONSPECIFIC IMMUNOSTIMULATION FOR SARCOMAS

It was with sarcomas, at the turn of the century, that the remission-inducing effect of bacterial products as immunostimulants was discovered (Coley, 1898; Coley, 1908). An abundance of anecdotal case histories has since then been assembled documenting the clinically beneficial effects of immunostimulation with toxins of streptococci and prodigiosus bacteria (now known as *Serratia marcescens*) in the treatment of soft tissue and bone (Ewing's) sarcomas (Nauts, 1974).

In a more recent clinical trial, killed *Corynebacterium parvum* vaccine was given in addition to chemotherapy to patients with nonlymphoid sarcomas. Of 12 patients receiving chemotherapy only, 65.2% were alive at 6 months and 43.5% were alive at 12 and 18 months, but all patients died by the 24th month. In the chemoimmunotherapy group consisting of 13 patients, 84% were alive at 6 and 12 months, 52.2% were alive at 18 months, and 38.8% were alive at 24 and 30 months; all patients were dead by the 36th month. A statistically significant difference of $P < 0.03$ had been claimed for these 2 groups of patients (Israel and Edelstein, 1975).

Sarcoma-Specific Active Immunization

IMMUNIZATION WITH SARCOMA CELLS AND EXTRACTS. — In uncontrolled clinical trials, single patients or small groups of patients were immunized with allogeneic cultured sarcoma cells or with X-irradiated autologous or allogeneic sarcoma cells with or without mixing the cells with BCG. Rejection of pulmonary metastases in a patient with osteogenic sarcoma (Mendoza et al., 1968), elevation in titers of antibodies cytolytic to sarcoma cells in the presence of complement (Wood and Morton, 1971), decrease of serum factors blocking cytotoxicity of lymphocytes directed to sarcoma cells (Currie, 1973), and increase of lymphocyte-mediated cytotoxicity and serum factors potentiating lymphocyte-mediated cytotoxicity to sarcoma cells (and sometimes also to carcinoma cells) (Sinkovics et al., 1974b; Sinkovics et al., 1975b) were demonstrated in the immunized patients. For example, after immunization with autologous X-irradiated sarcoma cells and BCG, 7 of 15 patients with sarcomas developed delayed hypersensitivity reactions to autologous sarcoma cells; this reaction was not evident before immunization (Morton, 1972).

Of 32 patients with soft tissue sarcomas, 6 patients (21%) survived 3 years, but of 27 patients with soft tissue sarcomas treated by conventional means plus immunotherapy with BCG and X-irradiated allogeneic sarcoma cells, 16 patients (59%) survived 3 years (Townsend and Eilber, 1975). The same treatment design, however, applied to patients with osteogenic sarcoma, failed; all 12 control patients died and only 3 of 17 patients (17%) immunized with BCG and X-irradiated allogeneic osteosarcoma cells survived (Eilber, Townsend, and Morton, 1975).

Patients with osteogenic sarcoma after the amputation of the involved extremity received immunotherapy with 1 of 3 types of autologous vaccines: 14 patients received cell-free and ultraviolet light-irradiated vaccine (UV vaccine); 17 patients received X-irradiated (^{60}Co) whole cell vaccine (X vaccine); and 5 patients received ^{60}Co-irradiated tissue culture grown tumor cells (TC vaccine). The clinical course of the immunized patients was compared with that of 145 historical control (119 adjusted historical control) patients with osteogenic sarcoma. In the TC vaccine group, 4 patients survived tumor-free 20–31 months. The clinical course of patients receiving the X vaccine was slightly (not significantly) worse than that of the control patients. Recipients of the UV vaccine fell into 3 subgroups: 6 patients developed metastases in 10 months (corresponding to the control series); 2 patients developed metastases, one by 20 and the other by 22 months (later than expected); and 4 patients remained tumor-free at 60 to 76 months. A Wilcoxon-Gehan analysis failed to show a significant difference between the control group and the UV vaccine group; however, there was a significant difference between the course of the 2 vaccinated groups in that patients in the whole cell vaccine group succumbed earlier than did patients in the lysed UV vaccine group, with the control curve lying in between. Thus, immunological manipulations appear to have some effect on the course of osteogenic sarcoma (Marcove *et al.*, 1973).

Three of 6 patients with sarcomas immunized with neuraminidase-treated tumor cells and BCG after surgical removal of metastases developed recurrent tumors (Gunnarson, McKhann, Simmons, and Gage, 1974). In another similar attempt at tumor-specific active immunization, 25 patients (including 6 with melanoma, 5 with gastrointestinal tumors, 4 with sarcomas, and 3 with breast carcinoma) received active immunization with neuraminidase-treated autologous tumor cells; while laboratory parameters improved (lymphocyte- and antibody-mediated cytotoxicity to tumor cells), only 6 patients experienced temporary stabilization of disease (Rosato *et al.*, 1974).

THE IMMUNIZING VALUE OF VIRAL ONCOLYSATES.—In a number of murine tumors, tumor cell membrane preparations derived from virus-infected cells were significantly more immunogenic than were membrane preparations of uninfected tumor cells. Animals immunized with membrane preparations or lysates of virus-infected cells readily rejected large doses of viable nonvirus-infected tumor cells, thus proving that strong tumor-specific immunity had been acquired by the immunized animals. It has been theorized that tumor antigens exist attached to a natural helper antigen; the natural helper antigen is labile and disintegrates when the cells are broken up. Viral antigenic units that bud through the cell membrane can serve as stable helper antigens to tumor antigens, thus replacing the labile natural helper antigen. Therefore, in cell membrane preparations or lysates of virally infected tumor cells, tumor antigens retain high immunogenic potency. In the preparation of tumor antigens from virally infected tumor cells, i.e. viral oncolysates, myxoviruses (influenza and Newcastle disease viruses) acted as helper antigens superior to other viruses (vesicular stomatitis virus). Purified virus preparations were less antigenic than preparations containing tumor cell membrane fragments, and cytoplasmic contents and preparations inactivated by ultraviolet light retained high tumor antigenicity, whereas formaldehyde-inactivated preparations were devoid of tumor antigenicity (Gillette and Boone, 1976).

Tumor enhancement has not as yet been reported in animals immunized with viral oncolysates and challenged with live tumor cells thereafter. In 1 system, Newcastle disease virus-infected murine sarcoma cells were rapidly rejected, but the surviving animals succumbed to Newcastle disease virus-induced encephalopathy. When anti-Newcastle disease virus mouse immune serum was administered to mice with Newcastle disease virus-infected sarcomas, enhanced tumor growth occurred in these mice (Sinkovics and Howe, 1969).

The high tumor-specific immunogenicity of viral oncolysates offered itself for tumor immunotherapy trials in man. The following investigators are known to have used virally prepared human oncolysates:

Drs. J. Lindenman and F. Cavalli at Inselspital, Bern, Switzerland administered allogeneic acute myelogenous leukemic cells infected with fowl plague virus to 22 patients without any detectable clinical benefit. However, the preparation was inactivated with formaldehyde (Sauter *et al.*, in press).

Drs. C. Boone (National Cancer Institute, Bethesda, Maryland) and E. Klein (Roswell Park Memorial Institute, Buffalo, New York) used intracutaneously inoculated autologous viral oncolysates and observed tumor-specific skin reactions (Boone, personal communication).

Drs. W. Cassel and D. R. Murray at the Emory University School of Medicine in Atlanta, Georgia, used autologous viral oncolysates prepared for melanoma cells infected with a mouse-adapted neurotropic Newcastle disease virus for the immunization of patients with advanced malignant melanoma. Increased lymphocyte-mediated cytotoxicity directed toward autologous cultured melanoma cells and stabilization of disease in some patients were observed (Cassel and Murray, personal communication).

Dr. R. C. Wallack at the Wistar Institute, Philadelphia, Pennsylvania, prepared viral oncolysates from various human tumors infected with vaccina virus. Stabilization of the status of some patients with disseminated tumors was reported (Wallack *et al.*, 1976).

Dr. A. A. Green at the St. Jude Children's Research Hospital, Memphis, Tennessee, applied autologous and allogeneic osteosarcoma cell viral oncolysates for the immunization of 12 children with osteogenic sarcoma; the viral oncolysates were inactivated with formalin (final concentration 1:10,000) and the infecting viruses were recently isolated A or B strains of influenza virus. (If less harmful myxoviruses were used, formalin inactivation of the vaccine could have been avoided.) In patients with advanced disease, the vaccine induced antibody production to virus and tumor cell antigens without increasing cell-mediated immunity. In patients with small tumor burden, both humoral and cellular immunity to autologous or allogeneic osteosarcoma cells was induced or augmented. The clinical effects of the vaccine remain to be determined (Green, Pratt, Webster, and Smith, 1976).

Finally, one of us (J.G.S.) has been using viral oncolysates for the treatment of patients with sarcomas and malignant melanomas during the past 3 years (Sinkovics *et al.*, 1974b; Sinkovics *et al.*, 1975b). Against malignant melanoma we use viral oncolysates prepared from our established melanoma cell line #2124. Patients with malignant melanoma were shown to circulate antibodies and lymphocytes that are highly reactive to this cell line (McMurtrey *et al.*, 1976). The harmless PR8 influenza A virus grown in the allantois cavity of fertilized chicken eggs is used to infect cultured #2124 cells at a high multiplicity. Within 4 days, a weak cytopathic effect is clearly discrenible. At this time, the cultured cells are mechanically removed and pelleted. The resuspended cells are treated with DNAse and homogenized in a Dounce apparatus. The cell homogenate is then further disrupted by ultrasound in ice water. The centrifuged sediment is saved and is resuspended in phosphate buffered saline in 1/10 of its original volume. The homogenate is then treated with ultraviolet light, and the preparation's bacteriological sterility is ascertained next. The sterile homogenate, referred to as viral oncolysate, is rapidly deep frozen in acetone and dry ice and is stored deep frozen in 0.5 ml aliquots at $-120°C$. The lysates are to be inoculated intracutaneously in 0.25 ml volume per site. It is estimated that the 0.5 ml volume is the product of 10^7 tumor cells.

Two treatment regimens have been in use for malignant melanoma. In the first regimen, methyl chloroethyl cyclohexyl nitrosourea (MeCCNU) and dimethyl triazeno imidazole carboxamide (DTIC) were given at 6-week intervals and 2 immunizations were given between courses of chemotherapy with scarified Chicago BCG (6×10^8 organisms) and 0.5 ml melanoma viral oncolysate. The immunizations are given on the same day, at the same regional anatomical site (so that the same regional lymph nodes will process both BCG and melanoma cell antigens) but separately and not at exactly the same site. The sites are the limbs and trunk. In the second regimen, the chemotherapy consists of vincristine, cyclophosphamide, actinomycin D, and DTIC for 5 days to be repeated at 28-day intervals. On days 17 and 24, immunotherapy is given with scarified Chicago BCG and melanoma viral oncolysates as described above. Patients with deeper than Clark's level 3 trunk lesions, with satellitosis or in-transit metastases, with regional lymph node metastases after surgical dissection, and with disseminated disease are eligible. The patient's general immune status is assessed by skin tests to recall antigens. Antibody- and lymphocyte-mediated immune reactions to cultured allogeneic and autologous (when available) tumor cells are tested only exceptionally because the National Cancer Institute contract that initially supported these studies was not funded in 1975. These clinical trials with patients having malignant melanoma appear very favorable at their preliminary evaluation (Tables 6–8) and form the basis of our similar chemoimmunotherapy trials with patients having metastatic sarcomas. In the 2 melanoma chemoimmunotherapy trials, 50% of those 12 patients who received both chemotherapy and BCG progressed, whereas of the 27 comparable patients receiving chemotherapy, BCG, and viral oncolysates (melanoma lysates) only 26 % progressed.

TABLE 6.—CHEMOIMMUNOTHERAPY FOR MALIGNANT MELANOMA

MeCCNU DTIC BCG > 1 YR		PROGRESSORS/ PATIENTS TREATED	% PROGRESSORS
Stage I	1 Stable		
	1 → IV progressed		
III	1 NED		
	1 → IV died		
IV	2 died	4/6	66

MeCCNU DTIC BCG MVO > 1 YR		PROGRESSORS/ PATIENTS TREATED	% PROGRESSORS
Stage I	1 NED (omitted from % calculation)		
II	1 NED		
III	10 NED		
	1 → IV progressed		
	1 → IV died		
IV	1 progressed		
	2 died	5/17	29

MeCCNU—methyl chloroethyl cyclohexyl nitrosourea
DTIC—dimethyl triazeno imidazole carboxamide
NED—no evidence of disease
MVO—melanoma viral oncolysate
BCG—Bacille Calmette-Guérin

TABLE 7.—CHEMOIMMUNOTHERAPY FOR
MALIGNANT MELANOMA

VCR CTX Act D DTIC BCG > 6 MO	PROGRESSORS/ PATIENTS TREATED	% PROGRESSORS
Stage I 2 NED		
III 2 NED		
1 → IV progressed		
IV 1 died	2/6	33
I 3 entered < 6 mo		
III 5 entered < 6 mo		

VCR CTX Act D DTIC BCG MVO > 6 MO	PROGRESSORS/ PATIENTS TREATED	% PROGRESSORS
Stage I 3 NED		
II 1 NED		
III 4 NED		
1 → IV progressed		
IV 1 NED		
1 progressed	2/11	18
I 1 entered < 6 mo		
III 3 entered < 6 mo		
IV 7 entered < 6 mo		

VCR—vincristine; CTX—cyclophosphamide; Act D—actinomycin D; BCG—Bacille Calmette-Guérin; MVO—Melanoma viral oncolysate.

The design of the sarcoma chemoimmunotherapy trial is as follows: Patients with metastatic sarcomas receive chemotherapy with vincristine, cyclophosphamide, Adriamycin, and DTIC for 5 days every 28 days; after 500 mg/m² Adriamycin has been given, instead of Adriamycin, actinomycin D is administered. Immunotherapy consists of 6 × 10⁸ viable units of Chicago BCG scarified on days 17 and 24 with or without intracutaneous inoculations of sarcoma cell viral oncolysates

TABLE 8.—CHEMOIMMUNOTHERAPY FOR STAGE III
(REGIONAL LYMPH NODE INVOLVEMENT AFTER SURGICAL
LYMPH NODE DISSECTION)
PATIENTS WITH MALIGNANT MELANOMA

TREATMENT REGIMENS	PROGRESSORS/ PATIENTS	% PROGRESSORS
MeCCNU DTIC BCG (1 yr)	1/2	
VCR CTX Act D DTIC BCG (6 mo)	1/3	
	2/5	40
MeCCNU DTIC BCG MVO (1 yr)	2/12	
VCR CTX Act D DTIC BCG MVO (6 mo)	1/5	
	3/17	18

For abbreviations see Tables 6 and 7

into the same anatomical region. The following established sarcoma cell lines are being used as viral oncolysates: culture #2291, malignant fibrous histiocytoma; culture #2322, chondroblastic osteosarcoma; culture #2454, chondrosarcoma; culture #3123, neurofibrosarcoma; culture #3743, cystosarcoma phylloides; culture #4929 rhabdomyosarcoma (see Table 3). Whether or not these cultures express cross-reacting sarcoma-specific antigens is an unsolved problem; however, incomplete data are affirmative. Therefore, either one, especially the highly antigenic cell line #2291 (Romero, Campos, and Sinkovics, 1975; Sinkovics, Kay, and Thota, 1975), or a mixture of these cell lines may be used for active sarcoma-specific immunizations in the future. Contemporary patients with metastatic sarcomas receiving chemotherapy only, form the control group in this trial: Of 48 patients, 10 are in complete remission (21%), 6 are in partial remission or in stable clinical status (13%), and 32 progressed, many to death (66%). Ten patients with metastatic sarcomas received combination chemotherapy and BCG scarifications only; 1 patient is in complete remission (10%), 5 patients are in partial remission or in stable clinical status (50%), and 4 patients progressed, some to death (40%). Fourteen patients with metastatic sarcomas received combination chemotherapy, BCG scarifications, and active immunizations with viral oncolysates (sarcoma lysates). Six patients are in complete remission (43%), 6 are in partial remission or in stable clinical status (43%), and 2 have progressive disease (14%). Thus, the group receiving chemoimmunotherapy with both BCG and sarcoma lysates appears to be in the most favorable clinical condition at 1 year (Table 9). It should be clearly recognized that this is a preliminary report and that these patients should be reanalyzed later in a stratified fashion so that known prognostic factors in each group can be determined.

TABLE 9.–CHEMOIMMUNOTHERAPY FOR METASTATIC SOFT TISSUE SARCOMAS 1974–76

CLINICAL STATUS IN OCT 76	CHEMOTHERAPY + BCG + SVO		CHEMOTHERAPY + BCG		CHEMOTHERAPY ONLY	
Number of patients	14	–	10	–	48	–
CR and NED	6	43%	1	10%	10	21%
PR and stable	6	43%	5	50%	6	13%
Progressors and dead	2	14%	4	40%	32	66%

BCG – Bacille Calmette-Guérin; SVO – Sarcoma viral oncolysates; CR – Complete remission; NED – No evidence of disease; PR – Partial remission.
All patients received chemotherapy° and surgery and/or radiotherapy as indicated.
° Intermittent, combination.

ADOPTIVE IMMUNOTHERAPY

The cross-transplant cross-transfusion design for adoptive immunotherapy has been used primarily for the treatment of malignant melanoma, but patients with various other tumors, among them sarcomas, were also included (Nadler, and Moore, 1969). Three patients with osteogenic sarcoma and 1 patient with synovial sarcoma received allogeneic leukocytes and plasma transfusions from other patients who rejected their sarcoma transplants; 2 patients with metastatic osteogenic sarcoma showed partial remission (Krementz *et al.*, 1974). H-L antigen-matched thoracic duct lymphocytes were transfused from siblings into 2 patients with osteosarcomas without clinical effect; the same procedure resulted in complete remission of 6 months' duration in another patient with ovarian carcinoma (Yonemoto, 1976).

Tumor-specific antigenicity of human osteosarcoma was demonstrated by a precipitin reaction between osteosarcoma extracts and rabbit immune sera; these rabbits were immunized with human osteosarcoma preparations and the immune sera were absorbed with normal human bone antigens (Neff and Enneking, 1975). The clinical course of 8 patients with metastatic osteogenic sarcoma was not changed by passive immunization with these rabbit immune sera or by active immunization with osteosarcoma antigens. The tumors of patients with osteosarcoma were transplanted into patients with osteosarcoma and other sarcomas. At the time of tumor rejection, lymphocytes were harvested from the tumor recipients and were transfused into the tumor donors. Patients receiving adoptive immunotherapy realized fewer metastases and longer survival than did historical controls, but the difference was not significant (Neff and Enneking, 1975); 33% of 32 immunized patients were tumor-free at 2 years, whereas 22% of 145 control patients (Memorial Sloan-Kettering Hospital series) were tumor-free at 2 years.

One of 2 identical twin young women developed widely spread (tumor cells in peripheral blood) rhabdomyosarcoma; the patient did not, but her healthy twin did, possess lymphocytes cytotoxic to cultured allogeneic sarcoma cells. Also, the healthy twin possessed unblocking serum factors. Remission was induced by combination chemotherapy, and thereafter the patient received repeatedly large transfusions of plasma and leukocytes from her healthy twin and was also immunized with X-irradiated allogeneic sarcoma cells. At this time, the patient displayed lymphocyte-mediated cytotoxicity to allogeneic, but not to autologous, sarcoma cells. After $3\frac{1}{2}$ months of remission maintained by immunotherapy only, the patient developed brain metastases and died. It was theorized that the patient's tumor expressed no or very weak tumor antigens and could grow in the presence of cytotoxic lymphocytes (Sinkovics, Cabiness, and Shullenberger, 1973).

TRANSFER FACTOR

It has been claimed that close relatives of patients with osteosarcoma develop lymphocytes specifically cytotoxic to cultured osteosarcoma cells. These healthy donors were used as a source of dialyzable transfer factor for the prophylactic treatment of postamputation patients with osteosarcoma or patients with metastatic osteosarcoma. Anecdotal individual case histories or histories of small groups of patients compared to historical controls were claimed to have benefited from transfer factor administration, i.e. metastases stabilized or presumably present micrometastases did not manifest themselves in clinically recognizable disease (Fudenberg, 1976). Of 5 postamputation patients receiving allegedly osteosarcoma-specific transfer factor, 4 remained tumor-free for 2 years (Byers et al., 1976). However, in another clinical trial, it was not possible to demonstrate osteosarcoma-specific immune reactions by a leukocyte adherence inhibition test. In this trial, the transfer factor donors were long-term tumor-free survivors of osteosarcoma. Three groups of patients with postamputation osteosarcoma were treated. One group of 9 patients received transfer factor only; 4 patients developed metastases and 5 patients survived tumor-free for more than 1 year. A second group of 23 patients received chemotherapy (methotrexate, Adriamycin, and vincristine) and transfer factor; 11 patients developed metastases and 9 patients are alive and tumor-free for more than 1 year. In this group, 3 non tumor-related deaths occurred (chemotherapy toxicity). A third group of 18 patients received only chemotherapy (methotrexate, Adriamycin, and vincristine). In this group, 9 patients developed metastases and 6 patients remained alive tumor-free; however, 3 non tumor-related deaths (chemotherapy toxicity) occurred (Ivins et al., 1976; Ritts et al., in press).

A young man with soft part alveolar sarcoma received transfer factor from his healthy identical twin. The patient's lymphocytes, after exposure to tumor homogenate, released migration inhibitory factor only after treatment with transfer factor; the healthy twin's lymphocytes were positive in this assay. During 6 months of treatment with transfer factor the patient's clinical condition stabilized, but tumor growth continued thereafter (Lo Buglio et al., 1973). A young woman with alveolar soft part sarcoma of the retroperitoneum also achieved stable disease status for 10 months after treatment with transfer factor preparation of the above described donor (Sinkovics *et al.*, 1974c). (These transfer factor preparations were the gift of Drs. A. Lo Buglio and J. A. Neidhart.) Later tumor growth became evident despite transfer factor administration.

INTERFERON

Human interferon can now be produced in large amounts in Sendai virus-infected cultures of leukocytes. In a clinical trial now being conducted in Sweden, patients with osteogenic sarcoma received, after amputation, 3×10^6 units of human interferon intramuscularly daily for 1 month and weekly for 1½ years thereafter. During the first 6 months the trial appeared very promising: none of the treated 12 patients developed metastases, but 15 of 33 control patients did. By 1 year, 3 of the treated patients (25%) had metastatic disease. At this point, the difference between treated and untreated patients was of borderline significance ($P < 0.05$) (Strander, 1975).

FUTURE PROSPECTS

ADJUVANT TRIALS. — The clinical setting with sarcomas favors the integration of immunotherapy into the conventional treatment regimens.

After the wide excision of primary or locally recurrent sarcomas, X-ray therapy of the tumor site controls the disease very well. Table 10 lists those patients who were attended by our Solid Tumor Service, Department of Medicine, for chemotherapy in combination with radiotherapy as administered by Dr. R. Lindberg (Lindberg, 1977, see pages 343–352, this volume). However, trunk and head and neck sarcomas could not be treated in combination chemoradiotherapy as well as could sarcomas of the limbs: the dose of radiotherapy by necessity had to be less in trunk lesions than that delivered to the extremities, and chemotherapy (especially with doxorubicin) caused unusually severe mucositis when given in combination with radiotherapy to sarcomas of the head and neck. Further, combination chemotherapy can permanently sterilize the gonads and deprive young, potentially curable patients of future parenthood. Also, combination chemotherapy may be carcinogenic in long-term survivors. Finally, adjuvant chemotherapy in cases of chemotherapy-resistant tumors (for example, vincristine and cyclophosphamide for neurofibrosarcoma or chondrosarcoma) can be immunosuppressive without antitumor effect; in these

TABLE 10.—CHEMORADIOTHERAPY FOR PATIENTS WITH
PRIMARY OR LOCALLY RECURRENT SARCOMAS AFTER
SURGICAL EXCISION OF THE TUMOR

| SARCOMA SUBTYPE | RADIOTHERAPY | | | CHEMORADIOTHERAPY[°] | | | |
	PATIENTS	NED	P	PATIENTS	NED	P	D
Epithelioid	1	1	–	–	–	–	–
Fibro	3	3	–	1	1	–	–
Giant cell							
soft parts	1	1	–	–	–	–	–
Leiomyo	1	1	–	–	–	–	–
Lipo	2	2	–	2	2	–	–
Malignant fibrous							
histiocytoma	5	4	1	1	1	–	–
Neurofibro	2	2	–	2	2	–	–
Pleomorph	–	–	–	2	2	–	–
Rhabdomyo	2	1	1	4	3	1	–
Synovial	1	–	1	3	1	1	1
Undifferentiated,							
unclassified	–	–	–	1	–	–	1
Total	18	15	3	16	12	2	2
		(83%)			(75%)		

[°]Vincristine, cyclophosphamide, Adriamycin/actinomycin D as treated and evaluated at the Solid Tumor Service, Department of Medicine, M. D. Anderson Hospital. (For a detailed account, see Lindberg *et al.*, 1977, pages 343–352, this volume.)
P = progressing disease; D = death due to disease.

cases, metastases may develop because the host-tumor relationship has been compromised by the chemotherapy. Therefore, adjuvant chemotherapy should be stratified according to sarcoma subtype and known chemotherapy sensitivity (for example, doxorubicin and DTIC for liposarcomas and fibrosarcomas; vincristine, cyclophosphamide, doxorubicin, actinomycin D, and DTIC for rhabdomyosarcoma, sequentially and in an intermittent fashion). For these reasons, considerations should be given to immunotherapy without chemotherapy for patients receiving surgical therapy and radiotherapy for primary or locally recurrent sarcomas. The efficacy of chemotherapy or immunotherapy of whatever modality (nonspecific immunostimulation and sarcoma-specific active immunization preferably with nucleoprotein-free, purified sarcoma antigens; transfer factor) should be proved in well-designed (randomized and prospective; stratified according to prognostic factors) clinical trials. If high grade sarcomas are included in the chemotherapy-radiotherapy group versus low grade sarcomas given radiotherapy only, it is to be expected that one will see more metastases in the prognostically worse chemotherapy-radiotherapy group.

In the adjuvant treatment of postamputation osteosarcoma, neither interferon nor transfer factor should be relied upon without chemotherapy, unless clear evidence (better than what is available now) in favor of these immunotherapeutic modalities is provided. However, these immunotherapeutic modalities could be applied combined with large-dose methotrexate and leukovorin rescue with or without Adriamycin and DTIC.

EWING'S SARCOMA. — This tumor is either of multicentric origin or metastasizes very early. Conventionally, primary and selected metastatic lesions are treated by radiotherapy; systemic chemotherapy is mandatory for the control of disease distant from the clinically evident primary site. Vincristine, cyclophosphamide, doxorubicin (Adriamycin), nitrosourea preparations, DTIC and, occasionally, mithramycin have been shown to be effective. Table 11 shows our more recent series of patients who received radiotherapy (Dr. R. Lindberg's service) and chemotherapy for 2 years with vincristine, cyclophosphamide, and doxorubicin; doxorubicin was replaced with actinomycin D after 400–450 mg/m² total dose of Adriamycin was delivered. Chemotherapy is given at 28-day intervals; this would permit immunotherapy on days 13, 17, and 24 between courses of chemotherapy. We intend to use live BCG by scarification and viral oncolysates prepared from our established Ewing's sarcoma cell line #1846 (Sinkovics *et al.*, 1975b) (Figs. 12–14).

METASTATIC SARCOMAS. — It has not been proved that immunotherapy significantly contributed to remission induction in the case of

TABLE 11. — EWING'S SARCOMA IN
YOUNG ADULTS* 1975–1976

Treatment: Radiotherapy to primary tumor
VCR   CTX   Adriamycin/actinomycin   D
intermittently for 2 years

Patients treated more than 1 yr	12
NED	7
PR	1
Stable	1
Progressing†	2
Dead with tumors	1

*Patients attended by Solid Tumor Service, Department of Medicine, M. D. Anderson Hospital.
†Further failure on MeCCNU and DTIC VLB and mithramycin.
NED = no evidence of disease; PR = partial remission; VCR = vincristine; CTX = cyclophosphamide.

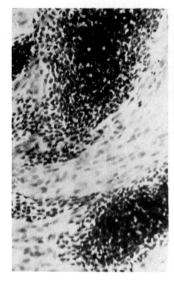

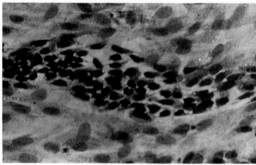

Fig. 12 (left). – Primary culture #1846 of Ewing's sarcoma shows colonies of tumor cells and an underlying sheet of fibroblast-like cells. Giemsa stain, ×25 objective, ×10 ocular.

Fig. 13 (above). – Small, densely stained tumor cells among fibroblast-like cells in primary culture #1846 of Ewing's sarcoma. Giemsa stain, ×40 objective, ×10 ocular.

metastatic sarcomas. Nevertheless, patients receiving combination chemotherapy for metastatic sarcomas should continue receiving immunotherapy with nonspecific immunostimulation (live BCG; killed corynebacteria) combined with sarcoma-specific active immunization (viral oncolysates; purified sacoma antigens) on days 13, 17, and 24 between 5-day courses of chemotherapy (Adriamycin and DTIC) to be given at 28-day intervals. Chemotherapy should be stratified according to cell types of sarcomas; for example, patients with rhabdomyosarcoma, leiomyosarcoma, and Ewing's sarcoma should also receive vincristine and cyclophosphamide. Chemotherapy should continue for 2 years, with actinomycin D replacing doxorubicin (Adriamycin) after 450–500 mg/m² total dose of doxorubicin has been reached.

Levamisole, thymosin, transfer factor, and 2 immune mediators of lymphocyte origin (interferon and lymphotoxin) will eventually be incorporated into controlled investigational trials.

KAPOSI'S SARCOMA. – Dependence of this tumor on the host's immune status (Hardy *et al.*, 1976; Myers *et al.*, 1974), and its response to delayed hypersensitivity reactions elicited in the skin (Klein *et al.*, 1974) have been clearly demonstrated. Kaposi's sarcoma is a devastating disease in Africa, but even in Western countries it is much more commonly metastatic than hitherto realized; the metastases, or multicentric origin of the tumor can be readily demonstrated by gastroscopy (Ahmed, Nelson, Goldstein, and Sinkovics 1975). This tumor re-

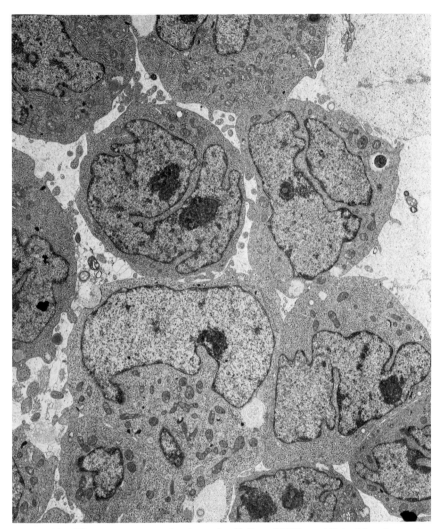

Fig. 14.—Electron microscopic view of cell line #1846 established by the senior author from a patient (MDAH #79610) with Ewing's sarcoma. Reduced from magnification ×15,000. (Courtesy of Dr. Bruce Mackay, Department of Pathology, M. D. Anderson Hospital.)

sponds to chemotherapy (Lanzotti, Campos, Sinkovics, and Samuels 1975; Sinkovics, 1976a) but elderly patients often cannot continue on prolonged regimens of chemotherapy. Intralesional immunotherapy (intralesional BCG) is probably effective in the treatment of injected lesions but carries the risk of systemic BCG infection. Perilesional scarifications of BCG often are not feasible because of severe edema of involved limbs. Since Kaposi's sarcoma afflicts the elderly who have naturally decreased immune competence, it would be essential to reinvestigate the presently available controversial data concerning the general (Dobozy *et al.*, 1973; Taylor *et al.*, 1971; Taylor and Ziegler, 1974) and tumor-specific immunocompetence of these patients (Master, Taylor, Kyalwazi, and Ziegler 1970). If immunoincompetence could be clearly demonstrated, Kaposi's sarcoma would be the tumor category in which thymosine or levamisole should be given controlled trials in order to determine whether restoration of immune competence would result in favorable tumor response.

Local modalities of immunotherapy that should be given trials, in addition to delayed hypersensitivity reactions already tried (Klein *et al.*, 1974), are intratumoral injections of lymphotoxin, intratumoral injection of human "recognition factor" and glucan (Mansell *et al.*, 1975), and non-living bacterial products (killed vaccines; lipopolysaccharides), so that "tumor necrosis factor" may be released from the macrophages infiltrating this tumor.

Addendum

One patient (Case 3, MDAH #89868) relapsed; he developed tumors in the abdomen and mediastinum. The abdominal tumor was excised; the mediastinum was irradiated. The patient receives immunotherapy with sarcoma viral oncolysates and BCG. One patient with Ewing's sarcoma (Table 11) relapsed 6 months after completing her 2 years of chemotherapy. She now receives additional doxorubicin with DTIC and radiotherapy to be followed by a nitrosourea and actinomycin D.

Of patients receiving chemoimmunotherapy for melanoma, 6 of 12 (50%) and 14 of 27 (52%) progressed in the group treated with chemotherapy plus BCG when analyzed in October 1976 and April 1977, respectively, with accrual of patients with over 6 months' treatment still continuing. In the group treated with chemotherapy, BCG, and melanoma viral oncolysates, 7 of 28 (25%) and 14 of 36 patients (39%) progressed when analyzed at these 2 points in time. According to analyses in October 1976 and February 1977, of 48 patients with metastatic sarcomas receiving chemotherapy only, 32 (67%) and 36 (75%) progressed, respectively. At these 2 points in time, 4 of 10 (40%) and 10 of 19 (53%) progressed, respectively, in the group treated with chemotherapy plus BCG (as accrual of patients treated for over 6 months continues). In the group treated with chemotherapy, BCG, and sarcoma viral oncolysates, 2 of 14 (14%) and 6 of 19 (32%) progressed, respectively. Therefore, longer follow-up of these patients now suggests that immunotherapy only temporarily delays the progression of disease.

Acknowledgments

The authors are grateful for essential financial support to the Kelsey-Leary Foundation and to the Dr. C. D. Howe Fund. Dr. C. C. Shullenberger has extended invaluable assistance in supporting this work. Dr. D. Gröschel performed the sterility testing of viral oncolysates. The technical assistance of Mesdames Frances Ervin and Doris Gaines is greatly appreciated. The authors thank Mrs. Karen Hill and Miss Donna Liling for secretarial assistance in the preparation of this manuscript.

The following clinical fellows, laboratory investigators, and house staff members contributed significantly to the data included in this report, either by patient care beyond the call of duty or by participation in laboratory research: Doctors Luis T. Campos, Frank Cormia, Francisco Gonzalez, H. David Kay, David K. King, Kevin K. Loh, Harikishan Thota, William Velasquez, and William C. Waterfield.

Abbreviations

BCG — Bacille Calmette-Guérin
DNAse — deoxyribonuclease
DTIC — dimethyl triazeno imidazole carboxamide
H-L antigen — normal leukocyte tissue type antigen
MeCCNU — methyl chloroethyl cyclohexyl nitrosourea
MDAH — M. D. Anderson Hospital and Tumor Institute
PHA — phytohemagglutinin
RNA — ribonucleic acid

REFERENCES

Ahmed, N., Nelson, R. S., Goldstein, H. M., and Sinkovics, J. G.: Kaposi's sarcoma of the stomach and duodenum: Endoscopic and roentgenologic correlations. Gastrointestinal Endoscopy, 21:149–152, May 1975.

Armine, A. R. C., and Sugar, O.: Suprasellar osteogenic sarcoma following radiation for pituitary adenoma. Journal of Neurosurgery, 44:88–91, January 1976.

Bekesi, G., Roboz, J., and Holland, J. F.: Therapeutic effectiveness of neuraminidase-treated tumor cells as an immunogen in man and experimental animals with leukemia. Annals of the New York Academy of Sciences, 277: 313–331, 1976.

Boddie, A. W., Jr., Urist, M. M., Chee, D. O., Holmes, E. C., and Morton, D. L.: Detection of human tumor-associated antigens by the leukocyte migration in agarose assay. International Journal of Cancer, 18:161–167, August 15, 1976.

Boone, C. W.: Personal communication.

Brooks, W. H., Roszman, T. L., and Rogers, A. S.: Impairment of rosette-forming T lymphocytes in patients with primary intracranial tumors. Cancer, 37: 1869–1873, April 1976.

Burk, K. H., Drewinko, B., Lichtiger, B., and Trujillo, J. M.: Cell cycle dependency of human sarcoma-associated tumor antigen expression. Cancer Research, 36:1278–1283, April 1976.

Byers, V. S., Levin, A. S., Hackett, A. J., and Fudenberg, H. H.: Tumor-specific cell-mediated immunity in household contacts of cancer patients. Journal of Clinical Investigation, 55:500–513, March 1975.

Byers, V. S., Levin, A. S., LeCam, L., Jonston, J. O., and Hackett, A. J.: Tumor-specific transfer factor therapy in osteogenic sarcoma: A two-year study. Annals of the New York Academy of Sciences, 277:621–627, 1976.

Campos, L. T., Sinkovics, J. G., Romero, J. J., Carrier, S., Cabiness, J. R., and Kay H. D.: Correlations and discrepancies of an *in vitro* assay for tumor immunity with clinical course. (Abstract #731). The Proceedings of the American Society of Clinical Oncology, 10:166, 1974.

Cassel, W., and Murray, D.: Personal communication.

Coley, W. B.: The treatment of inoperable sarcoma with the mixed toxins of erysipelas and B. prodigiosus. Journal of the American Medical Association, 31:389–456, 1898.

Coley, W. B.: The treatment of sarcoma by mixed toxins of erysipelas and B. prodigiosus. Boston Medical Surgical Journal, 158:175–182, 1908.

Costanzi, J. J.: Chemotherapy and BCG in the treatment of disseminated malignant melanoma: A southwest oncology group study. In Terry, W. D. and Windhorst, D., Eds.: *Immunotherapy of Cancer: Present Status of Trials in Man*, NCI Conference, 1976. (Abstract #7) New York, New York, Raven Press. (In press.)

Cunningham, T. J., Schoenfeld, D., Walters, J., Nathanson, L., Cohen, M., and Patterson, B.: A controlled study of adjuvant therapy (BCG, BCG-DTIC) with stage I and II melanoma. In Terry, W. D. and Windhorst, D., Eds.: *Immunotherapy of Cancer: Present Status of Trials in Man*, NCI Conference, 1976. (Abstract #1) New York, New York, Raven Press. (In press.)

Currie, G. A.: Effect of active immunization with irradiated tumor cells on specific serum inhibitors of cell-mediated immunity in patients with disseminated cancer. British Journal of Cancer, 28:25–35, July 1973.

Currie, G. A., and McElwain, T. J.: Active immunotherapy as an adjunct to chemotherapy in the treatment of disseminated malignant melanoma: A pilot study. British Journal of Cancer, 31:143–156, February 1975.

Cuttner, J., Glidewell, O., and Holland J. F.: A comparative study of the value of immunotherapy with MER as adjuvant to induction and two maintenance chemotherapy programs in acute myelocytic leukemia. In Terry, W. D. and Windhorst, D., Eds.: *Immunotherapy of Cancer: Present Status of Trials in Man*, NCI Conference, 1976. (Abstract #34) New York, New York, Raven Press. (In press.)

Dobozy, A., Husz, S., Hunyadi, J., Berkó, G., and Simon, N.: Immune deficiencies and Kaposi's sarcoma. (Letter) Lancet, 2:265, September 15, 1973.

Eilber, F. R., Morton, D. L., Holmes, E. C., Sparks, F. C., and Ramming, K. P.: Adjuvant immunotherapy with BCG in treatment of regional lymph node metastases from malignant melanoma. New England Journal of Medicine, 294:237–240, January 29, 1976.

Eilber, F. R., Nizze, J. A., and Morton, D. L.: Sequential evaluation of general immune competence in cancer patients: Correlation with clinical cancer. Cancer, 35:660–665, March 1975.

Eilber, F. R., Townsend, C., and Morton, D. T.: Osteosarcoma. Results of treatment employing adjuvant immunotherapy. Clinical Orthopaedics, 3: 94–100, 1975.

Engstrom, P. F., Paul, A. R., Catalano, R. B., Mastrangelo, M. J., and Creech, R. H.: Fluorouracil vs flourouracil + Bacillus Calmette-Guerin in colorectal adenocarcinoma. In Terry, W. D., and Windhorst, D., Eds.: *Immunotherapy of Cancer: Present Status of Trials in Man*, NCI Conference, 1976. (Abstract #48) New York, New York, Raven Press. (In press.)

Fudenberg, H. H.: Dialyzable transfer factor in the treatment of human osteosarcoma: An analytical review. Annals of the New York Academy of Sciences, 227:545–557, 1976.

Gainor, B. J., Forbes, J. T., Enneking, W. F., and Smith, R. T.: Specific antigen stimulated lymphocyte proliferation in osteosarcoma. Cancer, 37:743–750, February 1976.

Gangal, S. G., Agasho, S. S., Nair, P. N. M., and Rao, R. S.: Cellular immunity in human osteogenic sarcoma. Indian Journal of Cancer, 10:295–301, September 1973.

Gillette, R. W., and Boone, C. W.: Augmented immunogenicity of tumor cell membranes produced by surface budding viruses: Parameters of optimal immunization. International Journal of Cancer, 18:216–222, August 1976.

Giraldo, G., Beth, E., Hirshaut, Y., Aoki, T., Old, L. J., Boyse, E. A., and Chopra, H. C.: Human sarcomas in culture. Foci of altered cells and a common antigen; induction of foci and antigen in human fibroblast cultures by filtrates. Journal of Experimental Medicine, 133:454–478, March 1971.

Glasgow, A. H., Nimberg, R. B., Menzoian, J. O., Suporoschetz, I., Cooperband, S. R., Smith, K., and Mannick, J. A.: Association of anergy with an immunosuppressive peptide fraction in the serum of patients with cancer. New England Journal of Medicine, 291:1263–1267, December 12, 1974.

Glicksman, A. S., and Toker, C.: Osteogenic sarcoma following radiotherapy for bursitis. Mount Sinai Journal of Medicine, 43:163–167, March–April 1976.

Golub, S., O'Connel, T. X., and Morton, D. L.: Correlation of *in vivo* and *in vitro* assays of immunocompetence in cancer patients. Cancer Research, 34: 1833–1837, August 1974.

Gonzalez, R., Tzobari, S., Sinkovics, J. G., Campos, L. T., and Howe, C. D.: Immunological evidences for the viral etiology of human mesenchymal neoplasms. (Abstract #247) Proceedings of the American Association for Cancer Research, 15:62, 1974.

Gonzalez-Vitale, J. C., Slavin, R. E., and McQueen, J. D.: Radiation-induced intracranial malignant fibrous histiocytoma. Cancer, 37:2960–2963, June 1976.

Green, A. A., Pratt, C., Webster, R. G., and Smith K.: Immunotherapy of osteo-sarcoma patients with virus-modified tumor cells. Annals of the New York Academy of Sciences, 227:396–411, 1976.

Gunnarson, A., McKhann, C. F., Simmons, R. L., and Gage T. B.: Metastatic sarcoma. Combined surgical and immunotherapeutic approach? Neuramin-idase-treated tumor cells as a tumor vaccine. Minnesota Medicine, 57: 558–561, July 1974.

Gutterman, J. U., Mavligit, G. M., Blumenschein, G., Burgess, M. A., Mc-Bride, C. M., and Hersh, E. M.: Immunotherapy of human solid tumors with Bacillus Calmette-Guerin: Prolongation of disease-free interval and survival in malignant melanoma, breast and colorectal cancer. Annals of the New York Academy of Sciences, 277:135–158, 1976.

Hardy, M. A., Goldfarb, P., Levine, S., Dattner, A., Muggia, F. M., Levitt, S., and Weinstein, E.: *De novo* Kaposi's sarcoma in renal transplantation. Case report and brief review. Cancer, 38:144–148, July 1976.

Haynes, H. A., and Fitzpatrick. T. B.: Cutaneous manifestations of internal malignancy. In Wintrobe, M. D., *et al.* Eds: *Harrison's Principles of Internal Medicine*. 7th edition. New York, New York, McGraw-Hill Publishers, 1974, pp. 2028–2035.

Hewlett, J. S., Balcerzak, S., and Gutterman, J.: Remission induction in adult acute leukemia by 10-day continuous intravenous infusion of ara-C, plus Oncovin and prednisone. In Terry, W. D., and Windhorst, D., Eds.: *Immunotherapy of Cancer: Present Status of Trials in Man*, NCI Conference, 1976. (Abstract #32) New York, New York, Raven Press. (In press.)

Hirshaut, Y., Pei, D. T., Marcove, R. C., Mukherji, B., Spielvogel, A. R., and Essner, E.: Seroepidemiology of human sarcoma antigen S_1. New England Journal of Medicine, 291:1103–1107, November 21, 1974.

Holmes, E. C.: Immunology and lung cancer. Annals of Thoracic Surgery, 21: 250–258, 1976a.

Holmes, E. C.: Personal communication, 1976b.

Israel, L., and Edelstein, R.: Nonspecific immunostimulation with *Corynebacterium parvum* in human cancer. In *Immunological Aspects of Neoplasia*. (The University of Texas System Cancer Center M. D. Anderson Hospital and Tumor Institute, 26th Annual Symposium on Fundamental Cancer Research). Baltimore, Maryland. The Williams & Wilkins Co., 1975, pp. 485–504.

Ivins, J. C., Ritts, R. E., Jr., Pritchard, D. J., Gilchrist, G. S., Miller, G. C., and Taylor, W. F.: Transfer factor *versus* combination chemotherapy: A preliminary report of a randomized postsurgical adjuvant treatment study in osteogenic sarcoma. Annals of the New York Academy of Sciences, 277:558–574, 1976.

Jacobs, D. M., and Kripke, M. L.: Accelerated development of transplanted mammary tumors in mice pretreated with the methanol extraction residue of BCG and prevention of acceleration by concomitant specific immunization. Journal of the National Cancer Institute, 52:219–224, January 1974.

Jones, S. E., Salmon, S. E., Moon, T. E., and Butler, J. J.: Chemoimmunotherapy of non-Hodgkin's lymphoma with BCG: A preliminary report for the Southwest Oncology Group. In Terry, W. D., and Windhorst, D., Eds.: *Immunotherapy of Cancer: Present Status of Trials in Man*, NCI Conference 1976. (Abstract #44) New York, New York, Raven Press. (In press.)

Kay, H.: Five year follow-up of the Medical Research Council's "Concord" trial of ALL immunotherapy. In Terry, W. D., and Windhorst, D., Eds.: *Immunotherapy of Cancer: Present Status of Trials in Man*, NCI Conference, 1976. (Abstract #40) New York, New York, Raven Press. (In press.)

Kay, H. D., Thota, H., and Sinkovics, J. G.: A comparative study on in vitro cytotoxic reactions of lymphocytes from normal donors and patients with sarcomas to cultured tumor cells. Clinical Immunology and Immunopathology, 5:218–233, April 1976.

Klein, E., Holtermann, O. A., Case, R. W., Milgrom, H., Rosner, D., and Adler, S.: Responses of neoplasms to local immunotherapy. American Journal of Clinical Pathology, 62:281–289, August 1974.

Kotz, R., Rella, W., and Salzer, M.: The immune status in patients with bone and soft tissue sarcomas. In Grundemann, E., Ed.: *Malignant Bone Tumors*. Berlin and New York, New York, Springer Verlag, 1976, pp. 197–205.

Krementz, E. T., Mansell, P. W. A., Hornung, M. O., Samuels, M. S., Sutherland, C. A., and Benes, E. N.: Immunotherapy of malignant disease: The use of viable sensitized lymphocytes or transfer factor prepared from sensitized lymphocytes. Cancer, 33:394–401, February 1974.

Kufe, D., Hehlman, R., and Spiegelman, S.: Human sarcomas contain RNA related to RNA of a mouse leukemia virus. Science, 175:182–185, January 14, 1972.

Lanzotti, V. J., Campos, L. T., Sinkovics, J. G., and Samuels, M. L.: Chemotherapy of visceral Kaposi's sarcoma. Archives of Dermatology, 111:1331–1333, October 1975.

Lindberg, R., Murphy, W. K., Sinkovics, J. G., Martin, R. G., Romsdahl, M. M., Jesse, R. H., and Russell, W. O.: Adjuvant chemotherapy in the treatment of primary soft tissue sarcomas. A preliminary report. *Management of Primary Bone and Soft Tissue Tumors* (The University of Texas System Cancer Center M. D. Anderson Hospital and Tumor Institute, 21st Annual Clinical Conference on Cancer). Chicago, Illinois, Year Book Medical Publishers, Inc., 1977, pp. 343–352.

Lo Buglio, A. F., Neidhart, J. A., Hilberg, R. W., Metz, E. M., and Balcerzak, S. P.: The effect of transfer factor therapy on tumor immunity in alveolar soft part sarcoma. Cellular Immunology, 7:159–165, April 1973.

Magrath, I. T., and Ziegler, J. L.: Failure of BCG immunostimulation to affect the clinical course of Burkitt's lymphoma. British Medical Journal, 1:615–618, March 1976.

Makk, L., Delorme, F., Creech, J. L., Jr., Ogden, L. L., Faddell, E. H., Songster, C. L., Clanton, J., Johnson, M. N., and Christopherson, W. M.,: Clinical and morphologic features of hepatic angiosarcoma in vinyl chloride workers. Cancer, 37:149–163, January 1976.

Mansell, P. W. A., Ichinose, H., Reed, R. J., Krementz, E. T., McNamee, R., and Di Luzio, N. R.: Macrophage-mediated destruction of human malignant cells *in vivo*. Journal of the National Cancer Institute, 54:571–580, March 1975.

Marcove, R. C., Miké, V., Huvos, A. G., Southam, C. M., and Levin, A. G.: Vaccine trials for osteogenic sarcoma. A preliminary report. CA – A Cancer Journal for Clinicians, 23:74–80, March–April 1973.

Master, S. P., Taylor, J. F., Kyalwazi, S. K., and Ziegler, J. L.: Immunological studies in Kaposi's sarcoma. British Medical Journal, 1:600–602, March 7, 1970.

Mastrangelo, M. J., Bellet, R. E., and Berd, D.: A randomized prospective trial comparing McCCNU + vincristine to MeCCNU + vincristine + BCG + allogeneic tumor cells in patients with metastatic malignant melanoma. In Terry, W. D., and Windhorst, D., Eds.: *Immunotherapy of Cancer: Present Status of Trials in Man*, NCI conference, 1976. (Abstract #8) New York, New York, Raven Press. (In press.)

McAllister, R. M., Nelson-Rees, W. A., Peer, M., Laug, W. E., Isaacs, H., Jr., Gilden, R. V., Rongey, R. W., and Gardner, M. B.: Childhood sarcomas and lymphomas. Characterization of new cell lines and search for type C virus. Cancer, 36:1804–1814, November 1975.

McLaughlin, A. P., III, and Brooks, J. D.: A plasma factor inhibiting lymphocyte reactivity in urologic cancer patients. Journal of Urology, 112: 366–372, September 1974.

McMaster, J. H., Ferguson, R. J., Weinert, C. R., Jr., and Dickens, D. R. V.: Cellular immunity to human osteosarcoma. (Abstract) Journal of Bone and Joint Surgery, 56A:863, June 1974.

McMurtrey, M. J., Campos, L. T., Sinkovics, J. G., Romero, J. J., Loh, K. K., and Romsdahl, M. M.: Chemoimmunotherapy for melanoma: Preliminary clinical data and difficulties with *in vitro* monitoring of tumor-specific immune reactions. In *Neoplasms of the Skin and the Malignant Melanoma* (The University of Texas Cancer Center M. D. Anderson Hospital and Tumor Institute, 20th Annual Clinical Conference on Cancer). Chicago, Illinois, Year Book Medical Publishers, Inc., 1976, pp. 471–484.

Mendoza, C. B., Jr., Moore, G. E., Watne, A. L., Hiramoto, R., and Jurland, J.: Immunologic response following homologous transplantation of cultured human tumor cells in patients with malignancy. Surgery, 64:897–900, November 1968.

Moertel, C. G., O'Connell, M. J., Ritts, R. E., Jr., Schutt, A. J., Reitemeier, R. J., Hahn, R. G., and Frytak, S. K.: A controlled evaluation of combined immunotherapy (MER-BCG) and chemotherapy for advanced colorectal cancer. In Terry, W. D., and Windhorst, D., Eds.: *Immunotherapy of Cancer: Present Status of Trials in Man*, NCI Conference, 1976. (Abstract #47) New York, New York, Raven Press. (In press.)

Morton, D. L.: Immunotherapy of human melanomas and sarcomas. National Cancer Institute Monograph, 35:375–378, December 1972.

Morton, D. L., Malmgren, R. A., Hall, W. T., and Schidlovsky, G.: Immunologic and virus studies with human sarcomas. Surgery, 66:152–161, July 1969.

Mukherji, B., and Hirshaut, Y.: Evidence for fetal antigen in human sarcoma. Science, 181:440–442, August 3, 1973.

Myers, B. D., Kessler, E., Levi, J., Pick, A., and Rosenfeld, J. B.: Kaposi's sarcoma in kidney transplant recipients. Archives of Internal Medicine, 133: 307–311, February 1974.

Nadler, S. H., and Moore, G. E.: Immunotherapy of malignant disease. Archives of Surgery, 99:376–381, September 1969.

Nauts, H. C.: Ewing's sarcoma of bone: End results following immunotherapy (bacterial toxins) combined with surgery and/or radiation. (Monograph #14) New York, New York, Cancer Research Institute, 1974, 108 pp.

Neff, J. R., and Enneking, W. F.: Adoptive immunotherapy in primary osteosarcoma. In Godden, J. O., and Sinks, L. F., Eds.: *Conflicts in Childhood Cancer*. New York, New York, Alan R. Liss, 1975, pp. 289–296.

Newlands, E. S., Oon, C. J., Roberts, J. T., Elliot, P., Mould, R. F., Topham, C., Madden, F. J. F., Newton, K. A., and Westbury, G.: Clinical trials of combination chemotherapy and specific active immunotherapy in disseminated melanoma. British Journal of Cancer, 34:174–179, 1976.

Otten, J.: Immunotherapy *versus* chemotherapy as maintenance treatment of acute lymphoblastic leukemia. In Terry, W. D., and Windhorst, D., Eds.: *Immunotherapy of Cancer: Present Status of Trials in Man*, NCI Conference, 1976. (Abstract #38) New York, New York, Raven Press. (In press.)

Paik, H. H., and Wilkinson, E. J.: Peritoneal osteosarcoma following irradiation therapy of ovarian cancer. Obstetrics and Gynecology, 47:488–491, April 1976.

Pinsky, C. M., Domieri, A. E., Caron, A. S., Knapper, W. H., and Oettgen, H. P.: Delayed hypersensitivity reactions in patients with cancer. In Mathé, G., and Weiner, R., Eds.: *Recent Results in Cancer Research: Investigation and Stimulation of Immunity in Cancer Patients*. New York, New York and Heidelberg, Springer Verlag, 47:37–41, 1974.

Pinsky, C. M., Hirshaut, Y., Wanebo, H. J., Fortner, J., Miké, V., Schottenfeld, D., and Oettgen, H. F.: Surgical adjuvant immunotherpay with BCG in patients with malignant melanoma. Results of a prospective, randomized trial. In Terry, W. D., and Windhorst, D., Eds.: *Immunotherapy of Cancer: Present Status of Trials in Man*, NCI Conference, 1976. (Abstract #2) New York, New York, Raven Press. (In press.)

Powles, R. L., Russell, J., Lister, T. A., Oliver, T., Whitehouse, J.M.A., Malpas, J., Chapuis, B., Crowther, D., and Alexander, P.: Immunotherapy for acute myelogenous leukemia: Analysis of a controlled clinical study 2½ years after entry of the last patient. In Terry, W. D., and Windhorst, D., Eds.: *Immunotherapy of Cancer: Present Status of Trials in Man*, NCI Conference, 1976. (Abstract #25) New York, New York, Raven Press. (In press.)

Pritchard, D. J., Ivins, J. C., and Ritts, R. E., Jr.: Immunologic aspects of human sarcomas. In Grundmann, E., Ed: *Malignant Bone Tumors*. Berlin and New York, New York, Springer Verlag, 1976, pp. 185–196.

Pritchard, D. J., Reilly, C. A., Jr., Finkel, M. P., and Ivins, J. C.: Cytotoxicity of human osteosarcoma sera to hamster sarcoma cells. Cancer, 34:1935–1939, December 1974.

Rebel, A., Bregeon, C., Basle, M., Malkani, K., Le Patezour, A., and Filmon, R.: Les inclusions des osteoclastes dans la maladie osseuse de Paget. Revue du Rhumatisme 42:637–641, 1975.

Ritts, R. E., Jr., Pritchard, D. J., Gilchrist, G. S., Ivins, J. C., and Taylor, W. F.: Transfer factor *versus* combination chemotherapy: An interim report of a randomized post-surgical adjuvant study in osteogenic sarcoma. In Terry, W. D., and Windhorst, D., Eds.: *Immunotherapy of Cancer: Present Status of Trials in Man*, NCI Conference 1976. (Abstract #23) New York, New York, Raven Press. (In press.)

Romero, J. J., Campos, L. T., and Sinkovics, J. G.: Complement fixing cytolytic antibodies in human sera directed against established human tumor cell lines. Clinical Research, 24:32a, January 1976.

Rosato, F. E., Brown, A. S., Miller, E. E., Rosato, E. F., Mullis, W. F., Johnson, J., and Moskowitz, A.: Neuraminidase immunotherapy of tumors in man. Surgery, Gynecology and Obstetrics, 139:675–682, November 1974.

Sauter, C., Cavalli, F., Lindenman, J., Gmur, J., Berchtold, W., Alberto, P., Obrecht, P., and Senn, H. J.: Viral oncolysis: Its application in maintenance treatment of acute myelogenous leukemia. In Terry, W. D., and Windhorst, D., Eds.: *Immunotherapy of Cancer: Present Status of Trials in Man*, NCI Conference, 1976. (Abstract #29) New York, New York, Raven Press. (In press.)

Sinkovics, J. G.: Discussion on Kaposi's sarcoma. In *Neoplasms of the Skin and Malignant Melanoma* (The University of Texas System Cancer Center M. D. Anderson Hospital and Tumor Institute, 20th Annual Clinical Conference on Cancer). Chicago, Illinois, Year Book Medical Publishers, Inc., 1976a, pp. 543–547.

Sinkovics, J. G.: Immunology of tumors in experimental animals. In *The Immunology of Malignant Disease*. Harris, J. E., and Sinkovics, J. G., authors, 2nd edition. St. Louis, Missouri, C. V. Mosby Company, 1976b. pp. 93–282.

Sinkovics, J. G., Cabiness, J. R., and Shullenberger, C. C.: Disappearance after chemotherapy of blocking serum factors as measured *in vitro* with lymphocytes cytotoxic to tumor cells. Cancer, 30:1428–1437, December 1972.

Sinkovics, J. G., Cabiness, J. R., and Shullenberger, C. C.: *In vitro* cytotoxicity of lymphocytes to human sarcoma cells. Bibliotheca Haematologica, 39: 846–851, 1973.

Sinkovics, J. G., Campos, L. T., Kay, H. D., Loh, K. K., Gonzalez, F., Cabiness, J. R., Ervin, F., and Gyorkey, F.: Immunological studies with human sarcomas: Effects of immunization and therapy on cell- and antibody-mediated immune reactions. In *Immunological Aspects of Neoplasia* The University of Texas System Cancer Center M. D. Anderson Hospital and Tumor Institute, 26th Annual Symposium on Fundamental Cancer Research). Baltimore, Maryland, Williams & Wilkins, pp. 367–401, 1975a.

Sinkovics, J. G., Campos, L. T., Kay, H. D., Gonzalez, F., Loh, K. K., Rosenberg, P., and Cabiness, J. R.: Chemotherapy of metastatic sarcomas: Clinical results and correlations with immune reactions to cultured sarcoma cells. In Daikos, G. K., Ed.: *Progress in Chemotherapy* (Proceedings of the 8th International Congress of Chemotherapy, Athens, Greece) 3:508–513, 1974a.

Sinkovics, J. G., Campos, L. T., Loh, K. K., Cormia, F., Velasquez, W., and Shullenberger, C. C.: Chemoimmunotherapy for three categories of solid tumors (sarcoma, melanoma, lymphoma): The problem of immunoresistant tumors. In Crispen, R., Ed.: *Neoplasm Immunity: Mechanisms* (1975 Chicago Symposium) 1976.

Sinkovics, J. G., and Harris, J. E.: Immunology and immunotherapy of human tumors. In *The Immunology of Malignant Disease*, Harris, J. E., and Sinkovics, J. G., authors. 2nd edition. St. Louis, Missouri, C. V. Mosby Company, 1976, pp. 410–578.

Sinkovics, J. G., and Howe, C. D.: Superinfection of tumors with viruses. Experientia, 25:733–734, August 1969.

Sinkovics, J. G., Kay H. D., and Thota, H.: Evaluation of chemoimmunotherapy regimens by *in vitro* lymphocyte cytotoxicity directed to cultured human tumor cells. Bibliotheca Haematologica, 43:281–284, 1976.

Sinkovics, J. G., Thota, H., Loh, K. K., Gonzalez, F., Campos, L. T., Romero, J. J., Kay, H. D., and King, D.: Prospectives for immunotherapy of human sarcomas. In *Cancer Chemotherapy: Fundamental Concepts and Recent Advances* (The University of Texas System Cancer Center M. D. Anderson

Hospital and Tumor Institute, 19th Annual Clinical Conference on Cancer). Chicago, Illinois, Year Book Medical Publishers, Inc., 1975b, pp. 417–443.

Sinkovics, J. G., and Mackay, B.: A multidisciplinary approach to the understanding and treatment of human sarcomas. In *Sarcomas.* Mackay, B., author. (Monograph in the Series of Major Problems in Pathology) Philadelphia, Pennsylvania, W. B, Sanders, (In press.)

Sinkovics, J. G., Shirato, E., Martin, R. G., Cabiness, J. R., and White, E. C.: Chondrosarcoma. Immune reactions of a patient to autologous tumor. Cancer, 27:782–793, April 1971.

Sinkovics, J. G., Williams, D. E., Campos, L. T., Kay H. D., and Romero, J. J.: Intensification of immune reactions of patients to cultured sarcoma cells: Attempts at monitored immunotherapy. Seminars in Oncology, 1:351–365, December 1974b.

Sinkovics, J. G., Williams, D. E., Kay, H. D., Campos, L. T., and Howe, D. K.: Clinical settings favorable for immunotherapy of sarcomas. In Interaction of Radiation and Host Immune Defense Mechanisms in Malignancy. Brookhaven National Laboratory, U. S. Atomic Energy Comission, 1974c, pp. 331–339.

Sokal, J. E., Aungst, C. W., Snyderman, M., and Gomez, G.: Immunotherapy of chronic myelocytic leukemia: Effects of different vaccination schedules. Annals of the New York Academy of Sciences, 277:367–383, 1976.

Soriano, F., Shelburn, C. E., and Gokcen, M.: Simian virus 40 in a human cancer. Nature, 249:421–424, May 31, 1974.

Stewart, S. E., Kasnic, G., Jr., and Draycott, C.: Activation of viruses in human tumors by 5-iododeoxyuridine and dimethylsulfoxide. Science, 175: 198–199, January 1972.

Strander, H., cited by Krim, M.: *International Workshop on Interferon in the Treatment of Cancer.* New York, New York, Memorial Sloan-Kettering Cancer Center, 1975, pp. 39–47.

Tarpley, J. L., Potvin, C., and Chretien, P. B.: Prolonged depression of cellular immunity in cured laryngeopharyngeal cancer patients treated with radiation therapy. Cancer, 35:638–644, March 1975.

Taylor, J. F., Jung, U., Wolfe, L., Deinhardt, F., and Kyalwazi, S. K.: Lymphocyte transformation in patients with Kaposi's sarcoma. International Journal of Cancer, 8:468–474, November 1971.

Taylor, J. F., and Ziegler, J. L.: Delayed cutaneous hypersensitivity reactions in patients with Kaposi's sarcoma. British Journal of Cancer, 30:312–318, October 1974.

Townsend, C. M., and Eilber, F. R.: Adjuvant immunotherapy for skeletal sarcoma. (Abstract #1162) Proceedings of the American Association for Cancer Research and the American Society of Clinical Oncologists, 16:261, 1975.

Twomey, P. L., Catalona, W. J., and Chretien, P. B.: Cellular immunity in cured cancer patients. Cancer, 33:435–440, February 1974.

Twomey, P. L., and Chretien, P. B.: Impaired lymphocyte responsiveness in osteosarcoma. Journal of Surgical Research, 18:551–554, May 1975.

Vogler, W. R., Bartolucci, A. A., Omura, G. A., Miller, D., Smalley, R. V., Knospe, W. H., and Goldsmith, A. S.: A randomized clinical trial of BCG in myeloblastic leukemia conducted by the Southeastern Cancer Study Group. In Terry, W. D., and Windhorst, D., Eds.: *Immunotherapy of Can-*

cer: Present Status of Trials in Man, NCI Conference 1976 (Abstract #26) New York, New York, Raven Press. (In press.)

Wallack, M. K., Steplewski, Z., Rosato, E., Gallagher, J., and Rosato, F.: A new approach in specific, active immunotherapy. (Abstract #297) Proceedings of the 67th Annual Meeting of the American Association for Cancer Research 17:75, 1976.

Wang, C. H., Sinkovics, J. G., Kay, H. D., Gyorkey, F., and Shullenberger, C. C.: Growth of permanent lymphoid cell cultures from human source: Tenth anniversary, Texas Reports on Biology and Medicine, 33:213–250, 1975.

Waxweiler, J. R., Stringer, W., Wagoner, J. K., Jones, J., Falk, H., and Carter, C.: Neoplastic risk among workers exposed to vinyl chloride. Annals of the New York Academy of Sciences, 271:40–48, 1976.

Williams, J. P., and Savage, P. T.: Liposarcoma of the kidney. British Journal of Surgery, 46:225–231, July 1958.

Wood, W. C., and Morton, D. L.: Host immune response to a common cell surface antigen in human sarcomas. New England Journal of Medicine, 284: 569–572, March 1971.

Yonemoto, R. H.: Adoptive immunotherapy utilizing thoracic duct lymphocytes. Annals of the New York Academy of Sciences, 277:7–19, 1976.

Young, H. F.: Inhibition of cell-mediated immunity in patients with brain tumors. Surgery and Neurology, 5:19–23, January 1976.

A Clinicopathologic Study: Preoperative Intra-arterial Adriamycin and Radiation Therapy for Extremity Soft Tissue Sarcomas

FREDERICK R. EILBER, M.D.*, COURTNEY M. TOWNSEND, JR., M.D.*, THOMAS H. WEISENBURGER, M.D.†, JOSEPH M. MIRRA, M.D.‡, and DONALD L. MORTON, M.D.*

*Division of Oncology, Department of Surgery,
†Department of Radiology, ‡Department of Pathology,
University of California Medical School, Los Angeles,
California; and Surgical Services, Sepulveda Veterans
Administration Hospital, Sepulveda, California

MALIGNANT SOFT TISSUE SARCOMAS of the extremities are extremely resistant to conventional methods of therapy. The reasons for this resistance are: there is no true tumor capsule; they tend to spread along fascial planes; the tumors are often very large at presentation; and they have a great propensity for metastases to distant sites, primarily the lungs.

A variety of surgical procedures ranging from simple excision and muscle group resection, to radical amputation have been employed. However, it is apparent that even with radical amputation, the local recurrence rate remains as high as 20–30% (Martin, Butler, and Albores-Saavedra, 1965).

The most effective means of local control to date have been achieved with the combination of complete surgical excision followed by high-dose postoperative radiation therapy (Suit, Russell, and Martin, 1973). Local tumor control has been reported in up to 87% of patients treated with this combination, if the primary was located distal to the elbow or knee. However, with more proximal lesions, the local control rate fell to 57%.

While local control is important for evaluating any method of treatment, it alone cannot be the yardstick by which therapeutic effectiveness is judged. Distant metastases, the single most important determinant of survival, occur in over 50% of patients with soft tissue sarcomas who have no evidence of local recurrence.

Recently, several investigators reported encouraging results in the treatment of patients with soft tissue sarcomas using adjuvant postoperative chemotherapy with Adriamycin or high-dose methotrexate and calcium leukovorin "rescue" either alone or in combination (Cortez *et al.*, 1974; Jaffe, Frei, Traggis, and Bishop, 1974; Rosen *et al.*, 1976; Townsend, Eilber, and Morton, 1976). Disease-free survival was significantly prolonged by the addition of systemically active postoperative chemotherapy.

Our study was performed to evaluate the toxicity and therapeutic effectiveness of intra-arterial infusion of Adriamycin followed by moderate-dose radiation therapy before operation as part of a program of multimodality therapy for patients with skeletal and soft tissue sarcomas of the extremities. Our purpose was to determine if it was possible to achieve preoperative in situ tumor destruction before adequate resection of tumor in order to preserve a functional extremity, and to determine if postoperative adjuvant chemotherapy would improve disease-free survival.

Patients and Methods

Forty-two patients with soft tissue sarcomas of an extremity were treated by the Division of Surgical Oncology, UCLA School of Medicine, between 1973 and 1976. The histologic classifications and types of therapy are listed in Table 1. Prior to treatment, all patients had the following studies performed: CBC, SMA-12, electrocardiogram, chest radiographs, whole lung tomography, bone scans, and arteriography of the primary tumor. The stage of the soft tissue sarcomas was determined from incisional biopsy tissue using the staging method of the American Joint Commission for Cancer Staging (Russell, 1976; Suit, Russell, and Martin, 1975). The number of patients in each stage, the

TABLE 1.—HISTOLOGICAL TYPE AND TREATMENT OF
PATIENTS WITH SOFT TISSUE SARCOMA

		TREATMENT CATEGORY	
		SURGERY +	IA CHEMO.
		ADJUVANT	XRT, SURG. +
HISTOLOGICAL TYPE	SURGERY	CHEMO.	ADJ. CHEMO.
Rhabdomyosarcoma	4	2	4
Undifferentiated sarcoma	4	1	5
Synovial cell sarcoma	3	2	1
Liposarcoma	3	1	5
Fibrosarcoma	3	—	1
Malignant fibrous histiosarcoma	1	—	—
Giant cell sarcoma	1	—	—
Neurofibrosarcoma	—	—	1
TOTAL	19	6	17

site of the tumor, and the type of treatment are presented in Table 2.

Nineteen patients were treated by surgical resection alone; 9 by radical amputation, and 10 by complete muscle group resection.

Six patients were treated by radical amputation and postoperative adjuvant chemotherapy: Adriamycin, 45 mg/M² given i.v. on each of 2 consecutive days. Fourteen days later, each patient received high-dose methotrexate, 200 mg/kg as a 4-hour infusion, followed 4 hours later by calcium leukovorin rescue (Fig. 1).

Sixteen patients were treated with preoperative Adriamycin chemotherapy and radiation therapy (Fig. 2). Percutaneous arteriography was performed by the Seldinger technique, and the catheter was left in place in the major vessel supplying the extremity for the Adriamycin infusion. All patients received a total dose of 90 mg of Adriamycin suspended in 30 ml of normal saline over 3 days (30 mg/24 hrs), by continuous infusion with a Harvard pump.

TABLE 2.—CLINICOPATHOLOGIC STAGE AND
TREATMENT CATEGORY OF SOFT
TISSUE SARCOMAS

		TREATMENT CATEGORY	
			IA-ADRIA.
		SURGERY†	XRT., SURG. +
STAGE	SURGERY°	ADJUVANT CHEMO.	ADJ. CHEMO.
I	2	—	—
II	8	—	—
III	5	3	9
IV	4	3	8

°9/19 patients' surgery was amputation.
†All patients' surgery was amputation.

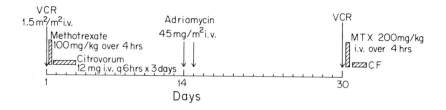

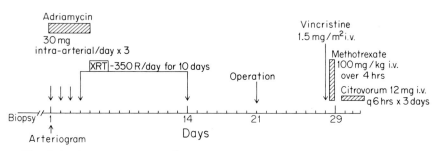

Fig. 1 (top).—Postoperative adjuvant chemotherapy regimen for soft tissue sarcomas.

Fig. 2 (bottom).—Preoperative therapy for soft tissue sarcoma of an extremity.

Radiation therapy was begun the day following the intra-arterial infusion of Adriamycin. A 6 MEV linear accelerator was used to deliver 3,500 rads to the midtumor plane in 10 equal fractions over 12–15 calendar days. Each day the complete anatomic region of the tumor (e.g., the entire thigh) was treated by PA and AP parallel opposed fields. Radical en bloc resection was performed 1 week after the completion of radiation therapy. The involved muscle group and the adjacent fascial planes were completely resected. Subadventitial dissection of the major vessels and nerves in the operative field was performed.

Operative specimens were examined using the pathologic staging system for soft tissue sarcomas based upon histologic grade and size of tumor. Other important factors for a determination of stage included invasion by the tumor of skin, bone, major vessels, or major nerves. All of these variables were considered before a final stage classification was assigned. This type of staging has been shown to more closely predict the biologic behavior of any given soft tissue sarcoma than does histologic examination alone (Russell, 1976).

To assess the effects of the Adriamycin/radiation therapy regimen on the histological characteristics and viability of the treated tumors, multiple representative sections of pretreatment and posttreatment

TABLE 3.—SOFT TISSUE SARCOMAS
PERCENT NECROSIS IN AMPUTATION SPECIMENS

		NECROSIS	
	# CASES	RANGE	AVERAGE %
Rhabdomyosarcoma	10	0–20	6.5
Liposarcoma	8	0–50	9
Malignant fibrous histiosarcoma	4	0–5	3.8
Undifferentiated sarcoma	7	0–30	8.5
TOTAL	29	(0–50)	7.2

specimens were examined by one of the authors (J. M. Mirra), who had no prior knowledge of the type of treatment. As a further control, slides from operative specimens of 29 tumors (4 – 10 for each histologic type) treated by operation alone and representative of the types of tumors treated by the present approach were also examined for evidence of cellular necrosis (Table 3). For all specimens, visual estimates of the amount of tumor cell necrosis present on each slide area were determined and averaged for the total number of slides reviewed, and the percentage of necrosis was calculated for each specimen.

Necrosis was defined as either the total lack, or severe diminution, of nuclear staining (smudging) by hematoxylin. In the nontreated tumors and in the pretreatment biopsy specimens, necrosis was characterized by a total loss of nuclear staining. In the posttreatment specimens, the nuclei were unstained or so pale, smudged, or misshapen that necrosis was obvious even though there was some hematoxylin staining. Viable, well-stained nuclei were always present on each slide so that an adequate staining technique was assured. Each en bloc operative specimen was carefully examined for evidence of viable tumor extending to the resection margins. Between 10 and 15 sections per patient were taken for this purpose. All slides were reviewed before the amount of necrosis was correlated with the type of treatment.

Results

Of the group of 19 patients treated by surgical resection alone, 5 of 19 (31%) developed local recurrence and of this group 13 of 19 (60%) developed distant pulmonary metastases (Figs. 3 and 4). Of the 6 patients who had amputation followed by adjuvant chemotherapy, 1 (16%) developed local recurrence and 3 (50%) developed distant metastases.

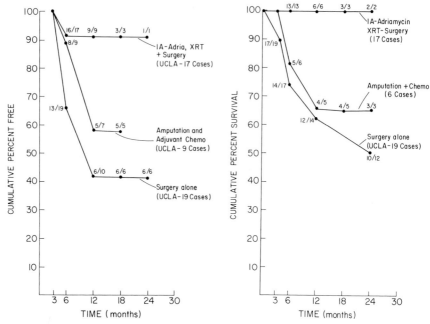

Fig. 3 (left).—Life-table analysis for the proportion of patients free of distant metastases. Vertical axis represents cumulative percentage of patients free of disease. Horizontal axis is time in months following operation. Numbers, separated by a slash (/), indicate number of patients who remained free of disease/number of patients at risk of developing recurrence during that time interval.

Fig. 4 (right).—Life-table analysis for survival in 3 patient groups. Vertical axis represents cumulative percentage of patients free of disease. Horozontal axis is time in months following operation. Numbers, separated by slash (/), indicate number of patients surviving/number at risk during that time interval.

The combination of intra-arterial Adriamycin and radiation produced sufficient shrinkage of tumor to allow radical en bloc resection and preservation of a functional extremity in 16 of 17 patients. The 1 failure occurred in a patient with an anaplastic spindle cell sarcoma arising in the subscapularis muscle. An intrascapulothoracic amputation was required for complete tumor removal with adequate margins. The remaining 16 patients with soft tissue sarcomas were treated by radical en bloc resection which removed the involved muscle group from origin to insertion and included the adjacent fascial planes. All 16 have functional, neurologically intact extremities. Furthermore, all 16 treated by the combination of drug and radiation remain free of local or distant recurrent disease from 4 to 34 months after operation (Fig. 4). The patient who underwent forequarter amputation developed pulmonary metastases 6 months after operation without any evidence of local recurrence of sarcoma.

The combination of Adriamycin and radiation therapy is not without complications. Five patients developed postoperative wound healing problems which required split-thickness skin grafting for coverage. One of these patients required ligation of the superficial femoral artery due to rupture in the depths of a septic wound, but now has a functional extremity. Only minimal systemic toxicity was noted during Adriamycin infusion. There were no instances of stomatitis, cardiac toxicity, or life-threatening infection. A single patient developed leukopenia below 2,000 cells/mm³, but he remained afebrile and no sepsis developed. Four patients of the total group developed skin erythema during infusion, but no full-thickness skin loss occurred. No interruption of radiation therapy was required due to complications.

Sixteen posttreatment specimens were available for histological examination (Table 4). Of the 16 patients, 5 demonstrated extensive necrosis characterized by liquefaction and hemorrhage with no visible residual tumor. In the remaining 11 specimens the amount of necrosis varied from 50%–95%.

Histological examination demonstrated pronounced effects of treatment when posttreatment specimens were compared to pretreatment specimens and to the 29 tumors treated by operation alone (Table 3). An average of 7.2% necrosis was noted for the specimens treated by operation alone, and 4.3% necrosis was noted for pretreatment specimens. After Adriamycin and radiation therapy, an average of 75% necrosis per specimen was noted. In 3 patients, tumor necrosis was at least 90%, and many of the remaining nuclei exhibited variable degrees of smudging associated with twisted, irregularly shaped chromatin, unlike the pretreatment specimens. These findings were

TABLE 4.—SOFT TISSUE SARCOMAS
PERCENT NECROSIS IN SPECIMENS FROM
PATIENTS TREATED WITH CHEMOTHERAPY AND
IRRADIATION THERAPY

| | # | NECROSIS | |
HISTOLOGICAL TYPE	CASES	RANGE %°	AVERAGE %
Rhabdomyosarcoma	5	60–100	87
Liposarcoma	5	60–100	80
Synovial cell sarcoma	1	90	90
Undifferentiated sarcoma	4	60–100	82
Fibrosarcoma	1	40	40
TOTAL	16	40–100	75

°5/16 specimens examined had no indentifiable tumor.

highly suggestive of irreversible, lethal dosage, but because faint hematoxylin staining was present, the specimens were not considered totally necrotic.

Histological observations of the 29 sarcomas treated by operation alone showed the usual range of cytologic features. Except for 1 specimen of a larger liposarcoma, the amount of necrosis rarely exceeded 30%. The necrotic foci usually showed total loss of nuclear and cytoplasmic detail. By comparison, the posttreatment specimens demonstrated a greater-than-50% necrosis, which could be characterized by cellular or nuclear "ghosts," or total necrosis. Any remaining nuclei that stained with hematoxylin were either unremarkable or demonstrated nuclear flattening. The chromatin was smudged, twisted, or had bubbly vacuolization. Mitoses were only seen in viable areas. Another significant finding in the treated tumor group was the absence or only minor evidence of necrosis in the surrounding normal tissue. There was apparent atrophy of skeletal muscle, but blood vessels almost always appeared viable.

Discussion

Our previous experience (Haskell *et al.*, 1974; Haskell, Eilber, and Morton, 1975; Morton *et al.*, 1976) and the experience reported in this paper indicate that intra-arterial infusion of Adriamycin followed by radiation therapy produces clinically apparent regression in sarcomas, sufficient to permit radical en bloc excision and limb salvage. However, in no instance was a 50% reduction in tumor size noted; therefore, by chemotherapeutic criteria, no objective response was seen.

Although ours was not a randomized study, the groups were comparable with respect to age, sex, stage, and site of tumor. In fact, the group of patients treated by operation alone had a lower and more favorable clinicopathologic stage. However, our data suggest that combination intra-arterial Adriamycin and moderate-dose radiation therapy do produce sufficient tumor cell necrosis and tumor size reduction to allow subsequent resection and limb salvage. This result, coupled with the observations (Suit, Russell, and Martin, 1973) that the radiation dose required to produce the same result would have to be 6,000 rads or greater, with its attendant potential problems of fibrosis, skin loss, and functional impairment of an extremity, made our decision to attempt the combination therapy preoperatively more reasonable.

Other investigators have described the clinical effects of combination, systemically administered chemotherapeutic agents or high-dose radiation therapy (McNeer, Cantin, Chu, and Nickson, 1968) for gross disease. However, there are few reports of histological examination of sarcomas after treatment with chemotherapy or radiation therapy. Rosen and his colleagues (1975, 1976) described necrotic primary and metastatic osteosarcomas after treatment with systemic chemotherapy alone or in a combination with radiation. Lee and Mackenzie (1964) reported tumor necrosis after high-dose (6,000–8,000 rads) radiation. The sequential histological examination of pre- and posttreatment specimens confirmed our clinical impression that direct, intra-arterial administration of Adriamycin combined with moderate doses of radiation could produce significant tumor cell necrosis in the majority of cases.

It is known that radiation damage to cellular DNA leads to cell death. However, not all cells are killed by this method, and DNA repair does occur after treatment (Byfield, 1974). Theoretically, then, the Adriamycin may exert its cytocidal effects through direct intercalation between DNA base pairs. This activity could interfere with the DNA reparative processes (Watring, *et al.*, 1974). Indeed, increased toxicity for normal and tumor cells has been produced both in vivo and in vitro when Adriamycin and radiation have been combined (Eltringham, Fajardo, and Stewart, 1975; Merrill *et al.*, 1975; Phillips and Fu, 1976). Previously irradiated sites have demonstrated recall phenomena after administration of Adriamycin (Donaldson, Glick, and Wilbur, 1974; Etcubanas and Wilbur, 1974), suggesting that susceptibility to this drug is increased in normal tissues after radiation. The question of whether these findings represent true synergism (radiosensitization) or merely the additive effects of 2 cytotoxic agents remains unanswered. Regardless of which mechanism is responsible for the increased effectiveness of the combination over single modalities alone, it is apparent from our study that this combination is not only clinically effective, but also produces histologic evidence of tumor cell necrosis.

Histological examination revealed that an average of 75% of the tumor cells treated by the combination of Adriamycin and radiation therapy were necrotic, and in 5 patients no viable tumor cells were present. While this result is impressive, it must be emphasized that viable tumor cells were present in the majority of patients treated. Therefore, the radical surgical resection must be performed with meticulous attention to technique. Preoperative treatment will not permit less than adequate operation.

There are several theoretic advantages for preoperative in situ tumor destruction. The decreased tumor size may permit limb salvage without an increased incidence of local disease recurrence. Tumor cell death, particularly at the periphery where most cell division takes place, should decrease the number of viable cells potentially dislodged by operative manipulation. Because the natural history of sarcoma has shown that the majority of patients developed metastatic disease within 2 years after operation, (Martin, Butler, and Albores-Saavedra, 1965) in all probability, microscopic, distant foci of cells are present at the time of original diagnosis. Therefore, the preoperative systemically active chemotherapeutic agent also functions against this occult disease. In addition, all patients receive postoperative adjuvant chemotherapy because their eventual outcome could depend upon the ability of the chemotherapeutic drugs to destroy distant subclinical metastasis.

Our results are encouraging indeed, despite the fact that most of these patients have been under treatment for less than 2 years. The degree of histologic cellular destruction of tumor is most impressive. This tumor destruction may have an in vivo correlate due to the fact that no local recurrences have been observed in these patients thus far. Whether this result represents cure or merely a delay in recurrence can only be answered by the results of a longer follow-up study. Nevertheless, even if this treatment regimen only represents a prolonged disease-free interval, the improved quality of life that a functional extremity affords one is, in itself, an improvement in care for these patients.

Summary

The combination of intra-arterial Adriamycin, moderate-dose radiation therapy, and radical, en bloc resection has been employed in the treatment of 17 patients with soft tissue sarcomas of the extremity. Preservation of a functional extremity has been accomplished in 16 of these 17 patients. Serial histological examination of pretreatment and posttreatment specimens showed that an average of 75% of tumor cells were necrotic, and in 5/15 specimens no viable cells were present; this is in contrast to 9% necrosis in 29 patients treated by operation alone. These results indicate that multimodality therapy prior to surgical resection is highly effective in causing in situ tumor cell destruction.

Acknowledgments

These investigations were supported by grants CA 12582 and CA 05262; NIH contract CB-53941 awarded by the National Cancer Institute (DHEW) and Medical Research Service of the Veterans Administration.

REFERENCES

Byfield, J. E.: The role of radiation repair mechanisms in radiation treatment failures. Cancer Chemotherapy Reports, (Part 1) 58:527–538, July–August 1974.

Cortez, E. P., Holland, J. F., Wang, J. J., Sinks, L. F., Blom, J., Senn, H., Bank, A., and Glidewell, O.: Amputation and adriamycin in primary osteosarcoma. New England Journal of Medicine, 291:998–1000, Nov. 7, 1974.

Donaldson, S. S., Glick, J. M., and Wilbur, J. R.: Adriamycin activating a recall phenomenon after radiation therapy. (Letter) Annals of Internal Medicine, 81:407–408, September 1974.

Eltringham, J. R., Fajardo, L. F., and Stewart, J. R.: Adriamycin cardiomyopathy: Enhanced cardiac damage in rabbits with combined drug and cardiac irradiation. Radiology, 115:471–472, May 1975.

Etcubanas, E., and Wilbur, J. R.: Uncommon side effects of Adriamycin (NSC-123127). Cancer Chemotherapy Reports, 58:757–758, 1974.

Haskell, C. M., Eilber, F. R., and Morton, D. L.: Adriamycin (NSC-123127) by arterial infusion. Cancer Chemotherapy Reports (Part 3) 6:187–189, October 1975.

Haskell, C. M., Silverstein, M. J., Rangel, D. M., Hunt, J. S., Sparks, F. C., and Morton, D. L.: Multimodality cancer therapy in man: A pilot study of Adriamycin by arterial infusion. Cancer, 33:1485–1490, June 1974.

Jaffe, N., Frei, E., III, Traggis, D., and Bishop, Y.: Adjuvant methotrexate and citrovorum-factor treatment of osteogenic sarcoma. New England Journal of Medicine, 291:994–997, Nov. 7, 1974.

Lee, S. E., and MacKenzie, D. H.: Osteosarcoma: A study of the value of preoperative megavoltage radiotherapy. British Journal of Surgery, 51: 252–274, April 1964.

Martin, R. G., Butler, J. J., and Albores-Saavedra, J.: Soft tissue tumors: Surgical treatment and results. In *Tumors of Bone and Soft Tissue* (The University of Texas M. D. Anderson Hospital and Tumor Institute at Houston, 8th Annual Clinical Conference on Cancer). Chicago, Illinois, Year Book Medical Publishers, Inc., 1965, pp. 333–347.

McNeer, G. P., Cantin, J., Chu, F., and Nickson, J. J.: Effectiveness of radiation therapy in the management of sarcoma of the soft somatic tissues. Cancer, 22:391–397, August 1968.

Merrill, J., Greco, F. A., Zimbler, H., Brereton, H. D., Laniberg, J. D., and Pomeroy, T. C.: Adriamycin and radiation: Synergistic cardiotoxicity. Annals of Internal Medicine, 82:122–123, 1975.

Morton, D. L., Eilber, F. R., Townsend, C. M., Jr., Grant, T. T., Mirra, J., and Weisenburger, T. H.: Limb salvage from a multidisciplinary treatment approach for skeletal and soft tissue sarcomas of the extremity. Annals of Surgery, 184:268–278, September 1976.

Phillips, T. L., and Fu, K. K.: Quantification of combined radiation therapy and chemotherapy effects of critical normal tissues. Cancer, Suppl. 37: 1186–1200, February 1976.

Phillips, T. L., Wharam, M. D., and Margolis, L. W.: Modification of radiation injury to normal tissues by chemotherapeutic agents. Cancer, 35: 1678–1684, June 1975.

Rosen, G., Murphy, M. L., Huvos, A. G., Gutierrez, M., and Marcove, R. C.: Chemotherapy, en bloc resection and prosthetic bone replacement in the treatment of osteogenic sarcoma. Cancer, 37:1–11, January 1976.

Rosen, G., Tefft, M., Martinez, A., Cham, W., and Murphy, M. L.: Combination chemotherapy and radiation therapy in the treatment of metastatic osteogenic sarcoma. Cancer, 35:622–630, March 1975.

Russell, W. O.: Staging of soft tissue sarcoma. In *Classification and Staging of Cancer by Site (Preliminary Handbook)*. Committee and Task Forces of the American Joint Commission for Cancer Staging and End Results Reporting, 1976, pp. 261–266.

Suit, H. D., and Russell, W. O.: Radiation therapy of soft tissue sarcomas. Cancer, Suppl. 36:759–764, August 1975.

Suit, H. D., Russell, W. O., and Martin, R. G.: Management of patients with sarcoma of soft tissue in an extremity. Cancer, 31:1247–1255, May 1973.

Townsend, C. M., Jr., Eilber, F. R., and Morton, D. L.: Skeletal and soft tissue sarcomas: Results of surgical adjuvant chemotherapy. (Abstract) Proceedings American Society Clinical Oncology, 17:265, 1976.

Watring, W. G., Byfield, J. E., Lagasse, L. D., Lee, Y. D., Juillard, G., Jacobs, M., and Smith, M. L.: Combination Adriamycin and radiation therapy in gynecological cancers. Gynecologic Oncology, 2:518–526, December 1974.

The Role of Surgery in the Management of Pulmonary Metastases

CLIFTON F. MOUNTAIN, M.D.
Department of Surgery, Section of Thoracic Surgery,
The University of Texas System Cancer Center M. D.
Anderson Hospital and Tumor Institute, Houston, Texas

KNOWLEDGE OF THE BIOLOGICAL BEHAVIOR of cancer, as it relates to metastasis, has influenced the development of a new conceptual approach to the role of surgery in the management of metastatic disease. The rationale for this approach is based on the study of fundamental characteristics of the host-tumor relationship as it has been observed in clinical and basic research investigations. Some of these considerations, as they bear upon surgical resection of pulmonary metastasis, are as follows:

(1) Many patients dying with pulmonary metastatic disease have the process confined to the lungs. The studies of Farrell (1935) of such patients having undergone autopsy showed that in 15% of the carcinomas and 25% of the sarcomas metastasis was limited to the lungs. Willis (1952), in his extensive work on the spread of tumors in the human body, makes similar observations.

(2) The potential for survival of patients with pulmonary metastasis following resection has been reported in the literature for nearly 40 years (Barney and Churchill, 1939). Overall survival rates from 25% to 40% have been cited (Martini, Bains, Huvos, and Beattie, 1974; Hutchison and Denner, 1972; Turnbull, Pool, Arthur, and Golbey, 1972; Feldman and Kyriakos 1972; Turney and Haight 1971; Choski, Takita, and Vincent 1972; and Cline and Young, 1970). In our review of 589 reported cases, there were 173 five-year survivors; the collective crude survival rate was 29% (Mountain, 1976).

(3) Survival curves for patients with resectable primary lung cancer and for patients treated surgically for pulmonary metastasis have been observed to be almost identical, even though the tumors treated vary in their structural type, rate of growth, and propensity for cure (Wilkins, 1976).

(4) The early studies of Shapiro and Fugmann (1957) of experimental animal solid tumor systems indicate a relationship between total tumor burden and response to drug therapy (Fig. 1).

(5) Cytokinetic studies have indicated that the cycle of tumor cells is related to tumor mass (Fisher, 1976). The work of Skipper and associates (Skipper, Schabel, and Wilcox, 1964) referable to the cell-kill hypothesis, and the kinetic studies of Muggia (1974), DeVita (DeVita, Young, and Canellos, 1975), Schabel (1969), and their colleagues, has reinforced these theories.

Evaluation of the contribution of surgery to the control of pulmonary metastasis requires acknowledgement of a number of variables that significantly affect end results. Most important among these are the criteria used for case selection. The intent of the surgery, whether definitive or reductive in nature, must be taken into account. Other variables relate to composition of the group. This includes: (a) frequency of the various morphologic types and primary tumor origins, (b) sensitivity of the tumor to available agents which may be employed as an adjunct to surgery, (c) sequencing of treatment modalities, (d) elements of time with respect to primary treatment and occurrence of pulmonary spread, (e) tumor doubling time, (f) periods of observations preceding resection, and (g) methods used in evaluation.

In the present study, an effort has been made to control some of these sources of variability in a subset of 257 consecutive patients undergoing definitive surgical resection. This selection of cases was

Fig. 1.—*Left*, Decreasing chemotherapeutic (6-MP) "cure" rates with increasing tumor size or age (4 experiments). *Right*, Complete regression of a 15-day-old 755 tumor by surgical tumor reduction (partial surgical excision) plus chemotherapy (6-mercaptopurine). (Courtesy of Shapiro and Fugmann, 1957.)

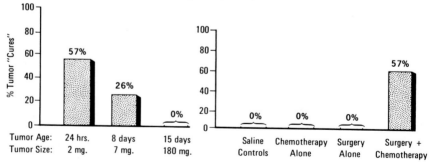

made to evaluate the contribution of surgery as a primary modality in the management of metastatic disease or as a primary modality followed by selective adjunctive therapy, where such treatment was applicable. In these particular cases, the pulmonary surgery by itself was considered to have the potential to remove all known tumor. One third of these patients had sarcomas, with the primary tumors originating in the skeletal system in 33 cases (34%) and in the soft tissues in 21 cases (21%) (Table 1).

The 54 patients with tumors of the soft parts and skeletal system constitute the data base for this report. Although all histologic patterns of disease were included, the majority of cases were those of osteogenic sarcoma or fibrosarcoma (Table 2). Included in the "other" group are cases of chondrosarcoma, leiomyosarcoma, lymphosarcoma, malignant chordoma, neurofibrosarcoma, and mixed mesodermal sarcoma. The distribution of cases was similar for all age groups, which contrasts sharply with data on a similar series of patients treated for carcinomatous lung metastasis.

Relatively simple criteria are employed in selecting cases for definitive surgery. Three basic questions must be answered. First, can the patient tolerate the contemplated surgery? Second, has the primary site of the tumor been definitively and successfully treated without evidence of residual or recurrent disease? Third, can all known meta-

TABLE 1.—PRIMARY SITE—
SARCOMA—FREQUENCY

PRIMARY SITE	NUMBER OF CASES	PERCENT
Skin	37	38
Soft parts	21	21
Skeletal system	33	34
Other	7	7

TABLE 2.—MORPHOLOGIC TYPE—FREQUENCY

CELL TYPE	NUMBER OF CASES	PERCENT
Melanoma	37	38
Ewing's sarcoma	4	4
Fibrosarcoma	11	11
Liposarcoma	6	6
Osteogenic sarcoma	21	22
Rhabdomyosarcoma	2	2
Synovial sarcoma	1	1
Other sarcoma	16	16

static disease be encompassed by the projected pulmonary resection? Regardless of the number or distribution of lesions within the lungs, if these 3 basic criteria can be fulfilled, surgical resection is recommended. Multiple and bilateral lesions are not deemed inoperable per se. Furthermore, subsequent lesions appearing sequentially are evaluated for surgery on the same basis as were those at first appearance. As long as the basic criteria apply, resection is advised. Following this policy, as many as 5 sequential thoracotomies have been performed in selected cases (Mountain, 1970 and 1976).

The diagnostic and evaluative process related to the selection of cases for surgical treatment identifies the presence of secondary spread and provides clinical assessment of the degree of spread for appropriate treatment selection. Careful screening for disseminated disease will eliminate from surgical consideration those patients with evidence of coexisting extrathoracic metastasis or those with diffuse seeding in the lungs.

In addition to the standard X-ray and biochemical studies, full chest tomograms and a liver scan are obtained routinely in sarcoma patients. Tomograms may reveal lesions not diagnosed on standard chest roentgenograms in about 15% of the cases. Mechanical lung function studies, arterial blood gas analysis, and ^{133}xenon scans are obtained to evaluate the ventilatory reserve.

The overall results of our experience through December 1973, with respect to definitive surgery, are shown in Figure 2. For sarcomas of primary origin in the skeletal system, the cumulative 5-year survival was 33%. For tumors originating in soft tissues, the cumulative 5-year survival was 18%. Survival was computed by the method of Gehan (1969), using the date of first thoracotomy as the starting point. A significantly better result was obtained in cases of osteogenic sarcoma, with a cumulative 5-year survival of 41%. In the pool of 22 cases representing small numbers of 9 other histologic presentations, the survival dynamics were similar to those for fibrosarcoma (Fig. 3). The relationship of these results to the primary treatment "cure-rate" should be kept in mind. The NCI Task Force Reports for this area of research indicate that chemotherapy will prevent metastasis in osteogenic sarcoma patients in 60% of the cases. Aggressive treatment by surgical resection, chemotherapy, and radiotherapy in the remaining 40% can increase the number who ultimately become disease-free (Jaffe and Watts 1976).

Another consideration in osteogenic sarcoma is that approximately half of the patients are dead within 3 months after the diagnosis of

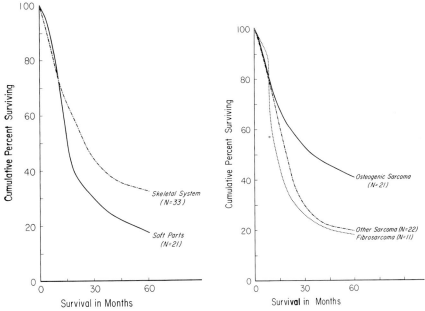

Fig. 2 (left). – Survival by primary site of patients with skeletal and soft parts sarcoma after surgical treatment of pulmonary metastasis.
Fig. 3 (right). – Survival by morphology of patients with skeletal and soft parts sarcoma after surgical treatment of pulmonary metastasis.

pulmonary metastasis, if the metastatic disease is not treated (Marcove and Lewis, 1973).

The interval of time elapsing between control of the primary and first recognition of pulmonary metastases has been observed by many to be related to survival; that is, the shorter the time, the worse the prognosis. In the present experience, this duration factor was observed to have quite different implications. In osteogenic sarcoma, pulmonary metastases are most often observed for the first time in the fifth or sixth month after resection of the primary disease (Sutow and Sullivan 1976). In this series, about one half of the pulmonary metastases were observed within 1 year of primary treatment (Fig. 4). The remaining cases were somewhat evenly distributed between the second through the fourth year time intervals with 17% first observed after 4 years. For the 25 patients observed and operated on within 12 months, the cumulative 5-year survival was 40%. Cumulative survival of those whose metastasis was detected in the second year fell to 5%,

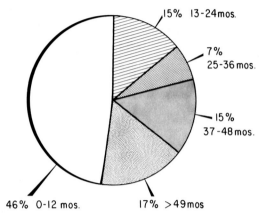

15% 13-24mos.

7% 25-36 mos.

15% 37-48mos.

46% 0-12 mos.

17% >49mos

Fig. 4.—Skeletal and soft parts sarcoma. Frequency by duration from primary treatment to first observed pulmonary metastasis.

with no 5-year survivors among patients whose disease was detected in the third and fourth years. Beyond 48 months, the survival rate increased to 20% (Table 3).

In an equivalent group of patients with carcinoma, survivors were more evenly distributed in these time intervals. The biology of these findings is not entirely clear, but this index of prognosis was not a factor in our selection of surgical cases. In such cases, the time interval between diagnosis and the appearance of pulmonary metastasis on chest X-ray film may not represent the spread of disease at a certain point in time, but rather the manifestation of occult disease which is already there (Jaffe and Watts, 1976). It is prudent, however, to observe the patient long enough for occult lesions to become clinically recognized, if the time between the primary treatment and the discovery of the first metastasis is short.

TABLE 3.—SKELETAL AND SOFT
PARTS SARCOMA SURVIVAL BY
DURATION FROM PRIMARY
TREATMENT TO FIRST OBSERVED
PULMONARY METASTASIS

DURATION (MONTHS)	% SURVIVING 5 YEARS
0–12	40
13–24	5
25–36	0
37–48	0
>49	20

Other biological characteristics, such as the tumor growth rate expressed as the tumor doubling time, appear to be directly related to survival. Present knowledge of the accelerating and retarding influences on the growth rate of cancer is incomplete, but the great variance within each cell type reflects the interdependence of the growth potential and the immune defense mechanisms of the host.

Morton and co-workers (1973) reported that measurement of the tumor doubling time appears to be a reliable means of selecting those patients who will benefit most from aggressive surgical treatment. Our findings in a previous study, based on examination of serial chest X-ray films, confirm that very rapid enlargement of pulmonary metastases is rarely associated with prolonged survival (Mountain, 1970). However, the predictive value of this variable remains to be definitively determined for various morphologies and was not used in the primary selection of surgical candidates for this study.

In the surgical approach, the least amount of tissue that encompasses all discernible metastatic disease is removed. A wedge or transsegmental resection is most commonly employed to conserve functional ventilatory reserve. This permits planned bilateral thoracotomy, when indicated, and allows for the resection of additional pulmonary nodules which may subsequently declare themselves. The usual peripheral location of metastases and the infrequent involvement of bronchi through the fourth order, make this choice of procedure feasible. Pneumonectomy is rarely justified. Following this program, the operative mortality is less than 2%.

Our studies, and those of others, give evidence that multiple sequential or synchronous bilateral metastases should not necessarily be considered inoperable. Figure 5 illustrates a survival comparison stratified by the number of thoracotomies. Thirty percent of the patients in the present study underwent more than 1 thoracotomy. In these cases, the number and distribution of metastases do not appear to adversely affect the survival rate in those patients in whom all residual malignant disease was apparently removed by more than 1 resection. Although some disagreement with this approach exists, many other surgical oncologists have reported the same conclusions (Martini, Bains, Huvos, and Beattie, 1974, Morton *et al.* 1973; and Spanos, Payne, Ivins, and Pritchard, 1976). Once we are committed to the program of resectional therapy, we persue an aggressive policy as long as the basic surgical criteria apply.

A comparison between the results of surgical treatment as a single modality and surgery plus planned postresection adjunctive chemo-

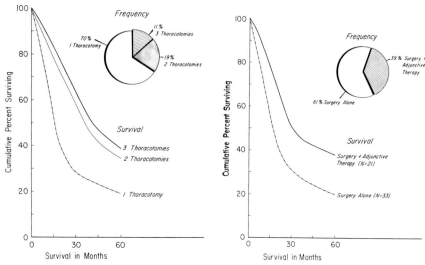

Fig. 5 (left). — Skeletal and soft parts sarcoma. Frequency and survival by number of thoracotomies.

Fig. 6 (right). — Skeletal and soft parts sarcoma. Frequency and survival by treatment regimen.

therapy is shown in Figure 6. Sixty-one percent (33 patients) had surgical therapy alone and 39% (21 patients) had surgical therapy plus adjunctive therapy. The cumulative 5-year survival rates were 19% and 38%, respectively. This work, accomplished on a retrospective basis, supports our expectation that the apparent success of surgical treatment of pulmonary metastasis can be enhanced through the use of combined therapy. In most instances, however, it seems advisable to establish that a tumor is sensitive to a planned chemotherapeutic and/or immunotherapeutic regime before committing a patient to a protracted program of adjunctive treatment.

This is particularly true in those cases where the primary therapeutic plan involved such adjunctive modalities and failed to control the disease. In this instance, where definitive resection of sarcomatous pulmonary metastases is deemed probable, it seems rational to initiate a brief trial of the proposed new adjuvant prior to pulmonary surgery. Basically, an in vivo sensitivity test is performed on a measurable lesion. In the absence of a complete and sustained response, the patient's tumor should be resected without undue delay. If the tumor is not totally insensitive to the adjunctive agents, they should be continued postoperatively in an effort to control or eradicate occult foci of disease.

REFERENCES

Barney, T. D., and Churchill, E. J.: Adenocarcinoma of the kidney with metastasis to the lung: cured by nephrectomy and lobectomy. Journal of Urology, 42:269–279, September 1939.

Choski, L. B., Takita, H., and Vincent, R. G.: The surgical management of solitary pulmonary metastasis. Surgery, Gynecology, and Obstetrics, 134:479–488, March 1972.

Cline, R. E., and Young, W. G., Jr.: Long-term results following surgical treatment of metastatic pulmonary tumors. The American Surgeon, 36:61–68, Februray 1970.

DeVita, V. T., Jr., Young, R. C., and Canellos, G. P.: Combination versus single agent chemotherapy: A review of the basis for selection of drug treatment of cancer. Cancer 35:98–110, January 1975.

Farrell, J. T., Jr.: Pulmonary metastasis: A pathologic, clinical roentgenologic study based on 78 cases seen at necropsy. Radiology 24:444–451, April 1935.

Feldman, P. S., and Kyriakos, M.: Pulmonary resection for metastatic sarcoma. Journal of Thoracic and Cardiovascular Surgery, 64:784–799, November 1972.

Fisher, B.: Factors that influence metastasis of tumors. In Najarian, J. S., and Delaney, J. P.: *Advances In Cancer Surgery.* New York, New York, Stratton Intercontinental Medical Book Corporation, 1976, pp. 119–126.

Gehan, E. A.: Estimating survival functions from the life table. Journal of Chronic Diseases, 21:629–644, February 1969.

Hutchison, D. E., and Denner, R. M.: Resection of pulmonary secondary tumors. The American Journal of Surgery, 124:732–737, December 1972.

Jaffe, N., and Watts, H. B.: Multidrug chemotherapy in primary treatment of osteosarcoma. An editorial commentary. Journal of Bone and Joint Surgery, 58A:634–635, July 1976.

Marcove, R. C., and Lewis, M. M.: Prolonged survival in osteogenic sarcoma with multiple primary metastasis. The Journal of Bone and Joint Surgery 55A:1516–1520, October 1973.

Martini, N., Bains, M. S., Huvos, A. S., and Beattie, E. J., Jr.: Surgical treatment of metastatic sarcoma to the lung. The Surgical Clinics of North America, 58:841–844, August 1974.

Morton, D. L., Joseph, W. L., Ketcham, A. S., Gellhoed, G. W., and Adkins, P. C.: Surgical resection and adjunctive immunotherapy for selected patients with multiple pulmonary metastasis. Annals of Surgery, 178:360–366, September, 1973.

Mountain, C. F.: Surgical management of pulmonary metastases. Postgraduate Medicine, 48:128–132, November 1970.

———.: The basis for surgical resection of pulmonary metastases. International Journal of Radiation Oncology, Biology, Physics, 1:749–753, May 1976.

Muggia, F. M.: Cell kinetic studies in patients with lung cancer. Oncology, 30:353–361, 1974.

Schabel, F. M., Jr.: The use of tumor growth kinetics in planning "curative" chemotherapy of advanced solid tumors. Cancer Research. 29:2384–2389, December 1969.

Shapiro, P. M., and Fugmann, R. A.: A role for chemotherapy as an adjuvant to surgery. Cancer Research, 17:1098–1101, December 1957.

Skipper, H. E., Schabel, F. M., and Wilcox, W. S.: Experimental evaluation of anticancer agents, XIII. On the criteria and kinetics associated with "curability" of experimental leukemia. Cancer Chemotherapy Reports (suppl), 35:1–111, February 1964.

Spanos, P. K., Payne, W. S., Ivins, J. C., and Pritchard, D. J.: Pulmonary resection for metastatic osteogenic sarcoma. Journal of Bone and Joint Surgery, 58A:624–628, July 1976.

Sutow, W. W., and Sullivan, M. P.: Childhood cancer. The improving prognosis. Postgraduate Medicine, 59:131–137, February 1976.

Turnbull, A. D., Pool, J. L., Arthur, K., and Golbey, R. B.: The role of radiotherapy and chemotherapy in the surgical management of pulmonary metastases. American Journal of Roentgenology, Radium Therapy, and Nuclear Medicine, 114:99–105, January 1972.

Turney, S. Z., and Haight, C.: Pulmonary resection for metastatic neoplasms. Journal of Thoracic and Cardiovascular Surgery, 61:784–794, May 1971.

Wilkins, E. W.: Solitary metastases in the lung. International Journal of Radiation Oncology, Biology, Physics 1:735–737, May 1976.

Willis, R. A.: *The Spread of Tumors in the Human Body*. London, England, Butterworth and Company, Ltd., 1952, 3rd Edition, 447pp.

A Clinicopathologic Discussion of Soft Tissue Neoplasms: Selected Case Material*

MODERATOR: ALBERTO G. AYALA, M.D.

Assistant Professor of Pathology, The University of Texas System Cancer Center M. D. Anderson Hospital and Tumor Institute, Houston, Texas

GUEST PANELIST: FRANZ ENZINGER, M.D.

Chief, Soft Tissue Branch, Armed Forces Institute of Pathology, Washington, D.C.

THE FINAL SESSION OF THE M. D. Anderson Hospital Twenty-First Annual Clinical Conference was the Ninth Annual Special Pathology Program. In addition to Dr. Ayala and Dr. Enzinger, the panel included the following staff members of The University of Texas System Cancer Center M. D. Anderson Hospital and Tumor Institute: H. Thomas Barkley, Jr., Robert S. Benjamin, Bruce Mackay, Richard G. Martin, and Luis de Santos. As in previous pathology programs, the panel discussion comprised a series of case presentations illustrating the clinicopathologic aspects of subjects covered by speakers during the previous sessions of the Annual Clinical Conference, and emphasized the multidisciplinary team approach to the management of cancer patients.

---

*Arranged by the Department of Pathology, The University of Texas System Cancer Center M. D. Anderson Hospital and Tumor Institute, and co-sponsored by the Texas Society of Pathologists.

CASE 1. ALVEOLAR RHABDOMYOSARCOMA

A 32-year-old white man noticed a "knot" at the angle of the right jaw in April 1971. It enlarged slowly, and antibiotic treatment was ineffective. On June 3, 1971, a biopsy was performed revealing an undifferentiated neoplasm in a cervical lymph node. The patient was then referred to M. D. Anderson Hospital for further evaluation. Results of physical examination were essentially negative except for a small scar in the right submaxillary area, beneath which there was a 5 cm indurated mass. On June 21, 1971, a re-excision of the submandibular area, along with an upper neck dissection, was performed. Residual tumor was present in the submaxillary gland and in several lymph nodes. Following surgery, radiotherapy was given to the surgical scar, the retropharyngeal and preauricular lymph nodes, and the supraclavicular areas. The course of radiotherapy was completed in August 1971. The patient died on November 8, 1971. An autopsy was not performed.

Dr. de Santos (Radiology). — Radiographic studies revealed a soft tissue mass adjacent to the body and angle of the mandible. The bone appeared to be essentially normal with no evidence of erosion. There was no evidence of calcification of any kind in the mass.

Dr. Mackay (Pathology). — Histologically, the excision specimen from the submaxillary gland showed small, round tumor cells infiltrating the gland predominantly in the spaces between the lobules. The nuclei of these cells appeared to be irregular, and some were quite bizarre in appearance. The tumor was traversed by branching and anastomosing trabeculae of connective tissue which subdivided the tumor into many irregular compartments. The tumor cells were located within these compartments and were lining the inner aspects of the connective tissue trabeculae (Fig. 1). Mitotic figures were seen throughout the tumor. The cells tended to lose contact with one another and to lie free within the spaces. The tumor cells contained PAS-positive material, which was removed by prior digestion with diastase, indicating the presence of cytoplasmic glycogen.

Viewed with the electron microscope, the nuclei of the tumor cells appeared particularly irregular in contour, with many of them having deep clefts. The chromatin material was well dispersed throughout the nucleus and occasional pyknotic nuclei were seen (Fig. 2). The nucleoli were prominent and often multiple. Slight thickenings of apposed cell membranes which hinted at the presence of intercellular attachments were also seen, although usually one does not find them in this tumor.

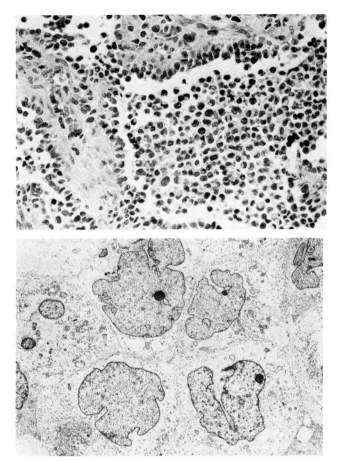

Fig. 1 (top).—Case 1. Fibrous partitions subdivide the tumor into irregular compartments filled with tumor cells. Most of the cells exhibit loss of cohesion, but a peripheral layer remains attached to the surrounding connective tissue. (×400.)

Fig. 2 (bottom).—Case 1. Low magnification electron micrograph showing the irregular nuclear contours. (×3,800.)

While many of the cells did not contain anything significant in the cytoplasm, a number contained sparse small bundles of cytoplasmic filaments. This particular tumor revealed no Z-band material. Characteristically, the filaments are relatively thick (140 angstrom units in diameter), with thinner filaments disposed between them, and the cytoplasmic ribosomes tend to line up in rows between the filaments (Fig. 3). These features indicate that they are skeletal muscle myofilaments. However, the proof of this is to find areas where the filaments

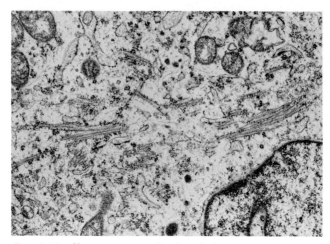

Fig. 3.—Case 1. Myofilaments were only identified in occasional cells. They formed small aggregates with cytoplasmic ribosomes. The filaments appear straight in longitudinal section, and their spatial relationship can be appreciated where they are transversely sectioned. Z band material was not present. (×48,000.)

are cut transversely and to observe the thick filaments and thinner filaments, with the latter arranged in hexagonal distribution around the former. This is the characteristic spatial organization of the myosin and actin filaments of skeletal muscle, confirming the diagnosis of rhabdomyosarcoma.

Dr. Barkley (Radiotherapy).—This patient received intensive radiotherapy. The patient was treated with parallel opposed fields to an area which included the parotid gland and the retropharyngeal nodes. An electron beam boost was also given to this area. The patient received approximately 6,000 rads tumor dose at 2.75 cm depth in 5 weeks. The lower neck was also treated, as is our habit when nodes or connective tissue in the upper neck have been involved.

Dr. Ayala (Pathology).—This patient was seen 5 years ago; at that time he did not receive chemotherapy. Dr. Benjamin will comment on the chemotherapy as it is used today in this type of case.

Dr. Benjamin (Developmental Therapeutics).—I think this is the type of patient who would likely have benefited from adjuvant chemotherapy along with radiotherapy, and I think were he to come in today, that would be our approach. Of course, there are many problems associated with giving chemotherapy together with radiotherapy, particularly to patients who have lesions in the head and neck area. There is a tremendous increase in the radiation-induced mucositis when radiotherapy is given together with Adriamycin, and we have had tremendous difficulty in maintaining these patients, often having to use hyperalimentation and extreme measures of supportive care. We still have not worked out a truly satisfactory way of giving the combined radiotherapy and chemotherapy.

Dr. Ayala. — I would now like to ask Dr. Enzinger to give his comments on this type of tumor.

Dr. Enzinger. — This is a typical case of alveolar rhabdomyosarcoma showing the characteristic features of this tumor, including a great variation of the histological pattern in various portions of the neoplasm. For this reason, careful sampling of the tumor and careful study of many portions of the neoplasm are exceedingly important for diagnosis. Study with the electron microscope is also most useful in poorly differentiated cases showing no apparent rhabdomyoblastic differentiation.

Typical of this tumor is the alveolar pattern, with trabeculae of fibrous connective tissue separating the loosely arranged, "floating" tumor cells. Another feature is the presence of scattered differentiated rhabdomyoblasts as well as multinucleated giant cells. The latter feature often helps in identifying the tumor in the absence of rhabdomyoblasts. Many of these cases — approximately 75% in our autopsy material — metastasize to regional lymph nodes, and it is important to be aware of this fact in planning therapy. The regional lymph nodes exhibit the typical histologic picture, and often the diagnosis of alveolar rhabdomyosarcoma can be made solely on the basis of the lymph node biopsy. In fact, sometimes the first manifestation of disease is lymph node metastasis, particularly when the primary tumor is located in the perirectal or head and neck area.

The most common type of rhabdomyosarcoma is the embryonal type, followed in frequency by the alveolar and then by the pleomorphic type. Benign tumors of rhabdomyoblasts are exceedingly rare and in our material amount only to about 1% of all cases. Although both embryonal and alveolar rhabdomyosarcoma are tumors of primitive rhabdomyoblasts, the 2 should be distinguished for clinical and diagnostic reasons. Embryonal rhabdomyosarcoma occurs most commonly in the head and neck region; the alveolar type more commonly affects the extremities. The age distribution also differs: embryonal rhabdomyosarcoma is primarily a tumor of young children, while alveolar rhabdomyosarcoma is mainly a tumor of adolescents and young adults between 10 and 25 years of age. In our study of about 100 cases of alveolar rhabdomyosarcoma, most tumors were of relatively small size when excised. However, even when the tumor measures only 1 or 2 cm in diameter, prognosis has to be guarded because even very small alveolar rhabdomyosarcomas are capable of metastasis. The median survival in our study (prior to combination chemotherapy and radiotherapy) was only 6 to 8 months. There was very little difference in the survival rates in regard to age, but older patients with alveolar rhabdomyosarcoma did slightly worse than those younger than 10 years of age. The stage of the tumor is obviously very important for prognosis. Those patients with localized lesions had a far better prognosis than those with regional lymph node metastasis at the time of the first treatment. In our study, 50% of the patients underwent autopsy. Of these 50%, 78% had metastases to regional lymph nodes and 74% had metastases to the lung and pleura, the latter being the most common site of metastases in all other soft tissue tumors.

Dr. Ayala. — Dr. Enzinger, do you see mixed patterns, ie., embryonal and alveolar rhabdomyosarcoma together?

Dr. Enzinger. — Yes, we do see occasional mixed patterns where some areas of the tumor are typical of embryonal and other areas are typical of alveolar rhabdomyosarcoma. This does occur, and we usually diagnose the case according to the predominant pattern.

Dr. Ayala. — I understand that most of the pleomorphic rhabdomyosarcomas are now being classified as fibrous histiocytomas. Could you comment on that?

Dr. Enzinger. — I believe that almost all cases formerly called "pleomorphic" or "adult" rhabdomyosarcoma are actually examples of malignant fibrous histiocytomas. I have never seen 1 case of a pleomorphic rhabdomyosarcoma with unequivocal cross striations in a patient older than 30 years of age. I have seen, however, pleomorphic rhabdomyosarcomas with cross striations in small children.

Perhaps I should say a few words here about the importance of the glycogen stain in differential diagnosis. In some poorly differentiated cases of rhabdomyosarcoma, it may be difficult to rule out a malignant lymphoma. This can be done quite reliably if glycogen can be demonstrated in the tumor cells. This stain is also helpful in ruling out neuroblastomas and malignant fibrous histiocytomas for intracellular glycogen is rare in either tumor.

CASE 2. EWING'S SARCOMA OF SOFT TISSUE

A 34-year-old white woman was first seen at M. D. Anderson Hospital on September 16, 1975, with a referral diagnosis of unclassified soft tissue sarcoma of her left anterolateral ankle. This lesion had been present for approximately 5 months. She underwent an excisional biopsy in August 1975, followed by cobalt radiotherapy (approximately 1,800 rads tumor dose) and was then referred for further evaluation and therapy. Results of physical examination were essentially negative except for a 5 cm leg scar overlying an area of swelling, with associated redness of the skin. Clincially, the lesion was believed to represent infection rather than tumor. The basic plan was to treat the area with 4,500 rads tumor dose over 4½ weeks. The patient did well until April 1976, when she noticed a mass over the posterior scalp. A biopsy from this mass was obtained and excision of the recurrent mass of the leg was performed. Pathological examination revealed a small round cell sarcoma in both locations. Radiotherapy was given to the mass, and the patient was placed on CY-VA-DIC chemotherapy. In September 1976, she developed lung and bone marrow metastases.

Dr. de Santos (Radiology). — In this case, radiology did not aid in the diagnosis, even though xeroradiography was used in addition to conventional radiography.

Dr. Mackay (Pathology). — This was a small cell tumor and the histological type was the same in both the leg and scalp accessions. There was no significant architectural organization; the cells were closely clumped, with areas of necrosis and hemorrhage (Fig. 4). There were some small spaces between the cells, but there was nothing to suggest, for example, rosette formation. The cells did not show much irregularity, and the nuclei were not pleomorphic when compared with the previous case. Nucleoli were small, and the chromatin material was diffuse. In some areas the cells appeared more elongated, but there were no truly fusiform cells. With the PAS stain it was possible to demonstrate some glycogen in the tumor cells.

Electron microscopy revealed that the tumor cells were closely apposed, although there were no significant invaginations or irregularities of the cell membranes, or any cell contact specializations (Fig. 5). In occasional areas, cell membranes were slightly thickened, but there were no true desmosomes. There was nothing remarkable about the organelles and no evidence of cytoplasmic myofilament formation (Fig. 6).

This appearance corresponds closely to what we expect to see in cases of Ewing's sarcoma of bone, particularly the regular profile of the nucleus, the finely dispersed chromatin material which makes the rather small nucleoli conspicuous, and the absence of significant features in the cytoplasm other than the presence of some glycogen.

There was no evidence of peripheral dendritic processes or small neurosecretory granules such as one would look for in a neuroblastoma, and the presence of glycogen ruled out reticuloendothelial neo-

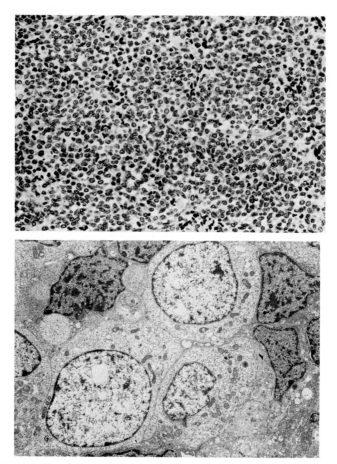

Fig. 4 (top).—Case 2. Compactly grouped, small round tumor cells without architectural organization. (×400.)

Fig. 5 (bottom).—Case 2. The nuclei are round or oval with smooth profiles. (×5,600.)

plasms. Therefore, our conclusion was that this is a small cell neoplasm of soft tissue with a striking resemblance to Ewing's sarcoma of bone.

Dr. Barkley (Radiotherapy).—Prior to referral to this hospital, the patient was given radiotherapy (2,016 rads) to a localized appositional field directed to the biopsy scar with small margins above and below. Our fields were enlarged and a parallel opposed field technique was designed to spare most of the ankle joint and to incorporate what we felt were adequate margins for this tumor, since we were under the impression that this was not a typical Ewing's sarcoma. The dose of

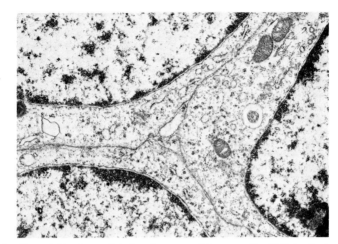

Fig. 6.—Case 2. Portions of 3 closely apposed tumor cells. Cell contact specializations were sparse and poorly developed, and membrane infoldings or microvilli were not seen. The cytoplasm contains free ribosomes, but other organelles were not numerous. (×23,000.)

4,500 rads which was given was somewhat less than would have been prescribed as the original treatment, but we were handicapped by the presence of an open, unhealed biopsy wound and by the previously administered radiation. Treatment provided for sparing some skin and muscle posteriorly, primarily the Achilles tendon, which is vital in terms of function.

After excision of the scalp lesion, this area was treated with the electron beam to a dose of 4,000 rads in 9 fractions. Subsequently, the patient has had other metastases and has been treated for relief of pain in the sacroiliac joint, the cranium, and a portion of the thoracic spine.

Dr. Ayala.—It was late in the course of the disease when the patient received chemotherapy. She was placed on CY-VA-DIC therapy. Doctor Benjamin, will you tell us about this regimen in connection with Ewing's sarcoma?

Dr. Benjamin (Chemotherapy).—CY-VA-DIC is a combination of 4 drugs: cyclophosphamide, vincristine, Adriamycin, and DIC or DTIC (dimethyl triazeno imidazole carboxamide). For Ewing's sarcoma, the partial remission rate is approximately 55%, while the complete remission rate is only 10% to 15%. Unfortunately, the patients that we see who are in this 10% to 15% complete remission group have very transient remissions. In this case, at the initiation of chemotherapy we had no tumor to evaluate, so it was impossible to say whether the patient was initially responding or not. Clearly, she had a very short period of disease-free survival, and, therefore, this is clearly a failure of chemotherapy.

Dr. Ayala.—Doctor Sinkovics was directly involved in the care of this patient and call tell us more about the case.

Dr. Sinkovics (Immunology).—This patient is still alive, but her condition is rapidly growing worse.

Our philosophy now in treating Ewing's sarcoma of bone and soft tissue is that radiotherapy directed to the primary site must be combined with chemotherapy from the beginning, because this disease is either multicentric in origin or metastasizes so early that treating the primary site alone with radiotherapy is inadequate. Originally, however, this tumor was unclassified and it was not diagnosed as Ewing's sarcoma until the recurrence and scalp metastases were excised.

This patient was referred to us from another institution where they elected to treat the primary tumor with radiotherapy; however, after an initial dosage, she was referred to us for completion of this therapy. We began treating the patient at the time that the scalp metastases occurred with the CY-VA-DIC regimen. This failed, and she developed further metastatic disease. At that time, we attempted control with an alternative regimen known to be effective in treating Ewing's sarcoma, namely, nitrosourea (methyl CCNU) in conjunction with actinomycin-D. This also failed. At present, the patient is receiving radiotherapy to some painful bone lesions, and we plan to start treating her with large-dose methotrexate and leucovorin rescue. There is little we can offer.

There was a claim published a few years ago in *Cancer* that mithramycin is effective in treating metastatic Ewing's sarcoma, and the article was documented with roentgenograms showing regression of large lung metastases. In the past 5 years, we have treated 5 patients with metastatic Ewing's sarcoma with mithramycin (sometimes in conjunction with vinblastine), and we have not seen a single response. This patient, therefore, will receive the investigational protocol of large-dose methotrexate and leucovorin rescue.

Dr. Ayala.—I would like to ask Dr. Enzinger to comment on this type of tumor, since he has recently published the results of a study of 39 cases which sheds new light on the diagnosis and treatment of Ewing's sarcoma of soft tissue.

Dr. Enzinger.—Our study seems to indicate that Ewing's sarcoma is not exclusively a bone tumor, but may also occur in the soft tissues. Of course, this tumor is still very difficult to diagnose because of its close resemblance to other types of round cell sarcoma. Many soft tissue tumors, including rhabdomyosarcoma, neuroblastoma, synovial sarcoma, and hemangiosarcoma, may be at times exceedingly poorly differentiated and may manifest themselves as solid round cell tumors. In order to reach a more specific diagnosis, it is necessary to prepare many sections of the tumor for histologic study and to use a variety of special stains, including a glycogen stain and a reticulum preparation.

The present tumor bears a close resemblance to Ewing's sarcoma of bone and is similar to the cases that were reported as malignant soft tissue neoplasm resembling Ewing's sarcoma.

One of the characteristics which helps to distinguish the tumor from a rhabdomyosarcoma is its uniform and almost monotonous cellular pattern and the absence of a fibrous stroma. Despite the poor differentiation of the tumor cells, there is little mitotic activity, much less so than, for instance, in a rhabdomyosarcoma. The tumor is rather vascular, but at first glance the vascular pattern is not very prominent because it is obscured by the proliferation of the tumor cells. The cells characteristically contain glycogen, the amount of which varies in different portions of the tumor. In general, glycogen is much more prominent at the periphery of the tumor than in the center of the lesion.

There is another feature of this tumor which should be noted. When the tumor outgrows its vascular supply and degenerates, the vascular pattern becomes increasingly prominent, a characteristic which probably accounts for the fact that Dr. Ewing originally called this tumor an "endothelioma." In fact, because of this feature, some of these cases have been misdiagnosed as malignant hemangiopericytoma. This vascular pattern, however, seems to be a secondary feature that is superimposed upon the primary round cell pattern.

The tumors that must be distinguished from Ewing's sarcoma include poorly differentiated synovial sarcoma, neuroblastoma, neuroepithelioma, malignant lymphoma, rhabdomyosarcoma, and poorly differentiated carcinoma. Neuroblastoma, synovial sarcoma, and malignant lymphoma can usually be ruled out if intracellular glycogen can be demonstrated. Differential diagnosis from rhabdomyosarcoma may be difficult because the age incidence of rhabdomyosarcoma is the same as that of extraskeletal Ewing's sarcoma. Rhabdomyosarcoma, however, usually shows a much greater variation in the size and shape of the tumor cells, and, more importantly, there are differentiated rhabdomyoblasts, with or without cross striations. Carcinomas can be ruled out in most cases on the basis of the patient's age. Most extraskeletal Ewing's sarcomas occur in the same age group as do

Ewing's sarcomas of bone, that is, they occur in patients between 12 and 25 years of age. The primary locations of this tumor are the paravertebral area, the chest wall, and the extremities.

Dr. Ayala.—We are honored to have here from the Mayo Clinic Dr. Edward Soule who belongs to the Intergroup Rhabdomyosarcoma Study Committee. He has been studying a number of small cell lesions, about which I will ask him to comment at this time.

Dr. Soule.—When we were studying rhabdomyosarcomas, we soon discovered that we were receiving a group of cases that were difficult to classify absolutely as being rhabdomyosarcoma. So we established a separate group which we called sarcoma, Type 1. At that time, we commented on the fact that they looked very much like a Ewing's tumor. We also saw another type which we called sarcoma, Type 2. These were probably large cell Ewing's sarcomas in which possibly some degenerative change had caused an abnormal appearance. A third group was undifferentiated and remained unclassified. It was our hope that at the end of the study we would learn something about the behavior, chemotherapy, and radiotherapy associated with these tumors which did not fit in the rhabdomyosarcoma group.

In other material at the Mayo Clinic, we have seen a number of these cases over the years and have set them aside. From the standpoints of cytological and morphological type, they look exactly like a Ewing's sarcoma of bone, but we have been very careful to exclude any lesion that involved bone. We have approximately 30 patients that we are still following. At present, approximately 35% of these individuals have survived, which is perhaps a better survival rate than that for Ewing's sarcoma of bone.

Dr. Sinkovics.—I would like to add that the survival rate of patients with Ewing's sarcoma of bone is improving. Since 1974, 12 patients have been treated with radiotherapy and chemotherapy from the time of diagnosis. An analysis made in October 1976 shows that 1 patient is dead, 2 patients have disease but are alive, and 1 patient is stable. However, in a group of 12 patients treated with radiotherapy and chemotherapy since diagnosis, there are 7 with no evidence of disease, and these are young adults and older, not pediatric patients.

CASE 3. MYXOID NEUROFIBROSARCOMA

A 43-year-old woman developed swelling in her left hip approximately 3 months prior to admission. Her physician performed a biopsy which was interpreted as showing a synovial sarcoma. She was then referred to M. D. Anderson Hospital for further evaluation and treatment. Roentgenograms taken at this hospital disclosed a large mass which had disrupted the left hip and joint, destroying the acetabular rim and left ischium and causing subluxation of the femoral head. Other studies were negative. Because of the extensive involvement with bone and soft tissues, it was believed that the best approach to treatment would be a left hemipelvectomy. Postoperatively, the patient developed a wound abscess and drainage to the vagina. Following healing, she was discharged and has had no further complaints over a 4-month period.

Dr. de Santos.—The radiograms of the left hip demonstrated a superior dislocation of the femoral head, with extensive erosion of the femoral neck and head and iliac bone secondary to a large soft tissue mass, best outlined on the tomograms, which extended within the pelvis and showed a small rim of calcification. A lytic defect was also present in the iliac bone. Although this tumor is an obviously malignant one from the radiological view, evidence of remodeling and erosion suggested that the tumor might have been there for a long time before showing the aggressive behavior.

Dr. Ayala.—There was, I believe, considerable difficulty in making a histological diagnosis on the basis of 2 biopsies, and because of the extensiveness of the lesion, surgery was contemplated. Dr. Martin, would you comment on the surgical approach?

Dr. Martin (Surgery).—With a tumor as extensive as this one, involving the bone, surgically, there is little to do other than a hemipelvectomy which, whenever possible, should be a modified hemipelvectomy, to save part of the pelvic bone. In this case, however, that was not feasible because of the extensive disease.

Dr. Ayala.—I would like to ask Dr. Mackay to review the pathological findings for us at this point.

Dr. Mackay.—The histologic appearance of this tumor was rather variable. The predominant pattern was that of a loose arrangement of branching tumor cells, the interstices of which were filled with myxoid-appearing material (Fig. 7). The tumor cells were elongated and appeared to have branching cytoplasmic extensions. In other areas, where the cellular pattern was more solid, there was not quite as much evidence of myxoid material, but again there were spindle-shaped tumor cells with fairly long cytoplasmic extensions. In some areas, there was some organization of nuclei into rows and a hint of palisading. In an even more solid zone of the tumor, there was a hint of a storiform type of arrangement, but this was not common throughout this particular tumor. Between the groups of nuclei there were considerable zones of pinkish material which are, for the most part,

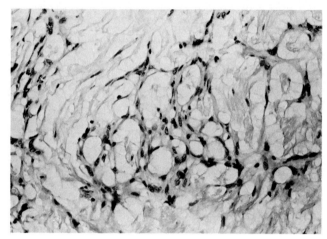

Fig. 7.—Case 3. In most areas of the tumor, considerable quantities of myxoid material separated the slender bands of tumor cells.

not intercellular collagen, but processes of the tumor cells seen on the electron micrographs. Some areas of the tumor exhibited close apposition of the cell membranes of these cytoplasmic extensions which were connected by some form of cell contact specialization with some resemblance to mature desmosomes, but lacking tonofilaments and the intermediate lines.

Another feature of this tumor, in addition to the processes, was the cell cytoplasm that was frequently seen to enclose little spaces enclosed by small tongue-like processes of the tumor cells (Fig. 8). Within the spaces there was basal lamina and collagen fibrils similar to the appearance that one sees in Schwann cells, producing mesaxons which are infolding axons in unmyelinated nerve formations. We have seen this appearance now in a number of tumors, and we certainly see it in benign neurogenic tumors. This fine structural appearance does not suggest any of the other soft tissue tumors with which I am acquainted, and this is evidence in favor of a neurogenic classification for this particular tumor. The ultrastructural evidence points toward this being, in fact, a myxoid malignant schwannoma.

Dr. Ayala.—I would like to ask Dr. Enzinger to give us his comments.

Dr. Enzinger.—This is a very unusual neoplasm, and I do not recall ever having seen a malignant schwannoma showing such a prominent myxoid component. I agree, however, that some areas, in particular the solid areas of the tumor, have a somewhat "neural" appearance

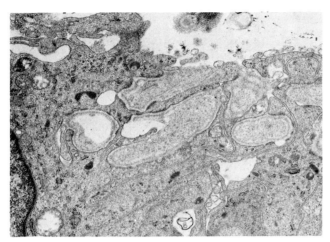

Fig. 8.—Case 3. The tendency of the tumor cells to develop small zones of stroma simulates mesaxon formation. (×22,000.)

and resemble areas of a malignant schwannoma. The electron microscopic findings, of course, support neural origin, and this case proves the value of electron microscopic studies of such rare tumors. Some mucin stains were done at the Armed Forces Institute of Pathology, but they were of little help in differential diagnosis. The mucoid material was alcian blue positive, but we did not have unstained slides to check whether or not this was removed by prior treatment of the sections with hyaluronidase, as one would expect in a neural tumor (in contrast to a chondrosarcoma, in which treatment with hyaluronidase does not affect the staining characteristics of the mucinous material). Therefore, I agree that a malignant neural tumor is more likely on the basis of the histology and the ultrastructural findings than, for instance, an atypical malignant chondroid tumor, another possibility which I had considered, in differential diagnosis.

Dr. Ayala.—In planning therapy, we are often asked to grade tumors. Dr. Enzinger, would you comment on the grading of such tumors.

Dr. Enzinger.—There is good evidence in the literature that grading of sarcomas is of importance in predicting the clinical behavior. For instance, in a recent review of fibrosarcomas from the Mayo Clinic (*Cancer*, 33:888–898, 1974), it was clearly shown that the grade of tumor is very important in predicting the clinical behavior and prognosis. However, we should not do this without first classifying or typing the tumor, because different types of sarcomas vary greatly in their behavior. If we compare, for instance, similar grades of liposarcomas and alveolar rhabdomyosarcoma, we will find that the natural behavior of these 2 tumors is entirely different and that we cannot base our judgment in regard to prognosis merely on the degree of cellular differentiation. Correct classification of the tumor and determination of its degree of differentiation, in addition to the clinical information, are prerequisites for reliable staging of a given tumor.

Dr. Ayala. — Any additional questions?

Question. — Is chemotherapy indicated?

Dr. Benjamin. — I think the answer is probably yes, although we do not know the answer to the question. We have done a study, but the results are very confusing. It shows that radiation therapy alone is having better results than we know radiation therapy alone can give, and that chemotherapy does not help. It is a dilemma. However, I think this patient certainly fits the criteria for entry in a study to determine the effects of radiation and chemotherapy. I think that, postoperatively, radiation would be contemplated and probably, because of the location of the tumor, it will be given in conjunction with chemotherapy.

Dr. Barkley. — I was afraid someone might raise this question. It has not been our habit to give postoperative radiation when surgery was extensive enough to give margins well beyond the limits of the tumor, such as in the case of amputation or hemipelvectomy. The important use of the radiation therapy program has been for local excision of the tumor with microscopic residuals. Perhaps Dr. Martin could tell us what sort of threat, in terms of local recurrence, the surgical procedure offers to this patient.

Dr. Martin. — There is an important factor that must be emphasized in a case of this type. If radiation is used postoperatively, after hemipelvectomy, the bowel will be damaged. There would be no protection whatsoever, and the bowel complications would be much more severe than the recurrent tumor which might possibly be excised.

Question. — What sort of things should be looked for before hemipelvectomy?

Dr. Martin. — We study the tomograms extensively, looking particularly at the symphysis and also at the sacral joint, both of which have to be free of tumor in order for us to do a successful hemipelvectomy. As I stated, we do not worry too much about the tumor protruding into the pelvic cavity because usually that is not a difficult problem. We also do a full chest tomogram to make certain that there is no metastasis; we do not want to do a hemipelvectomy if the patient has pulmonary metastasis. I think those are the main criteria.

Routinely, in these cases we do a bone survey. As a rule, we use neither the bone scan nor lymphangiograms. We remove all the regional lymph nodes at the time of hemipelvectomy. If it is a tumor that metastasizes to the lymph node, then a lymphangiogram is usually obtained.

Question. — Did the pictures taken show areas of calcification? How did this tumor look grossly? Was it circumscribed?

Dr. Mackay. — No, it did not seem to be circumscribed, it seemed to be infiltrating surrounding tissues. There was predominantly a myxoid tumor with some solid cellular areas, but we did not see calcification.

Dr. Ayala. — Are there any comments?

Question. — In the myxoid schwannoma case, did the electron microscopy show any specialized organelle in the cytoplasm, such as microtubules or specialized filaments.

Dr. Mackay. — Yes, it did. The frequency of microtubules in malignant schwannomas is quite variable. Sometimes they are found in most of the cells, sometimes they are difficult to find. In this particular case, they were not nearly as numerous as we frequently find, but they were present.

Dr. Ayala. — Are there any additional questions or comments?

Dr. Romsdahl (Surgery). — The discussion we were just having relates to using information from the pathologist, such as degree of differentiation, in determining whether the patient should receive adjuvant chemotherapy. Certainly, there are special problems that pathologists have in grading these types of sarcomas. Perhaps most use criteria other than a specific grade in selecting those patients who are to be on an adjuvant program.

Dr. Enzinger. — In many cases the pathologist can grade a tumor reliably, but sometimes judgment and experience may be the cause of some differences in opinion. The goal is to establish a uniformly applicable basis for judging the grade of the tumor. We are still far from reaching this goal, and there is considerable work to be done before grading can be accomplished on a widely acceptable, uniform, and, hopefully, objective basis.

CASE 4. EXTRASKELETAL MYXOID CHONDROSARCOMA

A 23-year-old white man discovered a "lump"in his right buttock 2 months prior to hospital admission. His personal physician performed a biopsy, following which the patient was referred to M. D. Anderson Hospital for further evaluation. Examination of the right buttock demonstrated a recent surgical incision, beneath which there was a large soft mass. Results of the remainder of the physical examination were negative. A wide excision of the right gluteal area was performed, revealing a large, 15 cm mass arising deep within the gluteal muscles. His postoperative course was unremarkable and he is presently undergoing local radiotherapy.

Dr. Ayala. — Dr. de Santos, could you show us the X-ray films at this time?

Dr. de Santos. — There are 2 modes of xeroradiography, positive and negative, and the negative mode is better for visualization of the soft tissues. In this case, there was a large, lobulated gluteal mass with normal underlying bony structures. Most of the tumor was fairly well-defined, but the fact that there was 1 area which was ill-defined, with little delineation between the tumor and the adjacent soft tissues, indicated malignant disease. Otherwise, there were no other radiographic findings; the adjacent femur was normal.

Dr. Ayala. — This mass was excised, and I would like to ask Dr. Martin to comment on this case.

Dr. Martin. — Tumors of the buttocks lend themselves well to surgical resection. A total gluteal resection was done in this case. Preoperative radiotherapy was contraindicated because the biopsy scar was draining. The tumor was growing and we did not want to wait for the wound to heal. Postoperative radiation was planned.

This case is a good example of the need for taking extreme care when doing a biopsy. Whenever possible, the individual who is going to be responsible for a resection should plan the biopsy site because when a biopsy is done immediately over the gluteal muscle, the skin flaps so vital in closing these wounds can be disturbed.

Dr. Ayala. — Dr. Mackay, would you review the histology.

Dr. Mackay. — Much of the tumor was composed of a myxoid-like matrix in which the tumor cells were scattered (Fig. 9). Many were small round cells without significant nuclear pleomorphism, but in some areas there was pleomorphism, and mitotic activity was easily detected. In some regions, the tumor was more cellular, with compactly arranged small cells infiltrating through connective tissue planes (Fig. 10). The myxoid material of the tumor appeared to stain positively with the alcian blue procedure. Zones of well-differentiated cartilage were present in many areas, and some osteoid was also being formed. Dr. Ayala is interested in this type of tumor and will give us his diagnostic assessment.

Dr. Ayala. — This case certainly is not the classical extraskeletal myxoid chondrosarcoma as described by Dr. Enzinger. Characteristically, these tumors contain much more myxoid background, and

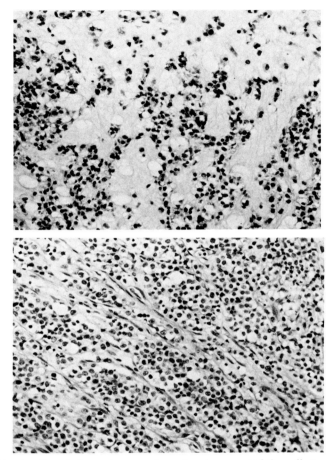

Fig. 9 (top).—Case 4. Stromal mucopolysaccharide separated the cells in many parts of the tumor. (×400.)

Fig. 10 (bottom).—Case 4. The small round tumor cells had little cytoplasm. They were compactly grouped in some areas. (×400.)

the cells are small, dark, and form a characteristically interlacing pattern. Perhaps in 6 cases seen at M. D. Anderson Hospital, the clinical pattern has been that of slowly growing lesions which metastasize to the lungs but allow the patients at least 3 or 4 years' survival even with these metastases. Of the six patients to date, 3 are surviving, and those 3 who have had metastases have had them for at least 3 years.

Dr. Enzinger has made a study of this tumor involving a larger series of cases, and he can tell us more.

Dr. Enzinger.—Chondrosarcomas in extraskeletal tissue are in many aspects different from chondrosarcomas in bone. Most of the extra-skeletal tumors are of the myxoid type and consist of typical chondro-blasts separated by mucinous material that shows the staining charac-teristics of sulfated mucopolysaccharides. Some of these tumors are poorly differentiated and almost approach the picture of a round cell sarcoma, as in the case under discussion. These cellular variants be-have more aggressively than the ordinary, richly myxoid chondrosar-coma, which is a relatively slow-growing tumor, but which nonethe-less does mestastasize, sometimes as late as 5 or even 10 years after the initial diagnosis.

Myxoid chondrosarcomas are multinodular and frequently there are isolated nodules outside the main tumor mass. If these nodules are left behind when the mass is excised, by "shelling out" or "enu-cleation," recurrence will ensue. Therefore, wide local excision is necessary to prevent local recurrence of the tumor.

Microscopically, the individual cells are separated by considerable amounts of mucoid material and, as is typical of chondroblasts, are arranged in branching rows and cords, often resulting in a lace-like pattern. Unlike a myxoid liposarcoma—and this tumor is frequently confused with myxoid liposarcoma—the tumor lacks the prominent plexiform capillary pattern. In fact, small vessels are hard to find in well-differentiated myxoid chondrosarcomas. Sometimes it is difficult to distinguish this tumor from a malignant mixed tumor of sweat gland origin, but the complete absence of acini or ductal structures usually helps to rule out this diagnosis. Hemorrhage and secondary changes are frequent, and often there is extensive fibrosis or massive deposits of hemosiderin.

Special stains help greatly in making the differential diagnosis be-tween myxoid liposarcoma and extraskeletal myxoid chondrosarcoma. The small chondroblasts almost always contain considerable amounts of glycogen. The mucinous material between the chondroblasts is not removed by prior treatment of the sections with hyaluronidase. In myxoid liposarcoma, however, the mucinous material no longer stains following treatment with hyaluronidase.

In 1971 we studied 33 patients with extraskeletal myxoid chondro-sarcoma. The tumor occurred mainly in adults ranging from 13 to 89 years; the principal location was in the extremities. Most were fairly large tumors, with a median size of 7 cm; 33% recurred, and 21 metas-tasized. Since publication of our article, we received additional fol-low-up material in some cases, and it appears that the actual recur-rence rate and the rate of metastasis is higher than was indicated by our figures. In our material there was 1 case in which the tumor metastasized to the lung and was excised; the patient is still alive without further metastasis 10 years later.

Dr. Ayala. – The patient is now undergoing radiotherapy. Dr. Barkley, could you comment on the postoperative therapy?

Dr. Barkley. – We do anticipate a high local recurrence rate in this type of tumor, and therefore this patient was considered a prime candidate for postoperative radiation. Again, the principle is to include the entire muscle group with margins for a dose of 5,000 rads and then to give a 1,000 rad boost to the tumor bed per se. In this situation we are dealing with rather large field sizes and a considerable depth, which will make the planning of the radiation somewhat more difficult than is common for an extremity, for instance.

CASE 5. LIPOSARCOMA VS. MALIGNANT FIBROUS HISTIOCYTOMA

A 40-year-old woman was referred to M. D. Anderson Hospital for further evaluation of lung metastases. The right kidney with a retroperitoneal mass had been removed and the mass diagnosed as liposarcoma 2½ years earlier. The patient did well until November 1973, 1 month before M. D. Anderson admission, when chest roentgenograms demonstrated metastatic disease in the lungs. Treatment with CY-VA-DIC was given during the next 7 to 8 months, eliciting partial response. Bilateral thoracotomies were then performed for resection of the metastases, which were interpreted as metastatic malignant fibrous histiocytoma. Recurrent disease appeared in the retroperitoneum, and in April 1975, the patient underwent tumor reduction. Pathologic interpretation was liposarcoma. When last seen, in October 1975, she had terminal disease with massive abdominal recurrence.

Dr. Ayala. – I would like to ask Dr. Mackay to review the pathology.

Dr. Mackay. – We do not have the slides of the initial abdominal tumor from which the diagnosis of liposarcoma had been made. Our material came from 2 thoracotomies and from the recurrence in the retroperitoneum. The first accession we received was from the right middle and upper lobes, and sections showed considerable variability in size and shape of the tumor cells. Many were rather small, and some showed a tendency toward spindling. A striking feature was the presence of larger cells, some of them multinucleated, with somewhat acidophilic cytoplasm that often was finely vacuolated (Fig. 11). The second accession, also from the right lung, showed similar features, with more evidence of elongated cells forming interweaving bundles and a suggestion of a storiform pattern.

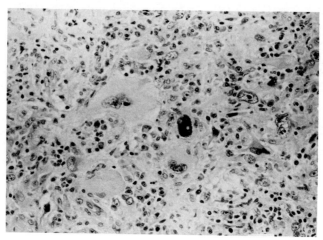

Fig. 11.—Case 5. Large cells with abundant cytoplasm were interspersed throughout the smaller mononuclear cells of the tumor. (×400.)

The recurrent abdominal tumor appeared to be thinly encapsulated, and the cut surface was whitish, with areas of necrosis and cyst formation towards the center. Surrounding the tumor there was a layer of fat in which some atypical cells were found, prompting the suggestion that the tumor might indeed be a liposarcoma rather than a malignant fibrous histiocytoma. However, we favored the latter diagnosis in view of the obvious storiform arrangement of cells in the abdominal neoplasm and the presence of the larger, often multinucleated cells.

Material for electron microscopy was available from all 3 specimens, and each showed a similar ultrastructural appearance, consistent with what we have seen in other malignant fibrous histiocytomas. By electron microscopy, one could appreciate the variation in size and shape of the tumor cells. Most contained plentiful granular endoplasmic reticulum, and, in some, the cisternae were distended with moderately electron-dense material. This can be found in malignant fibrous histiocytomas as well as in liposarcomas, but in the former, there usually are not large numbers of cytoplasmic lipid droplets; that was the situation in the case we are discussing. Some of the large multinucleated cells could be seen with the electron microscope to have very irregular nuclei (Fig. 12), but the cytoplasmic features were predominantly those of large pleormorphic fibroblasts.

Dr. Enzinger.—This case is somewhat similar to cases we have seen previously. The slides of the tumor removed from the retroperitoneum show the picture of a well-differentiated, sclerosing liposar-

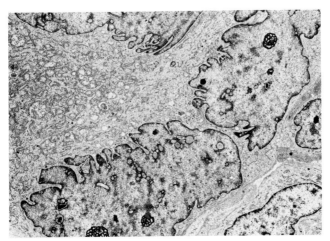

Fig. 12.—Case 5. Part of a multinucleated giant cell illustrating the jagged nuclear profiles. Granular endoplasmic reticulum was plentiful in this cell, but lipid droplets were infrequent. (×4,500.)

coma, including cells with atypical nuclei characteristic of lipoblasts. The sections from the lung and the retroperitoneum, which were removed later, show the typical picture of malignant fibrous histiocytoma.

The obvious question in this case is whether this tumor is a liposarcoma or a malignant fibrous histiocytoma. In the past, we have seen a number of tumors in which there was obvious overlapping of lipoblastic features and features characteristic of malignant fibrous histiocytomas. From this, there seems to be little doubt that intermediate forms between these 2 types of sarcoma exist and that liposarcoma and malignant fibrous histiocytoma are closely related neoplasms. In our material, we have classified such tumors according to most differentiated area, i.e., if there were lipoblasts, we classified them as liposarcoma.

Dr. Ayala.—Dr. Benjamin is there any chemotherapy for this type of tumor?

Dr. Benjamin.—Yes, there is. This patient came to us with disseminated disease in November 1973, had a response to chemotherapy, and lived for 2 years. She did not have a complete response to chemotherapy, but we were able to make it complete by using adjuvant surgery; the adjuvant concept is proving more successful as time goes on. Certainly this patient's survival was far longer than that which we would have expected for a patient who had only a partial remission with chemotherapy. Survival in this case was obviously not good enough, but it was quite impressive compared to the usual expected course.

It is tempting for me to suggest that perhaps the residual pulmonary lesions were more like malignant fibrous histiocytoma than liposarcoma because the liposarcomatous elements were more responsive to the chemotherapy than those suggesting malignant fibrous histiocytoma. Since Adriamycin has a cumulative dose limitation, it had to be discontinued; however, it was only long after this discontinuation that the more differentiated elements came back.

Question.—I would like to ask just 1 question of Dr. Enzinger. These tumors show a significant component of a small cell tumor. Have you seen myxoid chondrosarcomas mixed with mesenchymal chondrosarcomas?

Dr. Enzinger.—No, I have not.

Case 6. Sarcoma, Cell Type Uncertain

This 59-year-old white woman was first seen here in January 1973, with the chief complaint of a "mass on the dorsum of the left foot." Approximately 10 years previously she had observed a small mass in that same location, which did not change over a period of many years. A sudden rapid growth occurred during 1972. An excisional biopsy was done in June 1972, and the tumor was classified as malignant fibrous histiocytoma. One month before admission she developed a recurrence and was referred to M. D. Anderson Hospital for further evaluation. Physical examination was essentially negative, except that the left foot demonstrated a surgical scar beneath which a nodule could be palpated. Her past history was noncontributory, except for mild diabetes mellitus. In February 1973, the lesion was re-excised. The tumor was reported as "sarcoma, type unclassified." She was then treated with radiotherapy, receiving 5,000 rads. In August 1974, she underwent further surgery for recurrent sarcoma. The second, third, and fourth toes of the left foot were amputated, and the pathology examination disclosed a sarcoma of uncertain type. Recurrent disease appeared rapidly and her left foot was amputated. Metastatic disease to the left groin was discovered a few months later, and a groin dissection was performed. A metastatic nodule at the left lung base was found in March 1976, and in May, the patient was started on chemoimmunotherapy with the CY-VA-DIC protocol. An additional unrelated problem was the development of an adenocarcinoma of endometrium in June 1974, which was treated with radiotherapy followed by hysterectomy.

Dr. Mackay.—We have a number of accessions from this patient, and I will consider them in sequence. The first material we received was from the dorsum of the left foot, in February 1973. This was a 5 cm multinodular tumor mass involving the soft tissues between the skin and the underlying bone. At this time, most of the tumor cells were more or less round, with quite plentiful cytoplasm that appeared rather eosinophilic (Fig. 13). There was little cellular pleomorphism, and most cells had a single nucleus: some nucleoli were quite prominent. A moderate number of mitotic figures were seen.

In June 1974, an endometrial curettage revealed adenocarcinoma of the endometrium with some squamous metaplasia, and the hysterectomy that followed radiotherapy did not reveal residual tumor. In August 1974, the second, third, and fourth toes of the left foot were removed, and there was a tumor nodule about 5 cm in diameter over the dorsum of the third toe. The tumor cells were grouped into nodules separated by narrow bands of connective tissue. In some areas, the cells were separating from one another: these cells tended to be spindle-shaped, (Fig. 14), and many were loosely attached to a branching network of fine connective tissue trabeculae. In February 1975, the forefoot was amputated and several tumor nodules were found in the specimen, one being only 1 cm from the resection surface. The tumor was pale and soft, and it was again located between the skin and the underlying bone. Histologically it was similar to the previous specimens, but some larger, multinucleated cells were present.

Tumor was then detected in the left groin, where it was infiltrating fibroadipose tissue; the cells appeared to be the same as those from the foot. Finally, quite recently, tumor recurred in the foot, and the morphology was unchanged.

Specimens for electron microscopy had been obtained from all the accessions, and they revealed a consistent ultrastructural pattern. The polygonal tumor cells had nuclei with rather irregular profiles, and numbers of lipid droplets were usually seen in the cytoplasm along with aggregates of fine filaments that gave the cytoplasm a rather dense appearance. The granular endoplasmic reticulum was inconspicuous at this stage, but as the tumor cells assumed a spindle shape, the cisternae became larger and more prominent. The stroma was scanty in the regions where the cells were packed together, and in the loose aggregates of spindle cells, much of the stroma looked structure-

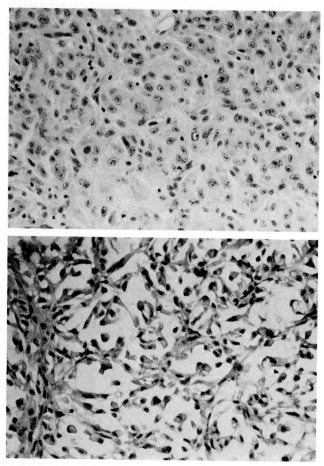

Fig. 13 (top).—Case 6. In the earlier accessions from this patient, areas of the tumor presented this histologic appearance. Round or ovoid cells of moderate size were closely grouped without attempts at architectural organization. (×400.)

Fig. 14 (bottom).—Case 6. The tumor cells tended to become spindle-shaped and separate, creating arborescent patterns. (×400.)

less in electron micrographs, with only sparse bundles of collagen fibrils.

This case posed a problem in diagnosis. I initially suggested that it might be an epithelioid sarcoma, but it certainly was not a typical example, and its transformation to a spindle-cell neoplasm did not support that first impression. Doctor Enzinger is going to discuss the differential diagnosis.

Dr. Enzinger.—We saw this patient in 1972, 1 year before she was first seen at M. D. Anderson Hospital. At the time, we made a diagnosis of malignant fibrous histiocytoma, feeling that the cellular appearance, the cellular pleomorphism, the absence of collagen, and the myxoid changes were more in keeping with the diagnosis of malignant fibrous histiocytoma than an epithelioid sarcoma, another diagnosis that we had considered. We also thought that this patient had an intermediate form between epithelioid sarcoma and malignant fibrous histiocytoma.

A few years ago, when Dr. Soule published his series on fibrous histiocytomas from the Mayo Clinic, he included among the fibrous histiocytomas several cases of epithelioid sarcoma; he suggested that epithelioid sarcoma is a variant of malignant histiocytoma. In the past, we have also seen a few cases which seem to be intermediate in appearance between these tumors, but I still do not know whether this resemblance is fortuitous or whether there is an actual relationship between these 2 lesions. Clinically, there are considerable differences in regard to age of incidence, location, etc. Perhaps Dr. Soule can comment on the cases that he has observed at the Mayo Clinic.

Dr. Soule. — In this particular case, I agree with Dr. Enzinger that the diagnosis is malignant fibrous histiocytoma. In this instance, the term "malignant histiocytoma" is meant to indicate that the cells are histiocytoid rather than spindle-shaped. If many sections are studied, multinucleated cells will be found. The tumor does not form compartments. As Dr. Enzinger stated, there does seem to be a relationship between malignant fibrous histiocytoma and epithelioid sarcoma; however, the exact nature of this relationship has not been determined.

Case 7. Hemangioma of Skeletal Muscle

A 57-year-old white man noted a lesion on the extensor surface of his right forearm approximately 4 months prior to hospital admission. No history of pain, lack of function, or absence of sensation was elicited. A biopsy was performed by his physician, who referred him to M. D. Anderson Hospital for further evaluation and treatment. Examination of the right forearm disclosed a 10 cm soft, fusiform swelling located on the extensor surface. Following angiographic studies, the lesion was resected.

Dr. de Santos. — The angiogram showed a tumor that was fairly deep, adjacent to the bone, and that was fed by a large branch of the dorsal interosseous artery. The venous phase in the anteroposterior projection showed an extension of the lesion that was fairly vascular.

Late in the arterial phase and early in the venous phase, there were multiple draining veins from the dorsal aspect of the forearm. There was no increase in the number of arteries to suggest a malignancy. Rather, some of the features were in keeping with the diagnosis of a benign vascular lesion such as an hemangioma. However, the angiographic features were not by any means specific and could actually indicate any other form of vascular lesion.

Dr. Martin.—The lesion in the case under discussion had been diagnosed elsewhere as being malignant. Our pathologists reviewed the case, and their report stated that the lesion was benign. For this reason, we took a conservative approach in order not to impair the function of the arm and hand. Therefore, we did not do a radical resection. The artery that was feeding the tumor was isolated and ligated. The area was explored and the abnormal tissue was resected. The patient has done well.

Dr. Mackay.—This lesion was not clearly circumscribed or encapsulated. Histologically, the predominant elements were skeletal muscle fibers and blood vessels (Fig. 15). Neither appeared malignant. A number of the skeletal muscle fibers showed degenerative changes, such as the presence of central nuclei and variability in caliber. Interspersed throughout the muscle were blood vessels of varying size and construction. In some areas, the lesion appears more solid than vascular, and there were occasional mitotic figures, but it was never thought

Fig. 15.—Case 7. The lesion was composed of skeletal muscle fibers, some of which showed degenerative changes, and numerous blood vessels that included small veins and arteries in addition to capillaries. (×400.)

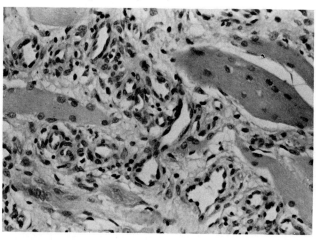

that this was other than a benign lesion. In the solid areas, there was a moderate admixture of fibroblasts indicating some sclerosis. Occasionally one could see an infiltration of lymphocytes outside the muscle fibers, and some fat was present within the muscle. The blood vessels were capillaries, small arteries, and small veins, and they all appeared benign. The diagnosis was mixed type of hemangioma of skeletal muscle.

Dr. Enzinger.—Angiosarcomas in the deep soft tissues, with the exception of postmastectomy or lymphangiosarcomas, are exceedingly rare; most such tumors are benign and represent variants of intramuscular hemangioma.

Intramuscular hemangioma shows a great variety of patterns, ranging from very cellular ones to very vascular ones that display dilated vascular spaces and suggest an arteriovenous shunt. A few years ago, we reviewed our cases of hemangioma, particularly in regard to the question whether or not the degree of cellularity is closely related to the behavior. About 20% of our cases recurred, but there was little correlation between the recurrence rate and the histological type. Even the very cellular tumors did not recur more often than those with markedly dilated cavernous vascular spaces.

Another interesting feature of intramuscular hemangiomas is the presence of considerable amounts of interstitial fat. When the muscle is immobilized, the muscle becomes atrophic and is slowly replaced by fat. These tumors should not be interpreted as angiolipomas or benign mesenchymomas, but should be considered as intramuscular hemangiomas with a prominent fatty component.

Still another feature of these tumors that is noteworthy is the proliferation of vessels around peripheral nerves. This should not be interpreted as evidence of intraneural or perineural invasion. Vascular proliferation within the nerve sheath is perfectly in keeping with the diagnosis of intramuscular hemangioma. Recanalized vessels in this tumor may also simulate intravascular invasion.

Distinction between intramuscular hemangiomas and diffuse angiomatosis may be difficult. In general, the 2 can be distinguished by the fact that diffuse angiomatosis involves not only muscle but also the subcutaneous tissue and sometimes even the underlying bone. Sometimes there is also overgrowth of bone resulting in a giant limb. Most examples of diffuse angiomatosis occur in small children, whereas most cases of intramuscular hemangioma occur in adult patients, usually between 18 and 35 years of age.

Dr. Ayala.—There is a question.

Question.—Dr. Enzinger would you comment on whether hemangiomas can be judged to be congenital and also whether this tumor can be caused by trauma.

Dr. Enzinger.—There are some cases of intramuscular hemangiomas reported in the literature (British Journal of Surgery, 23:245–251, 1935) which supposedly have followed trauma or have been thought to be secondary to trauma. To establish a causal relationship in these cases, however, is very difficult because a history of trauma is such a common event in soft tissue tumors. A relationship is possible, but I know of no way by which this can be established beyond doubt.

In regard to the congenital origin of the tumors, it must be emphasized that intramuscular hemangiomas are rarely seen before the patient reaches adolescence. It is possible that there is an underlying vascular malformation which expands with advancing growth. But if this is so, I know of no sound evidence in support of this concept.

CASE 8. PROLIFERATIVE MYOSITIS

A 55-year-old white man reported a small mass of several months' duration in his right lateral chest wall. An ill-defined nodule, arising in an intercostal muscle and attached to the parietal pleura, was excised. Following resection of the nodule, the patient has remained well for 4 years with no further problems.

Dr. Mackay.—We received sections and a tissue block from this lesion, because the resection had been performed at another hospital. The sections showed bundles of skeletal muscle fibers of normal size and appearance, but separated into irregular groups; in the intervening zones, there were loosely arranged round or ovoid cells with 1 or sometimes 2 nuclei and prominent nucleoli (Fig. 16). These cells had moderate amounts of eosinophilic cytoplasm with a finely granular appearance. The surrounding matrix contained slender wavy bundles of collagen. Although some tumor cells lay close to the muscle fibers, no transitional forms could be detected. There was a tendency for the cells to assume a spindle shape, and in some areas these fusiform cells were oriented into loose bundles. The predominant and characteristic pattern was, however, one of scattered plump cells whose cytoplasm simulated that of the skeletal muscle fibers, a resemblance prompting the designation of a lesion of this type as proliferative myositis.

Dr. Enzinger.—This case, a typical example of proliferative myositis, falls into the group of pseudosarcomatous lesions. It is a benign lesion which causes concern because of the presence of large immature-appearing basophilic cells which infiltrate muscle tissue.

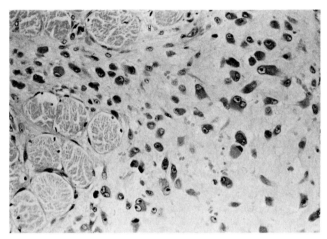

Fig. 16.—Case 8. Loosely arranged plump cells with cytoplasm similar to that of the surrounding skeletal muscle fibers. (×400.)

However, judging from the large number of cases we have studied, this is a reactive proliferative process which is cured by simple local excision.

Grossly, most of the lesions resemble scar tissue and usually measure between 2 and 4 cm in diameter. The surgeon is usually much less concerned about the gross appearance of the lesion than the pathologist is about its morphologic picture. Microscopically, there is marked proliferation of large cells with basophilic cytoplasm and prominent nucleoli in between atrophic muscle fibers. I am not sure whether these cells are modified fibroblasts or histiocytes, but from their ultrastructural appearance, fibroblastic origin seems more likely. A morphologically similar lesion may also occur in the subcutis (proliferative fasciitis). Both the intramuscular and the subcutaneous variants of this process are reactive rather than neoplastic cellular proliferations and are benign, despite the mitotic activity and the bizarre appearance of the constituent cells.

Most of the deep lesions occur in the large muscles of the shoulder area, the chest wall, or the thigh. Lesions of this type in young patients are exceedingly rare.

Dr. Mackay.—Unfortunately, we did not have material from this lesion for electron microscopy. It has been suggested in the literature that the cells may be derived from muscle since they have cytoplasmic filaments.

Dr. Enzinger.—It has been reported that some of the cells contain

prominent endoplasmic reticulum and a considerable amount of fila-
mentous material and that they may be muscle cells. It seems more
likely to me, however, that these are in the realm of myofibroblasts,
especially since we have never seen any evidence of rhabdomyoblastic differentiation, i.e., cross striations in these cells.

Acknowledgment

The narrative summary of this panel discussion was prepared by
Ms. Connie Reischer, Research Analyst, Department of Pathology.

Index